Care of the Obese in Advanced Practice Nursing

Lisa L. M. Maher, DNP, ARNP, FNP-BC, received her BS in wellness from Waldorf College in Forest City, Iowa, in 2003, her BSN from Allen College in Waterloo, Iowa, in 2005, and her MSN from Graceland University in Independence, Missouri, in 2008. In 2011, she received her DNP from the University of Iowa in Iowa City. She is board certified as a family nurse practitioner (FNP) through the American Nurses Credentialing Center (ANCC). She is the current president of the Cedar Valley (Iowa) chapter of Preventive Cardiovascular Nurses Association (PCNA) in Waterloo, Iowa.

Dr. Maher has been employed as a nurse practitioner (NP) at the Cedar Valley Cardiovascular Center since 2008. She specializes in treatment of general cardiology, sleep apnea, weight loss, and risk factor modification. She started the Cedar Valley Center for Lifestyle Medicine Clinic in 2008 and the Cedar Valley Cardiovascular Center Sleep Clinic in 2009.

Care of the Obese in Advanced Practice Nursing

Communication, Assessment, and Treatment

Lisa L. M. Maher, DNP, ARNP, FNP-BC

SPRINGER PUBLISHING COMPANY

NEW YORK

Springer Publishing Company, LLC
11 West 42nd Street
New York, NY 10036
www.springerpub.com

Acquisitions Editor: Joseph Morita
Production Editor: Kris Parrish
Composition: Westchester Publishing Services

ISBN: 978-0-8261-2357-2
e-book ISBN: 978-0-8261-2358-9

15 16 17 18 / 5 4 3 2 1

The author and the publisher of this work have made every effort to use sources believed to be reliable to provide information that is accurate and compatible with the standards generally accepted at the time of publication. Because medical science is continually advancing, our knowledge base continues to expand. Therefore, as new information becomes available, changes in procedures become necessary. We recommend that the reader always consult current research and specific institutional policies before performing any clinical procedure. The author and publisher shall not be liable for any special, consequential, or exemplary damages resulting, in whole or in part, from the readers' use of, or reliance on, the information contained in this book. The publisher has no responsibility for the persistence or accuracy of URLs for external or third-party Internet websites referred to in this publication and does not guarantee that any content on such websites is, or will remain, accurate or appropriate.

Library of Congress Cataloging-in-Publication Data

Maher, Lisa L. M., author.
  Care of the obese in advanced practice nursing : communication, assessment, and treatment / Lisa L. M. Maher.
    p. ; cm.
  Includes bibliographical references.
  ISBN 978-0-8261-2357-2 (hard copy : alk. paper) — ISBN 978-0-8261-2358-9 (ebook)
  I. Title.
  [DNLM: 1. Obesity—nursing. 2. Advanced Practice Nursing—methods. 3. Obesity—therapy. WD 210]
  RC628
  616.3'980231—dc23

                                                                              2015029702

Printed in the United States of America by Bradford & Bigelow.

*This book is dedicated to current and future advanced practice nurses.
Continue to educate with compassion.
This book is also dedicated to Brook, my loving husband.*

Contents

Preface

An extensive body of scientific literature supports prevention of obesity with a multidisciplinary approach. Advanced practice nurses (APNs) are at the forefront of patient diagnosis, assessment, treatment, and education. APNs are known for their increased patient time as well as their effective patient communication. These talents and skills can drive continued efforts for a reduction in chronic disease—especially obesity.

This book is written with the hope of inspiring continued efforts toward not only the prevention but also the treatment of this growing disease. Pediatric and adult obesity is addressed with regard to prevention, assessment, and treatment. Medical therapy based on a lifestyle medicine approach—nutrition, exercise, psychological, pharmacological, and surgical recommendations—is discussed. The following evidence-based clinical guidelines, focused on treatment of obesity and its comorbid conditions, support the recommendations for treatment using a multidisciplinary approach:

- *The American Heart Association (AHA), the American College of Cardiology (ACC), and the Obesity Society (TOS): Guideline for the Management of Overweight and Obesity in Adults*
- *National Institutes of Health (NIH), National Heart, Lung, and Blood Institute (NHLBI), and North American Association for the Study of Obesity: The Practical Guide Identification, Evaluation, and Treatment of Overweight and Obesity in Adults*
- *Institute of Medicine Guidelines for Obesity Management*
- *Institute for Clinical Systems Improvement: Prevention and Management of Obesity for Adults (2011 & 2013)*
- *Guidelines From the American Academy of Pediatrics (AAP) for the Prevention and Treatment of Childhood Obesity*
- *Prevention and Treatment of Pediatric Obesity: An Endocrine Society Clinical Practice Guideline Based on Expert Opinion*
- *Diet and Lifestyle Recommendations Revision 2006: A Scientific Statement From AHA Nutrition Committee*
- *Guide to the Assessment of Physical Activity: Clinic and Research Applications: A Scientific Statement From the AHA*
- *American College of Sports Medicine (ACSM)'s Exercise Management for Persons With Chronic Disease and Disabilities*
- *2014 Evidence-Based Guideline for the Management of High Blood Pressure in Adults: Report From the Panel Members Appointed to the Eighth Joint National Committee (JNC 8)*

- *JNC 7: The Seventh Report of the Joint National Committee on Prevention, Detection, Evaluation, and Treatment of High Blood Pressure*
- *2013 ACC/AHA Guideline on the Treatment of Blood Cholesterol to Reduce Atherosclerotic Cardiovascular Risk in Adults: A Report of the ACC/AHA Task Force on Practice Guidelines*
- *The National Cholesterol Education Program (NCEP; Adult Treatment Panel [ATP] III) Guidelines for Cholesterol Management*
- *Guidelines From the American Diabetes Association (ADA) for the Management of Diabetes*
- *2013 ACC/AHA Guideline on Lifestyle Management to Reduce Cardiovascular Risk*
- *2013 ACC/AHA Guideline on the Assessment of Cardiovascular Risk*

Obesity is a growing epidemic, one that is undertreated and misunderstood by many medical professionals. This disease is one of the fastest growing nationwide. Obesity is chronic, multifactorial, and complex. In more recent years, alarms have sounded regarding the pervasiveness of obesity in the United States, mostly because of the researched links found between obesity and increased health risks. According to numerous studies, more than 97 million people in the United States are either overweight or obese. Obesity is linked to hypertension (HTN), dyslipidemia, coronary artery disease (CAD), type 2 diabetes mellitus (T2DM), obstructive sleep apnea (OSA), bone or joint problems, pseudotumor cerebri, polycystic ovary syndrome (PCOS), and social or psychological problems (poor self-esteem or stigmatization). Long-term diseases related to obesity may include cardiovascular disease (CVD), cerebral vascular accident (CVA), osteoarthritis (OA), and several forms of cancer.

Abridged provider time during routine office visits is among the top-stated patient concerns with weight loss. Along with lack of time, patients also felt that providers lacked concern in addressing weight management/loss. These statements with regard to obesity, preventive health care, and quality patient care prompted the development of guidelines for clinical practice. This book focuses on prevention, provider recognition, and treatment of obesity with goals toward improving the overall quality of life.

The transition from current health care practice to a prevention focus has a tremendous effect on health care. Addressing current health practices before it is too late is essential. Total medical costs associated with obesity were estimated at $147 billion in 2006, whereas medical costs for an obese person are estimated at $1,429 higher per year than for a nonobese individual. The costs associated with obesity continue to climb and so do patients' fears of seeking help and treating obesity. APNs must be aware of these fears and address them appropriately. Patients as well as providers must realize that in today's culture it is difficult to eat less and engage in more physical activity.

I became interested in the study and treatment of obesity within my first year of practice as an NP. I work in general cardiology and continuously educate on the importance of risk factor modification. Visit after visit, I would give the same advice: Work on weight loss before your next appointment. Patients would smile politely, walk out the door, and return to the next visit at the same weight or, many times, even heavier. The frustration of poor patient outcomes with weight loss led to further research on the topic and became the focus of my doctoral project, *Establishing a Formal Business Plan for a Weight-Loss Clinic: A Capstone Project,* which was organized as follows:

- Purpose: Laying the foundation for establishment of a preliminary structure for an NP-led weight-loss clinic
- Outcome: Development of a formal business plan and evidence-based guidelines for weight loss and management of people with chronic health conditions
- Findings: Establishing a weight-loss clinic helps individuals focus on prevention and treatment of obesity while improving overall quality of life

This project included the following methodology:

- Set in a large outpatient care setting in a northeast Iowa city
- Provides specialty cardiovascular practice
- Serves a total of 15,717 patients yearly
- Employs five board-certified cardiologists, five board-certified ARNPs, a registered dietitian, and an exercise specialist with a master of science (MSN) degree in health promotions
- Accepts new patients with cardiac disease and risk factors for cardiac disease through either internal or outside referrals

This research led to the development of a separate clinic located within the cardiology practice that specialized in weight loss for patients with CVD or cardiovascular risk factors, the Center for Lifestyle Medicine (CLM).

As of November 1, 2015:
- Out of 474 total patients, there were 102 active patients
  - Patients considered active are those who have been seen at least five times
- Average patient age: 63.24 years
- Maximum body mass index (BMI): 61.52
- Minimum BMI: 27.00
- Average BMI: 41.86

Of the active patients:
- Average weight loss: 18.63 pounds
- Highest individual weight loss: 102.7 pounds or 32% total body weight
- Total pounds lost by active patients: 1,901 pounds

This model has been successful in my current patient practice setting. I have received both internal and external referrals, which have aided in the growth of my patient population. I am passionate about my work and believe in improving patient health. Since its initial establishment, the clinic has grown to include an outside referral to a counselor specializing in weight loss. The clinic continues in operation today. Not all the patients I work with have success with weight loss; however, I continue to work with them on avoiding further weight gain. This can be a very frustrating process, both for myself and, especially, for the patient. I revel in my patients' weight loss, even for amounts as small as 10 pounds. This is the most rewarding part of the job! I hope my personal patient experiences can guide the APNs to successful provider–patient relationships that lead not only to weight loss but also to trusting and rewarding experiences.

Although I work in a general cardiology practice, I developed this book to assist various practice settings, especially general practice. Patients in many clinics struggle with weight loss, and all of these patients need our help. Although these patients may not present with a chief complaint of obesity, weight can and should be addressed at every visit. All APNs play a crucial role in the fight against obesity.

This book is unique, because there are no current textbooks on the market that are aimed at communication, assessment, and treatment goals of the obese patient from the perspective of an APN. Part I, "Introduction," focuses on the disease of obesity in the United States and worldwide. The current trends and causes of obesity are addressed in detail. Obesity terms and numerous definitions used are also discussed. Finally, this section describes the multifaceted roles of the APN.

Part II, "Communication," describes nursing at its best. It focuses on common "dos and don'ts" with regard to the overweight or obese patient. A section on therapeutic communication is also provided. Real patient stories are shared to allow appreciation of the patient's perspective.

Part III, "Assessment," focuses on the technical aspects of obesity—genetics and pathophysiology. The addiction of obesity and eating disorders are discussed. Physical assessments of both adult and pediatric patients from the APN point of view are seen. Exercise and dietary assessment and recommendations with examples will be of interest to clinicians.

Part IV, "Disease Management," focuses on the numerous comorbid conditions associated with obesity. This includes the assessment and treatment of each disease in both the pediatric and adult populations. Diseases addressed in the adult population include HTN, dyslipidemia, CVD, diabetes mellitus (DM), obesity and the pulmonary system, OA, PCOS, and metabolic syndrome. Obesity in combination with pediatric HTN, dyslipidemia, DM, OSA, and asthma is also addressed. Prevention efforts for obesity, as well as methods to avoid weight cycling, are discussed.

Part V, "Treatment," involves the treatment of many comorbid conditions related to obesity. Pharmacological therapy, surgical therapy, and medical management with diet and exercise are addressed. The adult and pediatric patients are discussed. Costs associated with this condition as well as insurance coverage are also of interest to the clinician. Finally, weight management resources and tools are provided.

A comprehensive case study that progresses into a SOAP (subjective, objective, assessment, plan)-note style appears at the end of the text. Also included are several tools that one can use and adapt to clinical practice.

The past 2 years have yielded many new guidelines to address obesity. These guidelines have been summarized to aid the APN in the assessment and treatment of obesity. A multidisciplinary approach is continuously addressed in *Care of the Obese in Advanced Practice Nursing: Communication, Assessment, and Treatment,* and this provides the greatest comprehensive approach to fighting this disease. APNs are in a perfect place to provide the critical care needed for these patients, now and into the future!

Lisa L. M. Maher

Acknowledgments

First, I would like to thank Joseph Morita and Springer Publishing Company for taking a chance on this small-town Iowa girl. You have provided me with the opportunity to share my passion with the nursing community and given me a voice in the fight against this disease.

I would also like to thank my professors at the University of Iowa DNP program who served on my doctoral project, especially Dr. Kerri Rupe, Dr. Jo Eland, Dr. Brenda Hoskins, and Dr. Patricia Clinton. Thank you for your support and encouragement.

I would also like to express my deep appreciation to my wonderful colleagues who continuously put up with my "crazy" and "outlandish" ideas. Special thanks to Dr. Kari Haislet, my mentor, friend, proofreader, and sounding board. I could not have made it through this process without you. To Abbie Scharder, thanks for your continuous laughter when I needed it the most. To my colleague, Abbie Schaa, who just agrees with me and "goes with the flow." To Ashley Hall, who drops anything to help me whenever and with whatever I need. And to Dr. Kalyana Sundaram, who gave me my first and only nurse practitioner job and continues to support my career growth.

Thanks to my friend and contributor, Jennifer Roth. Your work on this book as well as the development of our clinic is much appreciated. You push me to be a better provider every day.

To my parents, Mark and Terri. Thanks for your continued love and support from the very beginning. To my family, especially Michael, Anne, and Jack; my in-laws, Mike, Kelli, Brady, and Bre; my grandparents, Jim, Joyce, and Lois; and all of my extended family—the aunt-brigade, uncles, and cousins. You will never know how much your love means to me. Thanks for the endless support and allowing me to spend numerous family events and holidays with my head buried in this book.

Finally, to my husband, Brook. Without you, this would not be possible. I love you!

Introduction

Obesity: The Epidemic, Trends, and Causes

Many factors contribute to obesity. Although it is a preventable disease, it is important to understand how this disease came to be one of the fastest growing nationwide. Referred to as a hormonal and multimetabolic disease state by the American Medical Association (AMA), obesity is a crucial public health issue. This chapter focuses on and addresses the obesity epidemic, trends, and causes.

THE EPIDEMIC

Obesity is a growing epidemic, one that is undertreated and misunderstood by many medical professionals. Obesity is chronic, multifactorial, and complex. Attributed to both genetic and environmental factors, obesity results from long-term positive energy imbalance and is associated with chronic low-grade inflammation (Wang & Nakayama, 2010). According to the WHO, which recognizes obesity as a chronic disease,

> Obesity is reaching epidemic proportions with more than 1 billion adults who are overweight, 300 million who have class I or II obesity and 30 million who have class III obesity, defined as a body mass index (BMI) greater than 40 kg/m^2 (also referred to as morbid obesity). (Christou & Efthimiou, 2009, p. 250)

Statistics show that rates of worldwide obesity have nearly doubled since 1980. Obesity in men, women, and children has increased: More than 200 million men, nearly 300 million women, and 43 million preschool children suffer from this disease. The overweight and obesity rates in children have shown a 60% increase since 1990. Even Europe, Africa, Asia, South and Central America, and the Western Pacific have shown an increase in the disease (Harvard School of Public Health, 2014g).

All-cause mortality is seen in those with higher body weights. Obese individuals may be discriminated against as well as suffer from social stigmatization (National Institutes of Health; National Heart, Lung, and Blood Institute; & National Institute of Diabetes and Digestive and Kidney Diseases [NIH/NHLBI/NIDDK], 1998). The widespread epidemic of obesity is directly linked to increased rates of chronic disease. This condition threatens the health care systems and world economies as well as individual lifestyle (Harvard School of Public Health, 2014e). Obesity is seen as a preventative disease with many comorbid associations. Obesity has been linked to hypertension (HTN), dyslipidemia, coronary artery disease (CAD), cardiovascular disease (CVD), and type 2 diabetes mellitus (T2DM). Chronic conditions also seen with obesity include obstructive sleep apnea (OSA), osteoarthritis (OA), polycystic ovary syndrome (PCOS), and metabolic syndrome (NIH/NHLBI/NIDDK, 1998).

Obesity Within the United States

Incidence and *prevalence* are common terms used in describing obesity statistics. According to Dictionary.com (2013a), *incidence* is defined as "the rate or range of occurrence or influence of something, especially of something unwanted." An example would be the high incidence of obesity in adults in the United States. *Prevalence* is defined as "the condition of being prevalent, or widespread" (Dictionary .com, 2013b). An example of prevalence is the spread of obesity worldwide.

In more recent years, alarms have sounded regarding the pervasiveness of obesity in the United States, mostly because of the links between obesity and increased health risks. The United States has the highest rates of both overweight and obesity in comparison to all high-income countries. One-third of the total population is obese; this is projected to rise to about 50% by the year 2030 (Harvard School of Public Health, 2014f). According to studies completed by the National Institutes of Health ([NIH]; NIH/NHLBI/NIDDK, 1998), 97 million people in the United States are either overweight or obese. The U.S. Department of Health and Human Services Centers for Disease Control and Prevention National Center for Health Statistics (HHS-CDC-NCHS) states that at least 78 million (35.7%) adults and approximately 12.5 million (16.9%) children and adolescents were considered obese from 2009 to 2010 (Ogden, Carroll, Kit, & Flegal, 2012). Data compiled by the Centers for Disease Control and Prevention (CDC) in 2010 and Jensen et al. (2013) state that 72.5 million or 35% of adults are obese (Institute for Clinical Systems Improvement [ICSI], 2011). The 35% of obese adults are part of a total 69% who are considered either overweight or obese (Jensen et al., 2013). Approximately 41 million women and 37 million men were considered obese; these numbers were based on 2009 to 2010 statistics with people aged 20 and older. The 12.5 million children and adolescents (aged 2–19) are further divided into the obese category with more than 5 million (15.0%) girls and approximately 7 million (18.6%) boys (Ogden et al., 2012). Approximately 31% of children, or one out of every three, are either overweight or obese (ICSI, 2011).

Although obesity continues to be highly prevalent, recent data from the National Health and Nutrition Examination Surveys estimate that overall rates of obesity have not differed significantly from 2003 to the present (Jensen et al., 2013). Although the overall prevalence of the disease has not differed, the past decade has shown a significant increase in obesity in both men and boys, as well as an increase in extreme obesity (BMI of 40 kg/m^2 or higher; ICSI, 2011; Ogden et al., 2012). This extreme obesity includes at least 6% of U.S. adults: "More than one quarter of all Americans ages 17–24 are unqualified for military service because they are too heavy" (ICSI, 2011, p. 5).

Varied results are seen in men and women. Older women were found to have a higher incidence of obesity in comparison to younger women. The incidence among men did not vary in age groups. Adolescents were found to have higher rates of obesity compared with preschool ages. Again, the prevalence of obesity has not differed in the past decade; however, the rates of men and boys have increased overall (Ogden et al., 2012). Groups with a high prevalence of obesity include ethnic minority groups, those of lower socioeconomic status, and those with less education (Jensen et al., 2013).

Obesity is also more common in certain ethnic groups. Non-Hispanic Blacks have the highest obesity rates at 49.5%. Mexican Americans, Hispanics, and non-Hispanic Whites also have high rates of obesity at 40.4%, 39.1%, and 34.3%, respectively. Interestingly, non-Hispanic Black and Mexican American men with a higher income level are more likely to be obese in comparison to those with a lower income, whereas women with a higher income are found to be less obese than those with a lower income. Women with a history of college education are also found to have a lower incidence of obesity, whereas their counterparts have no significant relationship with the education level and prevalence of obesity (Centers for Disease Control and Prevention [CDC], 2013).

The prevalence of obesity is widespread in the United States. According to the CDC 2012 statistics, Colorado continues to have the lowest statewide obesity rate, at 20.5%. The District of Columbia, Hawaii, Massachusetts, Montana, New Jersey, New York, Utah, Vermont, and Wyoming also have relatively low obesity rates, between 20% and 25% (Box 1.1).

The heaviest state is Louisiana, at 34.7%. The highest rates of obesity are found in the Midwest and South at 29.5% and 29.4%, respectively; in contrast, the lowest rates are found in the Northeast (25.3%) and West (25.1%). Those states with the highest prevalence of obesity at greater than or equal to 30% include Ohio (30.1%), Iowa (30.4%), Tennessee (31.1%), Michigan (31.1%), Kentucky (31.3%), Indiana (31.4%), South Carolina (31.6%), Oklahoma (32.2%), Alabama (33.0%), West Virginia (33.8%), Arkansas (34.5%), and Mississippi (34.6%) (Box 1.2; CDC, 2013).

BOX 1.1 LEAST OBESE STATES

Colorado, 20.5%	Vermont, 23.7%
District of Columbia, 21.9%	Montana, 24.3%
Massachusetts, 22.9%	Utah, 24.3%
Hawaii, 23.6%	New Jersey, 24.6%
New York, 23.6%	Wyoming, 24.6%

BOX 1.2 HEAVIEST STATES

Louisiana, 34.7%	Indiana, 31.4%
Mississippi, 34.6%	Kentucky, 31.3%
Arkansas, 34.5%	Michigan, 31.1%
West Virginia, 33.8%	Tennessee, 31.1%
Alabama, 33.0%	Iowa, 30.4%
Oklahoma, 32.2%	Ohio, 30.1%
South Carolina, 31.6%	

The Costs of Obesity

In the United States, obesity is second only to tobacco in the number of deaths caused per year; however, obesity is soon expected to exceed tobacco in the number of deaths caused per year (Harvard School of Public Health, 2014f). The increasing number of people suffering from obesity will result in a rise in overall health care costs. Total medical costs associated with obesity were estimated at $147 billion in 2006; another estimate states that costs of obesity reached more than $190 billion in 2005 (Harvard School of Public Health, 2014f; ICSI, 2011). Medical costs for an obese person are estimated at $1,429 higher than those for a nonobese individual. The costs associated with obesity continue to climb, and so do patients' fears of seeking help and treating obesity. The ICSI (2011, p. 17) states that patients become overwhelmed when thinking about losing weight: "It is discouraging if they think they have to quit eating all of their favorite foods and/or do hours of grueling exercise. It is even more challenging if they have a high level of stress in their lives." Providers must be aware of these fears and address them appropriately. Patients as well as providers must realize that in today's culture it is difficult to eat less and engage in more physical activity. The transition from current health care practice to a prevention focus will have a tremendous effect on health care. Addressing current health practices before it is too late is essential!

TRENDS

Trends exist in how people try to achieve weight loss and maintain a healthy weight. Fads—including "fad diets"—and trends are everywhere. Many products promise a "quick fix" for weight loss, which is far from the truth. Celebrity-endorsed diets, portion-control diets, organic diets, diet delivery, and sweet and savory diets are all part of today's trends.

Many weight-loss products use celebrities to promote their products. Celebrities with their "good looks" and "flawless bodies" make these products seem perfect. However, many of the celebrities have neither tried nor used these products themselves. Portioned diets are another current trend. These portioned diets are common and are usually prepackaged foods that may be picked up in stores or shipped directly to the consumer's home. These products are aimed at helping one stay within the recommended caloric range; however, once back to normal eating patterns, one can easily slip back into old habits. Organic diets are also part of the current weight-loss trends. They may be expensive for some; however, they can provide nutritional value. Diet delivery is another continuing trend. Nutrisystem, Diets to Go, Bistro MD, and eDiets.com are such dietary delivery systems. Again, users usually see results; however, the secret to long-term success is shifting from the product to more "normal" eating patterns. Sweet and savory diets, such as "The Cookie Diet," are used to tempt those with a sweet tooth, but a cookie-only diet lacks nutritional value and variety.

According to the CDC, many of these products lack nutritional value, may be unhealthy, and cause failure in the long run. The "best" diet to be on is not a short-term diet, but rather one that balances healthy dietary and nutritional value choices and promotes physical activity (CDC, 2011). The simple equation—calories in versus calories out—continues to provide the most efficient long-term success. There are healthy resources that exist to promote long-term growth and success. One such program is Healthy People 2020.

Healthy People 2020

Healthy People 2020 was launched on December 2, 2010. Focusing on 10-year goals, this agenda focuses on improving the nation's health. The vision of Healthy People 2020 is "A society in which all people live long, healthy lives" (U.S. Department of Health and Human Services, National Institutes of Health, & National Heart, Lung, and Blood Institute [HHS/NIH/NHLBI], 2011). The mission has several objectives, including to "Identify nationwide health improvement priorities; increase public awareness and understanding of the determinants of health, disease, and disability and the opportunities for progress; provide measurable objectives and goals that are applicable at the national, state, and local levels; engage multiple sectors to take actions to strengthen policies and improve practices that are driven by the best available evidence and knowledge; identify critical research, evaluation, and data collection needs" (HHS/NIH/NHLBI, 2011). Goals are aimed at prevention, health improvement, creating healthy environments, and promoting quality of life across all life spans. Four foundational health measures of progress are being used to track the progress of Healthy People 2020. These measures include (1) General Health Status, (2) Health-Related Quality of Life and Well-Being, (3) Determinants of Health, and (4) Disparities (HHS/NIH/NHLBI, 2011).

Several prevention efforts are partnered with the U.S. Department of Health and Human Services (HHS). This strategy is in support of Healthy People. These partnerships include the Tobacco Control Strategic Action Plan; HHS Initiative on Multiple Chronic Conditions; Action Plan for the Prevention, Care, and Treatment of Viral Hepatitis; Health Care-Associated Infection (HAI); Public Health System, Finance, and Quality Program; HHS Action Plan to Reduce Racial and Ethnic Health Disparities; National Prevention Strategy; National HIV/AIDS Strategy; National Drug Control Strategy; Let's Move Campaign; President's Food Safety Working Group; Global Health Initiative; U.S. National Vaccine Plan; National Action Plan to Improve Health Literacy; and HHS Environmental Justice. These organizations are helping with the fight against obesity. With the multitude of organizations involved, the message is able to be received by many different sectors of society (Box 1.3).

Healthy People 2020 topics and objectives related to obesity and chronic obesity conditions include Access to Health Services Health Services; Diabetes; Educational, and Community-Based Programs; Global Health (New); Health-Related Quality of Life and Well-Being (New); Heart Disease and Stroke; Mental Health and Mental Disorders, Nutrition and Weight Status; Physical Activity and Sleep Health (New). Specific goals are addressed within each category. The goal of Access to Health Services is to "improve access to comprehensive, quality health care services" (HHS/NIH/NHLBI, 2011). Coverage, services, timeliness, and workforce are four topic areas of focus in order to achieve a healthy life for all. Preventative services are included in this goal. This stresses the importance of obesity control. The objective of Educational and Community-Based Programs, another topic that is addressed, is to "increase the quality, availability, and effectiveness of educational and community-based programs designed to prevent disease and injury, improve health, and enhance quality of life" (HHS/NIH/NHLBI, 2011). The goal of Global Health, a new category within the topics and objectives, is to "improve public health and strengthen U.S. national security through global disease detection, response, prevention, and control strategies" (HHS/NIH/NHLBI, 2011). Another new category under topics and objectives is Health-Related Quality

BOX 1.3 LINKS TO HHS PREVENTION STRATEGIES

Tobacco Control Strategic Action Plan:
www.hhs.gov/ash/initiatives/tobacco/index.html

HHS Initiative on Multiple Chronic Conditions:
www.hhs.gov/ash/initiatives/mcc/index.html

Action Plan for the Prevention, Care, and Treatment of Viral Hepatitis:
www.hhs.gov/ash/initiatives/hepatitis/index.html

Health Care-Associated Infection (HAI):
www.health.gov/hai/prevent_hai.asp

Public Health System, Finance, and Quality Program:
www.hhs.gov/ash/initiatives/quality/index.html

HHS Action Plan to Reduce Racial and Ethnic Health Disparities:
http://minorityhealth.hhs.gov/npa/templates/content.aspx?lvl=1&lvlid=33&ID=285

National Prevention Strategy:
www.surgeongeneral.gov/priorities/prevention/strategy/

National HIV/AIDS Strategy:
www.whitehouse.gov/administration/eop/onap/nhas

National Drug Control Strategy:
https://whitehouse.gov/ondcp/national-drug-control-strategy

Let's Move Campaign:
www.letsmove.gov

President's Food Safety Working Group:
www.foodsafetyworkinggroup.gov

Global Health Initiative:
www.ghi.gov

U.S. National Vaccine Plan:
www.hhs.gov/nvpo/vacc_plan

National Action Plan to Improve Health Literacy:
http://health.gov/communication/hlactionplan/pdf/Health_Lit_Action_Plan_
  Summary.pdf

HHS Environmental Justice:
www.hhs.gov/environmentaljustice

of Life and Well-Being. The mission of this category is to "improve health-related quality of life and well-being for all individuals" (HHS/NIH/NHLBI, 2011). Nutrition and Weight Status is also covered thoroughly under the Healthy People 2020 objective. The goal of this category is to "promote health and reduce chronic disease risk through the consumption of healthful diets and achievement and maintenance of healthy body weights" (HHS/NIH/NHLBI, 2011). Physical Activity, another Healthy People 2020 objective, is also essential to aiding in weight loss. This mission is to "improve health, fitness, and quality of life through daily physical activity" (HHS/NIH/NHLBI, 2011).

Chronic diseases related to obesity include diabetes mellitus (DM), heart disease and stroke, mental health and mental disorders, and sleep health. DM is a

Healthy People 2020 topic. The objective is "reduce the disease and economic burden of DM and improve the quality of life for all persons who have, or are at risk for, diabetes mellitus" (HHS/NIH/NHLBI, 2011). Heart Disease and Stroke is another topic. The 2020 goal is to "improve cardiovascular health and quality of life through prevention, detection, and treatment of risk factors for heart attack and stroke; early identification and treatment of heart attacks and strokes; and prevention of repeat cardiovascular events" (HHS/NIH/NHLBI, 2011). Mental Health and Mental Disorders are also addressed in the topics and objectives. This objective is to "improve mental health through prevention and by ensuring access to appropriate, quality mental health services" (HHS/NIH/NHLBI, 2011). The last category that relates to obesity is a new category, Sleep Health. This goal is to "increase public knowledge of how adequate sleep and treatment of sleep disorders improve health, productivity, wellness, quality of life, and safety on roads and in the workplace" (HHS/NIH/NHLBI, 2011).

Again, the objectives for Healthy People 2020 incorporate an entire section designated to Nutrition and Weight Status. This goal is the most specific with a direct correlation with weight loss and obesity. Healthier food access, health care and worksite settings, weight status, food insecurity, food and nutrient consumption, and iron deficiency are the specific objective categories. The interventions listed for 2020 encompass weight support through a variety of settings, including health care settings. Objectives listed under health care and worksite settings and weight status are as follows:

> Increase the proportion of primary care physicians who regularly measure the BMI of their patients; increase the proportion of physician office visits that include counseling or education related to nutrition or weight; increase the proportion of worksites that offer nutrition or weight management classes or counseling; increase the proportion of adults who are at a healthy weight; reduce the proportion of adults who are obese; reduce the proportion of children and adolescents who are considered obese; and prevent inappropriate weight gain in youth and adults. (HHS/NIH/NHLBI, 2011)

These objectives clearly define the needs and goals for the next 10 years.

First Lady Michelle Obama helped launch the Let's Move campaign in 2009. This program, which was aimed at children, was started because of the increase in childhood obesity and the even higher rates in African American and Hispanic communities. During the launch, Mrs. Obama stated, "The physical and emotional health of an entire generation and the economic health and security of our nation is at stake" (Let's Move, 2014). The initiative is dedicated to helping children lead healthier lives. This program strives to help children start healthy habits at a young age and continue these healthy behaviors throughout their lives. Supporting parents by providing healthy choices with affordable food options, providing healthy food choices at school, and promoting physical activity are the main goals of this initiative (Let's Move, 2014).

CAUSES

At its most simple definition, obesity results when someone ingests more calories than he or she expends. Although this seems relatively simple, there are many factors that influence body weight: heredity and genetic components, prenatal and postnatal choices, early lifestyle influences, poor dietary choices, sedentary lifestyle, technology, lack of sleep, environmental changes, and globalization (Harvard School of Public Health, 2014e).

Genetic Influences

Genetic influences with regard to obesity are present in simple forms of physiology and development. Genetic research is ongoing and has been for several decades. The Human Genome Project is in the forefront of the continuing advancements in molecular biology. This research has found that single-gene obesity is present as a result of several genetic factors. As research continues, multiple genes have been identified as causes of obesity. With the advancement in research and continued investigation and discovery of the role of genetics in obesity, it is important not to dwell on the gene as a deterrent, but rather to continue to promote positive health and lifestyle changes:

> What's increasingly clear from these early findings is that genetic factors identified so far make only a small contribution to obesity risk—and that our genes are not our destiny: Many people who carry these so-called "obesity genes" do not become overweight, and healthy lifestyles can counteract these genetic effects. (Harvard School of Public Health, 2014c)

It is also clear that genes and the gene environment play a significant role in understanding the obesity process. Monogenic mutations or a spontaneous mutation in a single gene have been closely related to several obesity hormones. Some of these include leptin, the leptin receptor, pro-opiomelanocortin (POMC), and melanocortin 4 receptor (MC4R). These hormones are vital in regulating appetite control and intake, as well as energy homeostasis.

Prader–Willi and Bardet–Biedl are syndromes in which obesity is considered a hallmark sign. These genetic syndromes occur with gene mutations or chromosomal abnormalities. Mental retardation and reproductive anomalies are also seen in these conditions. Some attribute obesity to a single gene; however, large population studies, animal models, twin studies, and human linkage studies show "common" obesity as polygenic or caused by multiple genes. Although body fat levels vary in people, some people are more prone toward higher body fat accumulation.

In the further assessment of the genetics of obesity, twin studies have provided insight. Data show that mean correlations for BMI for monozygotic twins are 0.74; dizygotic twins, 0.32; siblings, 0.25; parent–offspring pairs, 0.19; adoptive relatives, 0.06; and spouses, 0.12. Data from more than 25,000 twin pairs and more than 50,000 biological and adoptive family members show that monozygotic twins suggest strong genetic influences in BMI. The downside of these data is the assumption that both monozygotic and dizygotic twins have a shared environment.

Genome-wide association studies are used to find gene variations that may be related to a particular disease, such as obesity. Hundreds of thousands of complete DNA sets are scanned to find these variations. *Gene variants* or *single-nucleotide polymorphisms* (SNPs) are defined as small sections of DNA that are changed in relation to disease risk. The fat mass and obesity-associated (FTO) gene was first identified in 2007 as the first obesity-related gene variant on chromosome 16.

People with the FTO gene have a 20% to 30% increased obesity risk than those without this gene variant. Chromosome 18 also has an obesity-associated gene variant. This chromosome is close to the MC4R gene, which is the same gene that is responsible for monogenic obesity. Currently, more than 30 candidate genes on 12 chromosomes have been identified by the genome-wide association in relation to BMI.

Genetic variations are not likely to be responsible for the rapidly rising obesity rates across the world, because gene mutations and polymorphisms take time. Our environment, including physical, social, political, and economic surroundings, influences overweight and obesity. Although many people carry the FTO gene, not all become overweight and/or obese. Monitoring caloric intake and exercise may counteract the gene-related risk.

A Danish 2008 study conducted with 17,058 participants demonstrated that those who carried the FTO gene in addition to being inactive had higher BMIs. This is in comparison to those without the gene who were inactive. Those who were physically active had no change in BMI, whether they were a carrier of the FTO gene or not.

Research combined the results of 45 adult and 9 child studies, with a total of 240,000 participants, and found that those who carried the FTO gene had a 23% higher risk of obesity compared with those who were not carriers. Again, those who were physically active had a 30% lower risk of obesity than inactive adult carriers.

Prenatal and Early Life

Just like genetics, early life influences, such as the prenatal environment and a child's early years, can also influence weight and obesity. Studies conducted as early as the 1980s demonstrated high birth weights were associated with chronic disease later in life, such as obesity, T2DM, HTN, CAD, and stroke. Several modifiable risk factors can shape fetal nutrition and the child's health status later in life. These factors include the mother's smoking habits and tobacco use during pregnancy, her weight gain during pregnancy, her blood sugar levels, and whether or not she develops gestational diabetes.

Ideally, smoking cessation should be recommended to the mother prior to conception; however, if this habit persists, it should be stopped as soon as possible. Children of mothers who smoke during pregnancy are more likely to be obese even though smoking during pregnancy has been shown to slow fetal growth rates. Maternal smoking has demonstrated up to a 50% higher risk of childhood obesity.

Since 1990, excessive weight gain during pregnancy has become more common. Women are also starting their pregnancy at heavier weights—overweight and/or obese—even prior to conception. Excessive weight gain has spurred further changes to the original Institute of Medicine (IOM) pregnancy-related weight gain guidelines (published in 1990). The new guidelines are as follows to include weight recommendations for prepregnancy BMIs: normal BMI (18.5–24.9), overweight BMI (25.0–29.9), and obese BMI (≥30). A weight gain of 25 to 35 pounds is recommended for those women with a normal prepregnancy BMI. Women in the prepregnancy overweight BMI category should gain only 15 to 25 pounds, and women in the prepregnancy obese BMI category should gain only 11 to 20 pounds (Box 1.4).

Weight gain, primarily composed of adipose or fat tissue, is common with pregnancy. The increased adipose tissue is directly correlated with relative insulin

BOX 1.4 PREPREGNANCY WEIGHT RECOMMENDATIONS

Normal Weight (BMI 18.5–24.9)
Recommended Weight Gain: 25–35 pounds

Overweight (BMI 25.0–29.9)
Recommended Weight Gain: 15–25 pounds

Obese (BMI ≥30)
Recommended Weight Gain: 11–20 pounds

Source: Harvard School of Public Health, 2014i.

resistance. Increased amounts of glucose across the placenta have the potential to expose the fetus to high glucose and insulin levels. These higher levels can lead to increased body fat at birth as well as later in life. Studies vary in conclusion as to whether the mother's treatment during gestational diabetes affects the child later in life and are ongoing (Harvard School of Public Health, 2014i).

Postnatal environmental influences are also present that contribute to a child's weight gain. These are addressed more thoroughly in Chapter 24.

Poor Dietary Choices

Many questions arise with regard to food and obesity. What to eat and drink? How many calories? Where should the calories come from? When to eat? When not to eat? How do we know what is right? One of the problems with current society is the jump to a quick fix. As cliché as it sounds, a calorie is a calorie. And with that, the best way to lose weight is to limit what is eaten (eat less) and to work hard to burn excess energy (exercise more). Research shows that foods and proper diets exist to fight heart disease, T2DM, and stroke.

Portion sizes continue to increase. This has been the trend since the 1970s, both at home and out, among both children and adults. Studies have shown that when people are routinely served more, they eat more. The same is true with beverages— when served more, one consumes more. Unfortunately, even though a person drinks more, this has no effect on appetite, as the person usually consumes more.

Fast food is also known for its larger portion size as well as its convenience, low prices, and high fat and sugar content. One study demonstrated that people who had higher consumption of fast food were on average more than 13 pounds heavier than people who less frequently consumed fast food. These individuals also had a higher waist circumference and increased triglycerides, as well as an increased risk for metabolic syndrome (Harvard School of Public Health, 2014b). Further research with regard to income, neighborhood, and potential individual traits that increase fast food consumption would be beneficial.

Inactivity and Sedentary Lifestyle

Energy imbalance is directly related to obesity. Again, the simple equation is that calories in should equal calories expended or burned for weight maintenance, while weight loss should focus on less caloric intake or more energy output. Age, body size, genetic makeup, and the amount of daily activity are important factors that influence how many calories are burned.

Physical activity, or the process of staying active, can aid in weight maintenance or weight loss. Again, in general, the current population is more inactive or sedentary now than in the past. Based on national statistics, one in every three people gets minimal physical activity. This also correlates with the trend that the populations of most countries are physically inactive regardless of their income status. This trend is surprising, because the number of sports and/or leisure activities has been increased slightly and/or is stable; however, the levels of daily physical activity have decreased due to decreased activity levels at work and home, advancement in technology, increases in transportation, and social changes.

The United States, the United Kingdom, and China provide several examples of decreasing activity among their populations. In 50 years, the percentage of Americans working in high-activity jobs decreased by 8%, from 30% in 1950 to 22% in 2000. The number of children in the United States who walk to school has also decreased. This number fell from 40% to 13% in 2001. In addition, the number of Americans driving cars has increased over a 40-year span. Whereas 67% drove cars to work in 1960, that number increased to 88% in 2000. The United Kingdom has seen similar trends in decreased activity, as now many households own second cars. The number of physically active jobs has also decreased from 43% in 1991/1992 to 39% in 2004. Similar to the United States and the United Kingdom, China has also seen a decrease in work-related physical activity; men have seen a decrease by 35%, whereas women have seen a decrease of 46%. Physical activity around the house, such as cooking, cleaning, and washing clothes, has also decreased by 66%. In China, transportation by car is up, as are the sales of new cars (Harvard School of Public Health, 2014h).

Technology

Watching television has become a favorite pastime of U.S. citizens and has been so for the past 25 years. Taking up more than half of Americans' leisure time, it is also a common pastime in several European countries and Australia. Five hours of television time per day is the U.S. average. Alongside this trend is the habit of eating while watching television, as well as the temptation offered by the food advertisements seen on television. This affects both what people eat and how much they consume; it also promotes sedentary behavior.

Increased television time is linked to increased weight. Excess weight gain is also seen in those children with televisions in their bedrooms. When children watch a lot of television, the habit continues into adulthood, as does the increased risk for obesity. A direct correlation exists between increased television-viewing time and rates of obesity among both children and adults (Harvard School of Public Health, 2014k). According to the Nurses' Health Study of 50,000 women, data show an increased risk of 23% of developing obesity and an increased risk of 14% of developing DM (Hu, Li, Colditz, Willett, & Manson, 2003). In contrast, reduced television time is associated with a reduction in obesity. Many organizations recommend no more than 2 hours per day of media and/or television time.

Strasburger (2011) has hypothesized that television can lead to obesity in many ways; these include poor diets, unhealthy snacking while watching television, a lack of physical activity due to increased television watching, and interference with sleep. Other studies show evidence that obesity is linked to food and drink marketing on television (Harvard School of Public Health, 2014k). The IOM states that thousands of food-related television advertisements, many associated with higher calories and nutrition-dense foods and beverages, are seen by children and youth. "Pester power" by children is thought to lead to parents buying these foods and drinks (IOM, 2006). Halford et al. (2008) and Harris, Bargh, and Brownell (2009) found that children watching cartoons with food commercials versus those watching cartoons with no or nonfood commercials ate 45% more snack food while viewing television.

Similar to television time, other sedentary behaviors, including computer use, video games, driving, and sitting while at work, have a direct correlation with obesity. However, these do not have the extensive research and studies that have been conducted on television watching. Limiting these activities is recommended to help with weight control. One such method is to replace the sedentary activities deemed "sit time" with physical activity or "fit time." Consider biking or walking to work, if possible, or spending time outdoors or in a park instead of watching television or playing video games. Parents are encouraged to limit sedentary activities such as television watching to 2 hours per day or less (Harvard School of Public Health, 2014k).

Sleep Habits

Too little or lack of sleep is a contributor to obesity. Those sleeping less than 7 to 8 hours per night are at higher risk for weight gain compared to those getting the recommended 7 to 8 hours per night. From 1998 to 2005, Americans getting 8 hours of sleep per night decreased by 9% from 35% to 26% (Harvard School of Public Health, 2014j). The Nurses' Health Study included 68,000 women over a 16-year period. This study showed that women sleeping 5 hours or less were 15% more likely to be obese compared with women sleeping 7 hours per night (Patel, Malhotra, White, Gottlieb, & Hu, 2006). A few studies have shown that getting too much sleep may be as harmful as getting too little sleep; however, research is still incomplete. This theory, referred to as "reverse causation," is thought to have correlating conditions associated with obesity, such as sleep apnea, lung disease, depression, or cancer.

Sleep deprivation is associated with weight gain, possibly because of increased food amounts and decreased energy burned. Increased food intake is caused by increased hunger, more time spent eating, and choosing less healthy diets. Increased hunger caused by sleep deprivation is due to higher levels of ghrelin and lower levels of leptin. Also, those sleeping less, especially during the night, tend to both eat and snack more. Snacking, irregular meal patterns, and eating out often are other traits seen in people with sleep deprivation. Decreased energy expenditure occurs through decreased physical activity as well as lowered body temperature. Lack of sleep is shown to have a direct correlation with lack of physical activity, as those people appear sleepier during the day. These individuals also display a drop of body temperature, which is thought to lead to decreased energy expenditure. Healthy sleep habits have positive effects, such as mood improvement, alertness, and enhanced quality of life (Harvard School of Public Health, 2014j).

Environmental Barriers

Our current manmade world, as well as our social surroundings, can hinder physical activity. Cities, neighborhoods, parks, and streets have an impact on our lives. These determine whether we play or ride our bikes outside. Our familial support, friends, and coworkers also determine how active we are.

Family can determine the levels of physical activity. Research shows that parents and social support are role models as well as facilitators in physical activity. This can be as simple as taking children to sporting practice, buying sporting equipment, or even offering praise and positive reinforcement. Time spent outdoors, sibling involvement, and family income can also determine physical activity levels.

Worksites can also promote physical activities. A majority of people's time is spent at work, thus determining their activity levels and eating patterns. Studies have shown that work environments that promote physical activity, such as using the stairs, offering gymnasium passes or onsite gymnasiums, or providing bicycle storage, lead to modest improvements in employees' weight. Schools, like worksites, can also make a positive impact on students' physical activity and healthier lifestyles, as well as on the community and neighborhood. For example, studies have shown that opening schoolyards after school hours made a positive impact on the community by increasing outdoor activities.

Making neighborhoods safer is also a priority in promoting an increase in physical activity. Sidewalks, bicycle paths, bike lanes, and streetlights are ways to do so. Gymnasiums, shops, and other facilities that are placed within walking distance are ways to promote an increase in healthier lifestyles (Harvard School of Public Health, 2014a).

Globalization

Globalization is defined as "the act of globalizing, or extending to other or all parts of the world" (Dictionary.com, 2014). The obesity epidemic has spanned the globe and spread into many developing countries. Over the past 2 decades, obesity has affected nearly 2 billion people, with this number expected to increase to as high as 3.3 billion by 2030.

The rapid rate of this disease has been fueled by food, technology, and the environment in which we live. Changes in food prices as well as world trade have made this possible. Also, the shift to wealthier nations is also responsible for this epidemic as money has a direct correlation with food. Urbanization is another factor linked to obesity. Finally, changes in cultural norms have caused a heavier world. Stress, sleep deprivation, shifting consumer preferences, and women entering the workforce are other changes in cultural norms (Harvard School of Public Health, 2014d).

Obesity is linked to numerous trends and causes and is truly a global epidemic. Limited activity, convenience foods, and technology are linked to our increased waistlines. Learning about the past will help us plan for the future, manage chronic disease conditions, and focus on prevention.

REFERENCES

Centers for Disease Control and Prevention (CDC). (2011). *Healthy weight—It's not a diet, it's a lifestyle!* Retrieved from http://www.cdc.gov/healthyweight/index.html

Centers for Disease Control and Prevention (CDC). (2013). *Overweight and obesity: Adult obesity facts.* Retrieved from http://www.cdc.gov/obesity/data/adult.html

Christou, N., & Efthimiou, E. (2009). Five-year outcomes of laparoscopic adjustable gastric banding and laparoscopic Roux-en-Y gastric bypass in a comprehensive bariatric surgery program in Canada. *Canadian Journal of Surgery, 52*(6), E259–E258. Retrieved from http://www.ncbi.nlm.nih.gov/pmc/articles/PMC2792387/

Dictionary.com. (2013a). *Incidence.* Retrieved from http://dictionary.reference.com/browse/incidence?s=t

Dictionary.com. (2013b). *Prevalence.* Retrieved from http://dictionary.reference.com/browse/incidence?s=t

Dictionary.com. (2014). *Globalization.* Retrieved from http://dictionary.reference.com/browse/globalization?s=t

Halford, J. C., Boyland, E. J., Hughes, G. M., Stacey, L., McKean, S., & Dovey, T. M. (2008). Beyond-brand effect of television food advertisements on food choice in children: The effects of weight status. *Public Health Nutrition, 11,* 897–904.

Harris, J. L., Bargh, J. A., & Brownell, K. D. (2009). Priming effects of television food advertising on eating behavior. *Health Psychology, 28,* 404–413.

Harvard School of Public Health. (2014a). *Environmental barriers to activity.* Retrieved from https://www.hsph.harvard.edu/obesity-prevention-source/obesity-causes/physical-activity-environment

Harvard School of Public Health. (2014b). *Food and diet.* Retrieved from https://www.hsph.harvard.edu/obesity-prevention-source/obesity-causes/diet-and-weight

Harvard School of Public Health. (2014c). *Genes are not destiny.* Retrieved from https://www.hsph.harvard.edu/obesity-prevention-source/obesity-causes/genes-and-obesity

Harvard School of Public Health. (2014d). *Globalization.* Retrieved from https://www.hsph.harvard.edu/obesity-prevention-source/obesity-causes/globalization-and-obesity

Harvard School of Public Health. (2014e). *Obesity causes.* Retrieved from https://www.hsph.harvard.edu/obesity-prevention-source/obesity-causes

Harvard School of Public Health. (2014f). *Obesity consequences.* Retrieved from http://www.hsph.harvard.edu/obesity-prevention-source/obesity-consequences

Harvard School of Public Health. (2014g). *Obesity trends.* Retrieved from http://www.hsph.harvard.edu/obesity-prevention-source/obesity-trends

Harvard School of Public Health. (2014h). *Physical activity.* Retrieved from https://www.hsph.harvard.edu/obesity-prevention-source/obesity-causes/physical-activity-and-obesity

Harvard School of Public Health. (2014i). *Prenatal and early life influences.* Retrieved from https://www.hsph.harvard.edu/obesity-prevention-source/obesity-causes/prenatal-postnatal-obesity

Harvard School of Public Health. (2014j). *Sleep.* Retrieved from https://www.hsph.harvard.edu/obesity-prevention-source/obesity-causes/sleep-and-obesity

Harvard School of Public Health. (2014k). *Television watching and sit time.* Retrieved from https://www.hsph.harvard.edu/obesity-prevention-source/obesity-causes/television-and-sedentary-behavior-and-obesity

Hu, F. B., Li, T. Y., Colditz, G. A., Willett, W. C., & Manson, J. E. (2003). Television watching and other sedentary behaviors in relation to risk of obesity and type 2 diabetes mellitus in women. *Journal of the American Medical Association, 289,* 1785–1791.

Institute for Clinical Systems Improvement (ICSI). (2011). *Health care guideline: Prevention and management of obesity (Mature Adolescents and Adults).* Retrieved from http://www.obesitycast.com/guidelinecasts/ICSI_Obesity.pdf

Institute of Medicine. (2006). *Food marketing to children and youth: Threat or opportunity?* Washington, DC: National Academies of Sciences Press.

Jensen, M. D., Ryan, D. H., Apovian, C. M., Ard, J. D., Comuzzie, A. G., Donato, K. A., & Yanovski, S. Z. (2013). 2013 AHA/ACC/TOS guideline for the management of overweight and obesity in adults: A report of the American College of Cardiology/American Heart Association task force on practice guidelines and the obesity society. *Circulation*. Retrieved from http://circ.ahajournals.org/content/early/2013/11/11/01.cir.0000437739.71477.ee.citation

Let's Move. (2014). *America's move to replace a healthier generation of kids*. Retrieved from www.letsmove.gov

National Institutes of Health, National Heart, Lung, and Blood Institute, & National Institute of Diabetes and Digestive and Kidney Diseases (NIH/NHLBI/NIDDK). (1998). *Clinical guidelines on the identification, evaluation, and treatment of overweight and obesity in adults* (NIH Publication no. 98-4083). Retrieved from http://www.nhlbi.nih.gov/guidelines/obesity/ob_gdlns.pdf

Ogden, C. L., Carroll, M. D., Kit, B. K., & Flegal, K. M. (2012). *Prevalence of obesity in the United States, 2009–2010* (NCHS Data Brief no. 82). Retrieved from http://wood-ridge.schoolwires.net/cms/lib6/NJ01001835/Centricity/Domain/175/Obesity%20Article.pdf

Patel, S. R., Malhotra, A., White, D. P., Gottlieb, D. J., & Hu, F. B. (2006). Association between reduced sleep and weight gain in women. *American Journal of Epidemiology, 164*, 947–954.

Strasburger, V. C. (2011). Children, adolescents, obesity, and the media. *Pediatrics, 128*, 201–208.

U.S. Department of Health and Human Services, National Institutes of Health, & National Heart, Lung, and Blood Institute (HHS/NIH/NHLBI). (2011). *Healthy People 2020*. Retrieved from http://www.healthypeople.gov/2020/default.aspx

Wang, Z., & Nakayama, T. (2010). Inflammation, a link between obesity and cardiovascular disease. *Mediators Inflammation, 2010*, 535918.

Definition of Obesity and Obesity Terms

Many terms are used when treating the adult overweight or obese patient. As these terms can be somewhat confusing, it is best to have a handle on as many as possible. This chapter defines many of the terms commonly used in obesity treatment, including *body mass index (BMI), underweight, normal weight, overweight, obesity, class I obesity, class II obesity, class III obesity,* and *superobesity.*

BMI (see Box 2.1) is defined as the total body mass (in kilograms) divided by the height squared (in meters) (Kemper, Stasse-Wolthuis, & Bosman, 2004). *Underweight* is defined as a BMI of less than 18.5 kg/m². *Normal weight* is defined as a BMI of 18.5 to 24.9 kg/m². At their most common and basic description, *overweight* and *obesity* are defined as having too much body fat (Harvard School of Public Health, 2014a). *Overweight* is defined as a BMI ranging from 25.0 to 29.9 kg/m², whereas *obesity* is defined as a BMI greater than or equal to 30 kg/m². *Obesity* is further divided into three categories: class I, class II, and class III. *Class I obesity* is defined as a BMI of 30.0 to 34.9 kg/m². *Class II obesity*, also known as severe obesity, is defined as a BMI of 35.0 to 39.9 kg/m² (Brethauer, Kashyap, & Schauer, 2013; National Institutes of Health, National Heart, Lung, and Blood Institute, National Institute of Diabetes and Digestive and Kidney Diseases [NIH-NHLBI-NIDDK], 1998). *Class III obesity*, also known as morbid obesity or severe obesity, is defined as a BMI greater than or equal to 40 kg/m² (Brethauer et al., 2013; Christou & Efthimiou, 2009). According to Brethauer et al. (2013), *superobesity* is defined as a BMI greater than or equal to 50 kg/m² (see Box 2.2).

An individual's weight distribution is also important to understand and define. Increased abdominal fat or trunk fat is classified as *android* obesity, whereas

---

BOX 2.1 BODY MASS INDEX

The total body mass (in kilograms) divided by the height squared (in meters)

English BMI Formula
    BMI = (weight in pounds)/(height in inches) × (height in inches) × 704

Metric BMI Formula
    BMI = (weight in kilograms)/(height in meters) × (height in meters)

BOX 2.2 BMI CLASSIFICATIONS (IN KG/M²)

Underweight less than 18.5

Normal weight 18.5 to 24.9

Overweight 25.0 to 29.9

Obese greater than or equal to 30.0
  Class I 30.0 to 34.9
  Class II 35.0 to 39.9
  Class III greater than or equal to 40.0

Superobese greater than or equal to 50.0

more fat located around the hips and thigh is defined as *gynoid* or *gynecoid* obesity (Pescatello, Arena, Riebe, & Thompson, 2014).

As with many terms, the definition of *obesity* in children cannot be considered a direct comparison to the definition of *obesity* in adults. The definition of *overweight* in children is a BMI of the 85th percentile to lower than the 95th percentile (Centers for Disease Control and Prevention [CDC], 2012). "Obesity in children was defined as a BMI greater than or equal to the age and sex-specific 95th percentiles of the 2000 CDC growth charts" (Ogden, Carroll, Kit, & Flegal, 2012, p. 6).

Two other common terms used with the treatment of obesity are *ideal body weight* (IBW) and *excess body weight* (EBW). IBW is defined by the Metropolitan Life Table as a BMI of 25 kg/m². EBW is defined as the amount of weight a person possesses over and above the IBW. Those with class I obesity have an IBW greater than or equal to 20%. Those in the category of class II obesity have an over IBW greater than or equal to 100%, whereas those in the superobese category have an over IBW greater than or equal to 250% (Brethauer et al., 2013).

Measurements are also important in the treatment of the obese patient. A wide variety of recommendations exists with regard to body measurements. There are no set numbers that set one person apart; however, measurements should be taken and compared individually to weight and BMI. Neck circumference (NC), chest circumference (CC), and waist and hip circumferences (WC, HC) are essential measurements to understand. Measurements should be taken with the patient standing upright, using a nonstretchable plastic tape measure. NC is measured to the nearest millimeter. NC measurements should be taken between the mid-cervical spine and mid-anterior neck. Men with a prominent Adam's apple or laryngeal prominence should have this measurement taken just below the prominence (Aswathappa, Garg, Kutty, & Shankar, 2013). CC is also used to determine weight loss. Chest measurements should be taken at the widest part of the upper torso below the level of the arms. WC should be taken after a gentle exhaling breath. The measurements should be taken to the nearest millimeter (mm) and reported in centimeters (cm) and millimeters. The tape measure should be placed at the midpoint between the iliac crest and costal margin in the mid-axillary line. HC should be measured in centimeters. The patient should continue standing erect with legs and feet together. The patient should be measured at the level of the greater trochanters for the best accuracy (Aswathappa et al., 2013). The *waist-to-hip ratio* (WHR) is a determinant of health risks associated with obesity. Low and moderate risks are defined in the WHR Chart (Box 2.3).

Abdominal obesity is defined as the extra fat found in the midsection or that of a centrally distributed fat mass of the abdomen. The Harvard School of Public Health guidelines generally describe abdominal obesity as greater than 35 inches

BOX 2.3 WHR CHART

Male	Female	Health Risk Based Solely on WHR
0.95 or below	0.80 or below	Low risk
0.96 to 1.0	0.81 to 0.85	Moderate risk

in a woman and 40 inches in a man (Harvard School of Public Health, 2014a). *Adipocytes* are simply defined as fat cells (Obesity in America, 2014).

Metabolism is another term used when talking about obesity. *Metabolism* is defined as "the aggregate of all chemical processes that take place in living organisms, resulting in growth, generation of energy, elimination of wastes, and other body functions as they relate to the distribution of nutrients in the blood after digestion" (Anderson, 2002, p. 1085). Factors that affect metabolic rate include body composition, growth, hormonal status, fasting/starvation, dieting, and alcohol, caffeine, and tobacco abuse.

Total body fat, total body water, and fat-free mass are used when describing the makeup of weight. *Total body fat* is defined as a percentage of weight that is derived of fat. Body fat guidelines are divided into categories of male and female and also sectioned into age groups. *The American Journal of Clinical Nutrition* provides guidelines on body fat. Healthy body fat percentages in women aged 20 to 39 ranged from 21% to 32%; whereas in men, they ranged from 8% to 19%. Women ranging from 40 years through 59 years of age have a healthy body fat percentage of 23% to 33%. Men in that same age range are recommended to stay between 11% and 21%. Women in the age range of 60 through 79 are recommended to stay between 24% and 35%, with men at 13% to 24% (McCoy, 2012). *Total body water* is defined as the water content of the human body. Fat-free mass is the total body mass minus the fat (Williams, 2014).

Basal metabolic rate (BMR) and the Harris–Benedict Formula are used when calculating weight loss. *BMR* is defined as "the amount of energy used in a unit of time by a fasting, resting subject to maintain vital functions" (Anderson, 2002, p. 184). Again, it is the calories burned in a 24-hour period by doing nothing, but maintaining bodily functions. This rate is expressed in the calories consumed per hour per square meter of body surface area (Anderson, 2002). There are many online calculators that will ask for weight and height; however, it is important to know the equation behind BMR. The BMR for women is calculated as follows: BMR = 655 + (9.6 × weight in kilograms) + (1.8 × height in centimeters) − (4.7 × age in years). The equation for men is BMR = 66 + (13.7 × weight in kilograms) + (5 × height in centimeters) − (6.8 × age in years) (see Box 2.4).

BMR is also used in the Harris–Benedict Formula, which is used to determine the daily energy expenditure. BMR is multiplied by the activity factor, which describes the level of activity. To use the formula, the BMR is multiplied by 1.2 for sedentary, 1.375 for lightly active, 1.55 for moderately active, 1.725 for very active, and 1.9 for extra active (BMI Calculator, n.d.; see Box 2.5).

The thermic effect of food (TEF) and activity thermogenesis (AT) are additional terms used in obesity treatment. These are the processes of the body used to burn calories. *TEF* is defined as the increase in energy expenditure that occurs with the digestion, absorption, and metabolism of food (see Box 2.6).

BOX 2.4 BMR EQUATIONS

English BMR Formula

Women: BMR = 655 + (4.35 × weight in pounds) + (4.7 × height in inches) – (4.7 × age in years)

Men: BMR = 66 + (6.23 × weight in pounds) + (12.7 × height in inches) – (6.8 × age in years)

Metric BMR Formula

Women: BMR = 655 + (9.6 × weight in kilograms) + (1.8 × height in centimeters) – (4.7 × age in years)

Men: BMR = 66 + (13.7 × weight in kilograms) + (5 × height in centimeters) – (6.8 × age in years)

BOX 2.5 HARRIS–BENEDICT FORMULA

Sedentary (little or no exercise):
Calorie Calculation = BMR × 1.2

Lightly Active (light exercise/sports 1–3 days/week):
Calorie Calculation = BMR × 1.375

Moderately Active (moderate exercise/sports 3–5 days/week):
Calorie Calculation = BMR × 1.55

Very Active (hard exercise/sports 6–7 days a week):
Calorie Calculation = BMR × 1.725

Extra Active (very hard exercise/sports and physical job or 2× training):
Calorie Calculation = BMR × 1.9

BOX 2.6 ENERGY REQUIREMENTS

Total energy expenditure = BMR (60%–70%) + TEF (5%–10%) + AT (15%–30%)

AT is the energy expended during active exercise and the energy expended with activities of daily living (ADLs)—referred to as nonexercise activity thermogenesis (NEAT). A metabolic equivalent (MET) describes the calories burned while one sits still for 1 minute. This is important to understand, as it can help the advanced practice nurse (APN) discuss physical activity with patients.

Although many refer to physical activity and exercise as one and the same, they are not and their definitions differ. *Physical activity* refers to any activity that burns calories. This includes the ADLs plus work and play. Exercise is more specific as a subcategory of physical activity; it is a structured activity done with the goal of improving physical fitness or health and is often thought of as a repetitive or planned activity. Some also refer to "leisure-time physical activity" or "recreational physical activity" as exercise (Harvard School of Public Health, 2014b). *Sedentary* is the opposite of physical activity and refers to either a lack of or very limited physical activity, or the condition of inaction (Anderson, 2002).

Many surgical terms and procedures are used when talking about obesity. *Gastric banding* is a surgical procedure that is used to limit the amount of food in the stomach. A band is used to section off the stomach, which creates a small pouch. This pouch helps delay the emptying of food, causing a feeling of satiety or fullness. *Laparoscopic adjustable gastric banding* is similar to gastric banding. This surgery promotes the use of an inflatable band around the upper stomach. This band can be adjusted to meet each patient's needs. A *vertical banded gastroplasty* is a surgical procedure in which a small pouch in the stomach is constructed. This pouch allows a narrow opening into the stomach and duodenum. *Gastric bypass* is a surgical procedure in which the food "bypasses" the duodenum to again promote that feeling of satiety (Obesity in America, 2014). Roux-en-Y gastric bypass (RYBG) uses what is called a "roux limb" to bypass most of the stomach and the upper portion of the small intestine. The pouch, which is about the size of an egg, is directly attached to the small intestine (Johns Hopkins Medicine, n.d.).

Definitions for the following diseases are described in Chapter 16. These chronic conditions include hypertension (HTN), dyslipidemia, cardiovascular disease (CVD), diabetes mellitus (DM), obstructive sleep apnea (OSA), osteoarthritis (OA), polycystic ovary syndrome (PCOS), and metabolic syndrome.

Prevalence and incidence are described in Chapter 1. To recap: *Incidence* is defined as "the rate or range of occurrence or influence of something, especially of something unwanted" (Dictionary.com, 2013). *Prevalence* is defined as "the condition of being prevalent, or widespread" (Dictionary.com, 2013a).

Diagnostic testing associated with obese conditions or diseases is also important to understand when considering the treatment process. An electrocardiogram (EKG) is a recording of the electricity conduction of the heart (Anderson, 2002). A *polysomnography (PSG)* is defined as "the polygraphic recording during sleep of multiple physiologic variables, both directly and indirectly related to the state and stages of sleep, to assess possible biological causes of sleep disorders" (Anderson, 2002, p. 1370).

Laboratory values are also vital to ensure the complete understanding of obesity. Laboratories commonly used in the treatment of obesity include complete blood count (CBC; see Box 2.7), comprehensive metabolic panel (CMP; see Box 2.8), thyroid-stimulating hormone (TSH), Free T3, Free T4, Lipid Panel (see Box 2.9), glycated hemoglobin (HbA1C), and vitamin D levels. A CBC, CMP, and Lipid Panel are split into the laboratories listed next. TSH, Free T3, and Free T4 are laboratories to check thyroid function, whereas an HbA1C laboratory gives an average blood glucose level over a 3-month period. Vitamin D

BOX 2.7 COMPLETE BLOOD COUNT (CBC)

- White blood cell count (WBC)
- Automated white cell differential
  - Granulocytes
  - Lymphocytes
  - Monocytes
  - Eosinophils
  - Basophils
- Red blood cell count (RBC)

- Hemoglobin (Hb)
- Hematocrit (Hct)
- Mean cell volume (MCV)
- Mean cell hemoglobin (MCH)
- Mean cell hemoglobin concentration (MCHC)
- Red cell distribution width (RDW)
- Platelet count

BOX 2.8 COMPREHENSIVE METABOLIC PANEL (CMP)

- Albumin
- Alkaline phosphatase
- Alanine aminotransferase (ALT)
- Aspartate aminotransferase (AST)
- Blood urea nitrogen (BUN)
- Calcium
- Carbon dioxide (CO_2)

- Chloride
- Creatinine
- Glucose test
- Potassium test
- Sodium
- Total bilirubin
- Total protein

BOX 2.9 LIPID PANEL

- Total cholesterol
- Low-density lipoprotein (LDL)
- High-density lipoprotein (HDL)
- Triglycerides

laboratories check for vitamin D deficiency.

Ethical principles help guide nursing practice when treating patients. The following terms and definitions are the basis of nursing practice: *autonomy, beneficence, nonmaleficence, justice, veracity,* and *fidelity*. *Autonomy* is defined as "self-directed freedom, especially moral independence" (Zaccagnini & Waud White, 2011, p. 320). *Beneficence* and *nonmaleficence* are oftentimes intertwined and at times difficult to balance. *Beneficence* is defined as "an action that is done for the benefit of others" (p. 322), whereas *nonmaleficence* is defined as "avoidance of harm" (p. 321). *Justice* is defined as being fair or impartial. Aristotle defines the principle of justice as follows: "Equals should be treated equally and unequals should be treated unequally" (p. 323). Merriam-Webster (2015b) defines *veracity* as "truth or accuracy" (n.p.). Finally, *fidelity* is "the quality or state of being faithful; accuracy in details; exactness" (Merriam-Webster, 2015a, n.p.).

This chapter defines many of the terms associated with obesity and treatment of obesity. It can be used as a reference for better patient understanding and treatment.

REFERENCES

Anderson, D. M. (Ed.). (2002). *Mosby's Medical, Nursing, & Allied Health Dictionary.* (6th ed.). St. Louis, MO: Mosby.

Aswathappa, J., Garg, S., Kutty, K., & Shankar, V. (2013). Neck circumference as an anthropometric measure of obesity in diabetes. *North American Journal of Medical Science, 5*(1), 28–31. doi: 10.4103/1947-2714.106188

BMI Calculator. (n.d.) Harris-Benedict equation. Retrieved from http://www.bmi-calculator.net/bmr-calculator/harris-benedict-equation/

Brethauer, S., Kashyap, S., & Schauer, P. (2013). *Obesity.* Cleveland Clinic. Retrieved from http://www.clevelandclinicmeded.com/medicalpubs/diseasemanagement/endocrinology/obesity/

Centers for Disease Control and Prevention. (2012). *Overweight and obesity: Basics of childhood obesity.* Retrieved from http://www.cdc.gov/obesity/childhood/basics.html

Christou, N., & Efthimiou, E. (2009). Five-year outcomes of laparoscopic adjustable gastric banding and laparoscopic Roux-en-Y gastric bypass in a comprehensive bariatric surgery program in Canada. *Canadian Journal of Surgery*, *52*(6), E259–58. Retrieved from http://www.cma.ca/multimedia/staticContent/HTML/N0/l2/cjs/vol-52/issue-6/pdf/pgE249.pdf

Dictionary.com. (2013). *Incidence*. Retrieved from http://dictionary.reference.com/browse/incidence?s=t

Dictionary.com. (2013a). *Prevalence*. Retrieved from http://dictionary.reference.com/browse/incidence?s=t

Harvard School of Public Health. (2014a). *Obesity definition*. Retrieved from https://www.hsph.harvard.edu/obesity-prevention-source/obesity-definition/

Harvard School of Public Health. (2014b). *Physical activity*. Retrieved from https://www.hsph.harvard.edu/obesity-prevention-source/obesity-causes/physical-activity-and-obesity/

Johns Hopkins Medicine. (n.d.). *Roux-en-Y gastric bypass weight-loss surgery*. Retrieved from http://www.hopkinsmedicine.org/healthlibrary/test_procedures/gastroenterology/roux-en-y_gastric_bypass_weight-loss_surgery_135,65/

Kemper, H. C. G., Stasse-Wolthuis, M., & Bosman, W. (2004). The prevention and treatment of overweight and obesity: Summary of the advisory report by the Health Council of the Netherlands. *Journal of Medicine*, *62*(1), 10–17. Retrieved from http://www.njmonline.nl/getpdf.php?id=157

McCoy, K. (2012). *Your body fat percentage: What does it mean?* NYU Langone Medical Center. Retrieved from http://www.med.nyu.edu/content?ChunkIID=41373

Merriam-Webster. (2015a). *Fidelity*. Retrieved from http://www.merriam-webster.com/dictionary/fidelity

Merriam-Webster. (2015b). *Veracity*. Retrieved from http://www.merriam-webster.com/dictionary/veracity

National Institutes of Health, National Heart, Lung, and Blood Institute, National Institute of Diabetes and Digestive and Kidney Diseases. (1998). *Clinical guidelines on the identification, evaluation, and treatment of overweight and obesity in adults* (NIH Publication No. 98-4083). Retrieved from http://www.nhlbi.nih.gov/guidelines/obesity/ob_gdlns.pdf

Obesity in America. (2014). *Understanding obesity: Glossary of terms*. Retrieved from http://obesityinamerica.org/understanding-obesity/glossary-of-terms

Ogden, C. L., Carroll, M. D., Kit, B. K., & Flegal, K. M. (2012). *Prevalence of obesity in the United States*, 2009–2010. NCHS Data Brief (82). Retrieved from http://wood-ridge.schoolwires.net/cms/lib6/NJ01001835/Centricity/Domain/175/Obesity%20Article.pdf

Pescatello, L. S., Arena, R., Riebe, D., & Thompson, P. D. (2014). *ACSM's guidelines for exercise testing and prescription* (9th ed.). Philadelphia, PA: Lippincott Williams & Wilkins.

Williams, L. (2014). *What is fat-free body mass?* Livestrong.com. Retrieved from http://www.livestrong.com/article/128552-fat-body-mass/

Zaccagnini, M. E., & Waud White, K. (2011). *The doctor of nursing practice essentials: A new model for advanced practice nursing*. Sudbury, MA: Jones and Bartlett.

The Many Roles of the Advanced Practice Nurse

Nursing is a broad term that encompasses many levels of education. Advanced practice registered nurses (APRNs) are nurses with a master's, post-master's, or doctorate level of education. Four roles encompassed under the definition of the *APRN* are certified nurse practitioners (CNPs), certified registered nurse anesthetists (CRNAs), certified nurse-midwives (CNMs), and clinical nurse specialists (CNSs). Each has its own context, but all share the commonality of nursing, especially advanced practice nursing. Although education similarities as well as accreditation and certification exist, uniform state regulations for APRN practice do not. States, with their governing licensing boards and statutes, provide state practice authority. The legal scope of the APRN is individually and independently determined by each state. Problems arise due to the lack of uniformity between states, making it difficult to provide care across state lines.

There are other nurses with advanced education who also enhance the role of APRNs. These nurses do not have direct patient care focus and, thus, do not require further licensure beyond that of the registered nurse (RN). Examples of advanced graduate nursing roles that are not included as an APRN function include education, administration, public health, research, and informatics. These nursing roles are essential for safe and quality patient care; however, they do not focus on direct patient care and are not the focus of this chapter.

The educational programs that APRNs graduate from are nationally accredited; therefore, their graduates are eligible for national certification and state licensure. These programs consist of graduate classes in advance pathophysiology or physiology, pharmacology, and health assessment. APRNs also meet certain criteria in education, including focus on "at least one of six population foci: family/individual across the life span, adult-gerontology, pediatrics, neonatal, women's health/gender-related or psych/mental health" (Advanced Practice Registered Nurse [APRN] Consensus Work Group & the National Council of State Boards of Nursing [NCSBN]-APRN Advisory Committee, 2008, p. 6). Those completing the educational criteria and graduation sit for a national certification examination (NCE). This certifying process is used to assess core competencies for each of the four specialty focus areas. The certification is accredited and requires continued competencies in one of the six specified foci. APRNs may specialize further, but they are not licensed exclusively within the specialty area. The APRN Regulatory Model strives to implement and support licensure, accreditation, certification, and education (LACE).

The definition of *APRN* was established with assistance from several nursing groups, including the American Nurses Association (ANA) and the National Council of State Boards of Nursing (NCSBN). According to them, an APRN is someone (APRN Consensus Work Group & the NCSBN-APRN Advisory Committee, 2008, pp. 7–8):

1. who has completed an accredited graduate-level education program preparing him or her for one of the four recognized APRN roles
2. who has passed an NCE that measures APRN, role, and population-focused competencies and who maintains continued competence as evidenced by recertification in the role and population through the national certification program
3. who has acquired advanced clinical knowledge and skills preparing him or her to provide direct care to patients, as well as a component of indirect care; however, the defining factor for **all** APRNs is that a significant component of the education and practice focuses on direct care of individuals
4. whose practice builds on the competencies of RNs by demonstrating a greater depth and breadth of knowledge, a greater synthesis of data, increased complexity of skills and interventions, and greater role autonomy
5. who is educationally prepared to assume responsibility and accountability for health promotion and/or maintenance as well as the assessment, diagnosis, and management of patient problems, which include the use and prescription of pharmacological and nonpharmacological interventions
6. who has clinical experience of sufficient depth and breadth to reflect the intended license
7. who has obtained a license to practice as an APRN in one of the four APRN roles: CRNA, CNM, CNS, or CNP

APRNs provide professional care across the health spectrum based on individual patient needs and educational experiences. Each role within the APRN scope of practice is different; however, care within the health wellness–illness spectrum is a priority. Roles within each specialty are further defined in the individual sections of CNP, CRNA, CNM, and CNS (APRN Consensus Work Group & the NCSBN-APRN Advisory Committee, 2008).

CERTIFIED NURSE PRACTITIONER (CNP)

A nurse practitioner (NP) is an autonomous, licensed, independent practitioner who uses skill sets of assessment, diagnosis, and treatment to manage patients' health care needs. CNPs order and interpret testing and laboratory values, as well as prescribe pharmacological agents. CNPs practice in a variety of settings, including family practice, acute or long-term care, ambulatory settings, and specialty practice clinics. Health promotion and disease management as well as treatment of acute and chronic diseases are among the CNPs' expertise areas (American Association of Nurse Practitioners [AANP], 2013). Care focused within the wellness–illness continuum is emphasized within the CNP practice. The NP treats patients with acute or chronic symptoms as having chronic diseases (APRN Consensus Work Group & the NCSBN-APRN Advisory Committee, 2008). Teaching, counseling, researching, and patient advocacy are other areas in which NPs excel (AANP, 2013).

CNPs are also responsible for taking and recording comprehensive medical histories, health assessments, and physical examinations; they also play a big role in the screening process. Diagnosis, treatment, and management are other assets of the CNP. In addition, CNPs provide prescriptions for durable medical equipment as well as refer patients to other providers and professional medical team members (APRN Consensus Work Group & the NCSBN-APRN Advisory Committee, 2008).

Education for NPs includes a master's, post-master's, or doctorate degree. Clinical courses focus on competencies in specialized practice for each NP track. Several NP tracks exist, including family nurse practitioner (FNP), adult nurse practitioner (ANP), gerontological nurse practitioner (GNP), pediatric nurse practitioner (PNP), acute care nurse practitioner (ACNP), and psychiatric mental health nurse practitioner (PMHNP). NPs are licensed at the state and national level through the certification process. The American Nurses Credentialing Center (ANCC) and AANP provide national certification. Again, each state determines the scope of the CNP for practice. Continued education courses are taken to maintain competency (AANP, 2013).

CERTIFIED REGISTERED NURSE ANESTHETIST (CRNA)

"Nurse anesthesia is the oldest organized specialty in nursing" (Hamric, Spross, & Hanson, 2000, p. 521). Standardized education as well as postgraduate training, continuing education, and credentialing are areas first explored by the CRNA. Apart from pioneering through APRN practice, CRNAs were also among the first to receive direct reimbursement for services rendered. The CRNA is autonomous and nowhere within the United States is it required that they be supervised by anesthesiologists (Hamric, Spross, & Hanson, 2000).

A CRNA is an RN with advanced education who provides comprehensive anesthesia care and treatment. Patients range across the human life span. CRNAs provide care to those in variable settings. Examples can include hospital or surgical suites, ambulatory surgical centers, obstetrical delivery rooms, pain management clinics or centers, as well as dental, plastic surgery, podiatry, and/or ophthalmology offices. Care may include acute or severe conditions, injury, or routine surgical patients (APRN Consensus Work Group & the NCSBN-APRN Advisory Committee, 2008).

The CRNA has various duties within the scope of practice. He or she is responsible for conducting and documenting a preanesthetic assessment and patient evaluation as well as for developing the plan for anesthesia. The CRNA also initiates the anesthetic technique. This may include general, regional, local, or sedation. Administration of anesthetics as well as monitoring the patient's physical status is also included in the scope of practice. The CRNA is responsible for managing the patient's ventilatory support and airway and pulmonary status throughout the procedure, as well as for providing postanesthesia care needs. Acute and chronic pain management implementation is also within the scope of practice. Finally, the CRNA is responsible for response to emergency situations (American Association of Nurse Anesthetists [AANA], 2010).

The average CRNA completes almost 2,500 clinical hours prior to graduation. Education for the CRNA includes a master's, post-master's, or doctorate degree (AANA, 2011). As of January 1, 2014, the National Board of Certification and Recertification for Nurse Anesthetists (NBCRNA) raised the passing standard for the NCE (The National Board of Certification and Recertification for Nurse Anesthetists [NBCRNA], 2013). This decision was made in recognition of the need for a greater knowledge and skills base secondary to the growing complexity in anesthesia care. The recertification process for CRNAs occurs every 2 years. Practice requirements as well as 40 continuing education hours must also be met (AANA, 2011).

CERTIFIED NURSE-MIDWIFE (CNM)

A CNM provides primary care to women throughout their life span. A CNM has historically been thought to primarily provide childbirth care; however, he or she provides more than just care through pregnancy. The CNM also provides family planning services, preconception counseling, prenatal care, postpartum care, and newborn care (for the first 28 days of life; APRN Consensus Work Group & the NCSBN-APRN Advisory Committee, 2008). Contraceptive and infertility care are also within the scope of practice (Hamric, Spross, & Hanson, 2000). Gynecological care, up to and including treating sexually transmitted diseases in both the woman and the partner, is provided by the CNM (APRN Consensus Work Group & the NCSBN-APRN Advisory Committee, 2008). Additional skills and procedures within the CNM practice include circumcision, vacuum extraction, colposcopy, endometrial biopsy, and elective termination of pregnancy (Hamric, Spross, & Hanson, 2000).

CNMs provide care in various settings. Hospitals, birthing centers, ambulatory settings, clinics, community public health clinics, and the home are possible care settings (APRN Consensus Work Group & the NCSBN-APRN Advisory Committee, 2008). No matter the place of service, four management aspects the CNM includes in service are independent management, consultation, comanagement or collaborative management, and referral (Hamric, Spross, & Hanson, 2000).

Education for the CNM includes a master's, post-master's, or doctorate degree. CNMs have education in two discipline areas—midwifery and nursing; however, education programs for the CNM and certified midwives are identical (American College of Nurse Midwives [ACNM], 2011, 2013). The Accreditation Commission for Midwifery Education (ACME) is the certifying body for CNM education programs. In the United States, 39 programs are accredited. In 2010, entry to CNM programs changed, requiring a graduate degree for entry. Similar to the CNP and CRNA specialties, CNMs are licensed and autonomous in practice (ACNM, 2013). They are certified by the national examination overseen by the American Midwifery Certification Board (AMCB). CNMs must be recertified every 5 years through the accreditation board and are also required to complete specific continuing education credits (ACNM, 2011). CNMs have prescriptive authority in all 50 states as well as in the District of Columbia and are considered primary care providers by the federal law. Insurance reimbursement for the CNM includes Medicaid, Medicare, and a majority of private insurances (ACNM, 2013).

CLINICAL NURSE SPECIALIST (CNS)

The role of the CNS involves a care continuum, including the patient, the nurse, and the system (APRN Consensus Work Group & the NCSBN-APRN Advisory

Committee, 2008). This role was initially created to keep APRNs in clinical practice through advocating and improving the overall patient care and satisfaction (Hamric, Spross & Hanson, 2000). The CNS is one "who, through study and supervised practice at the graduate level (master's or doctorate), has become expert in a defined area of knowledge and practice in a selected clinical area of nurse" (American Nurses Association [ANA], 1980, p. 23). The CNS integrates each distinctive part of the care continuum to provide better patient outcomes and improve nursing care. The dimensions of the expert clinician, researcher, educator, and consultant are integrated for sustained integrity; however, the scope must be differentiated within the distinct roles to maintain clear responsibilities and contributions. Competencies, including direct clinical practice, consultation, teaching and coaching, scientific inquiry, clinical and professional leadership, ethical decision making, and collaboration, are used within the four dimensions (Hamric, Spross, & Hanson, 2000).

Mentoring is a key element involved in the CNS role. Mentoring is used to create empowering environments for nurses to excel in patient care. Evidence-based practice as well as ethical decision making improves overall patient care within the various health care settings. Other responsibilities of the CNS include diagnosis of disease management and health/illness states. They are also accountable for health promotion and prevention of illness. Finally, they are responsible for risk behavior management on an individual basis as well as within families, group settings, and communities (APRN Consensus Work Group & the NCSBN-APRN Advisory Committee, 2008).

Education for the CNS includes a master's, post-master's, or doctorate degree. After graduation, the CNS is prepared to take the ANCC-CNS examination (Johns Hopkins School of Nursing, 2014).

APRNs can use their education and practice experience to provide the best care environment for the overweight and/or obese patient. Each of the four APRN roles can serve the patient in unique and different ways. Each role must know that the care of the obese individual is within his or her scope of practice and may require a comprehensive and collaborative approach to total patient treatment.

REFERENCES

American Association of Nurse Anesthetists (AANA). (2010). *CRNA scope of practice.* Retrieved from https://www.aana.com/aboutus/Documents/scopeofpractice.pdf

American Association of Nurse Anesthetists (AANA). (2011). *Education of nurse anesthetists in the United States—at a glance.* Retrieved from http://www.aana.com/ceandeducation/becomeacrna/Pages/Education-of-Nurse-Anesthetists-in-the-United-States.aspx

American Association of Nurse Practitioners (AANP). (2013). *Scope of practice for nurse practitioners.* Retrieved from https://www.aanp.org/images/documents/publications/scopeofpractice.pdf

American College of Nurse Midwives (ACNM). (2011). *Definition of midwifery and scope of practice of certified nurse-midwives and nurse midwives.* Retrieved from http://www.midwife.org/ACNM/files/ACNMLibraryData/UPLOADFILENAME/000000000266/Definition%20of%20Midwifery%20and%20Scope%20of%20Practice%20of%20CNMs%20and%20CMs%20Dec%202011.pdf

American College of Nurse Midwives (ACNM). (2013). *Essential facts about midwives.* Retrieved from http://www.midwife.org/Essential-Facts-about-Midwives

American Nurses Association. (1980). *Nursing: A social policy statement.* Kansas City, MO: Author.

APRN Consensus Work Group & the National Council of State Boards of Nursing-APRN Advisory Committee. (2008). *Consensus model for APRN regulation: Licensure, accreditation, certification & education.* Retrieved from https://www.ncsbn.org/Consensus_Model_for_APRN_Regulation_July_2008.pdf

Hamric, A. B., Spross, J. A., & Hanson, C. M. (2000). Advanced nursing practice (2nd ed.). Philadelphia, PA: W. B. Saunders Company.

Johns Hopkins School of Nursing. (2014). *Clinical nurse specialist.* Retrieved from http://nursing.jhu.edu/academics/programs/masters/clinical

The National Board of Certification and Recertification for Nurse Anesthetists. (2013). *Standard setting announcement.* Retrieved from http://www.nbcrna.com/certification/SiteAssets/Pages/default/NBCRNA%20Standard%20Setting%20Handout.pdf

Case Study 1

This case study builds upon information acquired in the introductory part of this book, Chapters 1 to 3:

- *Chapter 1: Obesity: The Epidemic, Trends, and Causes*
- *Chapter 2: Definition of Obesity and Obesity Terms*
- *Chapter 3: The Many Roles of the Advanced Practice Nurse*

Mrs. A is a pleasant, Caucasian, 60-year-old woman. She presents as a new patient to your office today. She reports no medical history. She has a family history of hypertension (HTN) (mother and father), diabetes (maternal grandmother and father), and coronary artery disease (CAD) (father died of a myocardial infarction [MI] at age 48). Her body mass index (BMI) is 40. She recently retired after 35 years of working as an administrative assistant. Since retiring, she reports that she loves reading, gardening, playing games on the computer, and watching her three favorite soap operas during the day. She states she is active—her activity includes taking care of her grandchildren—but admits that she does not engage in regular exercise. She reports that she eats healthy, but does not eat breakfast. She also states that she does not really like fruit. She reports that for the most part she is happy; however, she does state that she feels more tired and sluggish lately. She also reports no motivation to get going in the morning. She affirms that she has some ups and downs, but states that she thinks this is normal in life.

Her vitals are reviewed:

Blood pressure: 150/84
Pulse: 72 bpm
Respirations: 12
Height: 5 feet, 4 inches
Weight: 235 pounds
BMI: 40.35 kg/m^2
Pulse oximetry: 94% on room air
Neck circumference: 17.5 inches
Waist circumference: 57 inches
Hip circumference: 57.5 inches
Waist-to-hip ratio: 0.99 inches

Medication list:

- One multivitamin daily
- One calcium tablet with vitamin D daily
- Tylenol one to two tablets prn (as needed)

Her physical examinations reveal:

General: Looks stated age, appropriate conversation, in no acute distress.
Head, Eyes, Ears, Nose, Throat (HEENT): PERRLA, extraocular muscles intact, conjunctiva normal, anicteric.
Neck: Supple, no jugular vein distension (JVD).
Skin: Warm, pink, dry.
Mucosa: No cyanosis, moist.
Cardiovascular: Normal S1 and S2. No murmur.
Lungs: Good bilateral air entry.
Abdomen: Obese, soft, and nontender. Normal bowel sounds. No rebound pain or rigidity.
Extremities: No edema, cyanosis, or clubbing.
Neurological: Alert and oriented ×3. No motor or sensory deficit.

Is she overweight or obese? What category does her BMI fall into?

How would you address her BMI?

Would you address her family history?

What cardiovascular risk factors does she have?

What has led to her obesity?

Is she a candidate for weight loss?

How would you present her with a plan for weight loss? What would this include?

What would you do about her BP? What treatment options would you present to her?

Would you make any additional referrals?

Would you consider any medications for this patient? If yes, what medications and why?

Would you order any testing? If yes, what testing and why?

What dietary advice would you provide?

What lifestyle changes would you suggest?

You also draw fasting blood work on her and find the following:

Basic Metabolic Panel (BMP)

Sodium: 135
Potassium: 3.7
Chloride: 101
Carbon dioxide (CO_2): 25
Blood urea nitrogen (BUN): 22
Creatinine: 1.0
Glucose: 135

Complete Blood Count (CBC)

White blood cells (WBCs): 6.5
Hemoglobin (Hb): 14.7
Hematocrit (Hct): 44.5
Platelets: 202

Thyroid-stimulating hormone (TSH): 2.0

Fasting Lipid Panel

Total cholesterol: 215
Triglycerides: 225
High-density lipoprotein (HDL): 35
Low-density lipoprotein (LDL): 130

Would you make any additional changes in her medications?

When would you repeat laboratory work?

When would you schedule her next follow-up appointment?

Would you involve any other advanced practice nurses (APNs) in her care?

What additional education, if any, would you provide?

Communication

Addressing Pediatric Obesity

"Obesity is insidious, often beginning in childhood and perpetuating with age, but its incidence is not age specific" (Buttaro, Trybulski, Bailey, & Sandberg-Cook, 2003, p. 60). Pediatric obesity is a growing problem worldwide. Both the incidence and prevalence of overweight and obese children have increased. Advanced practice nurses (APNs) should realize that one must address weight at an early age. A multidisciplinary approach and parental involvement should drive this plan. In some instances, family counseling may be needed, especially in the case of overweight and/or obese parents. This issue is not one that should be taken lightly, as it is a delicate and sensitive subject for all those involved. Active listening skills should also be utilized.

Pediatric or childhood obesity affects children and adolescents and is a serious condition that must be addressed. It is determined when the child is above his or her weight for the appropriate age and height. As with adult obesity, childhood obesity occurs mainly due to lifestyle issues and is a result of too many calories consumed versus too few calories expended; however, some genetic disease and hormonal disorders also can lead to obesity (Mayo Clinic, 2014).

RISK FACTORS

Some children have larger than average body frames, whereas other children progress through the various stages of development with different amounts of fat. Risk factors that increase a child's likelihood of becoming overweight and/or obese can include any of the following: diet, lack of exercise, psychological factors, family history or family factors, or socioeconomic factors. Burns, Dunn, Brady, Barber Starr, and Blosser (2004) list maternal smoking while pregnant, bottle feeding, binge eating in response to body image and low self-esteem, and depression as other factors that can contribute to childhood obesity. Children learn from their parents; those who model poor eating and engage in minimal exercise also contribute to the rising trend. "A young child whose mother has a BMI of 27 or more is a risk for obesity" (Bergmann et al., 2003, as cited in Burns et al., 2004, p. 248). Psychosocial factors and family dysfunction, as well as children who have suffered from abuse, neglect, or overcontrolling parents, are likely to increase the incidence of childhood obesity (Burns et al., 2004). All risk factors should be addressed during a pediatric visit with the child and family members.

Encouraging healthy foods and snacks is important. Many children eat one or two meals and/or snacks at school. February 24, 2014, marked for the first time in 15 years that changes were made to the school lunch program. These changes were announced by First Lady Michelle Obama and U.S. Department of Agriculture Secretary Tom Vilsack. The National School Lunch Program was established in 1966 and is a federally assisted meal program serving low-cost or free lunches to school children (The U.S. Department of Agriculture Food and Nutrition Service, 2014). "The idea here is simple—our classrooms should be healthy places where kids aren't bombarded with ads for junk food," said First Lady Michelle Obama. "Because when parents are working hard to teach their kids healthy habits at home, their work shouldn't be undone by unhealthy messages at school" (The White House, 2014). In collaboration with the new school wellness standards, the United States Department of Agriculture (USDA) announced the launch of its new website—School Nutrition Environment and Wellness Resources. This website provides information for school districts and food marketing practices.

Children who suffer with weight gain should engage in physical activity. Parental instruction and family activity time are also helpful. School involvement and physical education or "gym class" are important, as they educate students on what types of activities to do while having a set time for activity. There continues to be controversy around physical education, especially as schools struggle with budget cuts and the growing need for "more" education. Some feel that physical education is not a needed class, whereas others strongly disagree, especially with the growing increase of obesity in children. There is a development toward inactivity as technology continues to trend. Inactive leisure activities, such as playing computer or video games and watching television, contribute to overweight and obesity.

Psychological factors can also lead to a child being overweight and/or obese. Some children use food to battle problems related to stress, whereas others tend to eat due to boredom. Some of these tendencies may be seen from parental examples.

Family history or family factors can also lead to weight problems. If a child has parents or other family members who are overweight or obese, he or she is also likely to suffer with unnecessary weight gain. Environment also plays a role in obesity, as this is where high-calorie foods are more readily available and many times physical activity is not encouraged. This is also where convenience foods play a role. Teaching parents to monitor the "junk" food the child eats will also help cut down on high-calorie items.

Socioeconomic factors also contribute to obesity. Convenience foods—those that are prepackaged—may also play a part in lower-income families. Fresh fruits and vegetables are more expensive and can easily deplete monetary funds more quickly than cheaper meals. Educating people on the fact that frozen foods are also a healthy option is essential. Promoting safe exercise facilities or recreation facilities is also important to address additional physical activity (Mayo Clinic, 2014).

GROWTH CHARTS

The definition of *obesity* in children cannot be considered a direct comparison to the definition of *obesity* in adults. Growth standards and growth charts are used in the pediatric and adolescent population to track growth. A series of percentile curves are used to get accurate body measurements. Growth charts are not used solely in practice; however, they are used to help form an accurate over-all clinical impression of the child's health. The Centers for Disease Control and Prevention (CDC) recommend use of the World Health Organization (WHO) growth charts for infants aged 0 to 2 years in the United States and use of the CDC growth charts to monitor growth for those children aged 2 years and older.

In 2006, the WHO released a new international growth standard statistical distribution of the growth of children aged 0 to 59 months. This growth is viewed as optimal and is used in six countries in the world, including the United States. These standards depict growth under optimal conditions, rather than including those countries that do not support optimal growth. The WHO recognizes the following standards in infants and children aged 0 to 2 years: "The WHO standards establish growth of the breast-fed infant as the norm for growth; The WHO standards provide a better description of physiological growth in infancy; and The WHO standards are based on a high-quality study designed explicitly for creating growth charts" (Centers for Disease Control and Prevention [CDC], 2010).

Clinic growth charts are divided into separate categories: infants, birth to 36 months; children and adolescents; and preschoolers, 2 to 5 years. These charts have grids scaled to metric units—kilograms (kg) and centimeters (cm). A secondary scale includes English units—pounds (lb) and inches (in). The chart for infants includes the recommended length and weight, head circumference, and weight-for-length for the child's age. The children and adolescent charts include the stature and weight-for-age, as well as the BMI-for-age. The preschooler charts include weight-for-stature. "BMI-for-age charts are recommended to assess weight in relation to stature for children ages 2 to 20 years. The weight-for-stature charts are available as an alternative to accommodate children ages 2 to 5 years who are not evaluated beyond the preschool years. However, all health care providers should consider using the BMI-for-age charts to be consistent with current recommendations" (CDC, 2010). The definition of *overweight* in children is a BMI of the 85th percentile to lower than the 95th percentile (CDC, 2012). "Obesity in children was defined as a BMI greater than or equal to the age and sex-specific 95th percentiles of the 2000 CDC growth charts" (Ogden, Carroll, Kit, & Flegal, 2012, p. 6).

QUICK TIPS—WHO CHARTS AND GROWTH CHARTS

The WHO Growth Charts and Data Tables:
www.cdc.gov/growthcharts/who_charts.htm#TheWHOGrowthCharts

Clinical Growth Charts:
www.cdc.gov/growthcharts/clinical_charts.htm

THE PROVIDER–PEDIATRIC PATIENT RELATIONSHIP

Approaching the subject of overweight and obesity with any patient is difficult, let alone a pediatric patient and family, which can prove even more complex, frustrating, time consuming, and costly. The topic should be addressed, just like with any adult patient, with compassion and honesty. As described in Chapter 5, therapeutic communication should be used with the patient and family. The child's age also determines the depth and wording of the conversation. With a child and family involved, family counseling may be beneficial to all. Including a dietitian as part of the treatment team is also beneficial to help with continued planning.

Pediatric obesity is a serious condition that requires immediate attention. The provider must establish an early relationship with the patient and family and work to gain trust. A thorough understanding of the disease and treatment process is essential for success.

REFERENCES

Burns, C. E., Dunn, A. M., Brady, M. A., Barber Starr, N., & Blosser, C. G. (2004). *Pediatric primary care: A handbook for nurse practitioners* (3rd ed.). St. Louis, MO: Saunders.

Buttaro, T. M., Trybulski, J., Bailey, P. P., & Sandberg-Cook, J. (2003). *Primary care: A collaborative practice* (2nd ed.). St. Louis, MO: Mosby.

Centers for Disease Control and Prevention (CDC). (2010). *Growth charts*. Retrieved from http://www.cdc.gov/growthcharts

Centers for Disease Control and Prevention (CDC). (2012). *Overweight and obesity: Basics of childhood obesity*. Retrieved from http://www.cdc.gov/obesity/childhood/basics.html

Mayo Clinic. (2014). *Diseases and conditions: Childhood obesity*. Retrieved from http://www.mayoclinic.org/diseases-conditions/childhood-obesity/basics/definition/con-20027428

Ogden, C. L., Carroll, M. D., Kit, B. K., & Flegal, K. M. (2012). *Prevalence of obesity in the United States, 2009–2010* (NCHS Data Brief no. 82). Retrieved from http://wood-ridge.schoolwires.net/cms/lib6/NJ01001835/Centricity/Domain/175/Obesity%20Article.pdf

The U.S. Department of Agriculture Food and Nutrition Service. (2014). *National school lunch program*. Retrieved from http://www.fns.usda.gov/nslp/national-school-lunch-program-nslp

The White House. (2014). *The White House and USDA announce school wellness standards*. Retrieved from http://www.whitehouse.gov/the-press-office/2014/02/25/white-house-and-usda-announce-school-wellness-standards

How to Initiate the Weight Conversation With Patients

According to a 2009 study, abridged provider time during routine office visits is among the top-stated patient concerns with regard to weight loss. Along with lack of time, patients also felt that providers lacked concern in addressing weight management/loss. These statements regarding obesity, preventive health care, and quality patient care were the impetus for the development of guidelines for clinical practice. This book focuses on prevention, provider recognition, and treatment of obesity with goals toward improving the overall quality of life (Christou & Efthimiou, 2009).

Stigmatization and discrimination are seen in three main areas of living: employment, education, and health care. Discrimination of the obese person is still viewed as "acceptable." Overweight individuals have been targeted by employers, teachers, and physicians; by strangers in public settings; and by the media. Overweight and obese individuals have stated concerns of being denied employment and promotions as well as receiving poor grades in school. Stories of discrimination of the obese have been shared by National Public Radio (NPR) as well as by social and print media. Dr. Kenneth Walker, in his nationally syndicated newspaper column, said "that for their own good and the good of the country, fat people should be locked up in prison camps" (Puhl & Brownell, 2001, p. 788).

WEIGHT DISCRIMINATION—PROVIDER

This negative view of obesity was seen not only by physicians but also by other medical professionals. As many as 24% of nurses stated they felt "repulsed" by obese people. In the past two to three decades, "obesity is becoming increasingly recognized as a 'social liability in Western society'" (Puhl & Brownell, 2001, pp. 788–789).

Klein, Najman, Kohrman, and Munro (1982) sampled more than 400 physicians on their feelings on social characteristics that elicited a negative response. Obesity was listed as the fourth most common category, out of dozens, behind only drug addiction, alcohol abuse, and mental illness. Obesity, along with the other negatively perceived conditions, was believed to be associated with noncompliance, hostility, poor hygiene, and dishonesty. Price, Desmond, Krol, Snyder, and O'Connell (1987) also examined 318 family physicians and their attitudes toward obesity. This study found that these physicians also felt negatively toward obese patients, stating that they lacked self-control and were lazy. These negative attitudes date back to 1969 in a study by Maddox and Liedermann. These physicians (100) viewed obese patients as inactive, weak-willed, unintelligent, and unsuccessful (Maddox & Liedermann, 1969).

Some research has also examined the perception of nurses and their views on obesity and treatment of obese patients. Hoppe and Ogden (1997) compiled a study of 586 nurses. Among these nurses, noncompliance was seen as the most likely reason for lack of weight loss. That same study also found that nurses rated ineffectiveness of weight-loss programs as the least likely reason for lack of success. Nurses also felt they were successful in giving weight-loss advice and admitted to spending less than 10 minutes while engaging in weight-loss discussions. A similar study also showed nurses' dislike for obese patients. Sixty-three percent of nurses stated they felt obesity could be prevented by self-control. They also felt that obese people were overindulgent, unsuccessful, lazy, and experienced unresolved anger (Maroney & Golub, 1992). Maroney and Golub (1992) also found that 31% of medical professionals would prefer not to care for an obese patient, whereas close to 50% stated they felt uncomfortable while providing care.

Many patients feel providers are discriminatory about weight and pass prior judgment when treating obesity (Chang, Asch, & Werner, 2010; Ferrante, Piasecki, Ohman-Strickland, & Crabtree, 2009; Wadden et al., 2000). It is true that some providers willingly admit and display negative attitudes toward obese patients. Some clinicians verbally express their dislike of caring for the obese patient, and some providers have even associated obese patients with feelings of discomfort, dislike, reluctance, awkwardness, or unpleasantness. Other providers find the treatment of obese patients lacking both gratification and professional rewards. Still other providers associate the obese patient with either low or little success (Chang et al., 2010).

A study of more than 1,200 physicians indicated poor obesity management. A self-reported questionnaire found that only 18% of physicians would address weight loss management with overweight patients, whereas 42% of physicians would address weight loss with those patients considered mildly obese. Another study by Price had similar results, with 23% of physicians not recommending any treatment for their obese patients, whereas other physicians felt that providing obesity counseling or talking about weight loss was considered "inconvenient." Some providers felt this was a bother, whereas others felt ambivalent about the issue. Physicians also stated lack of time, insufficient medical training, and lack of reimbursement as difficulties in treating and counseling for weight loss (Puhl & Brownell, 2001). Despite how a majority of providers felt, "the primary care physician who provides sensitive and compassionate care for severely obese patients without denigrating them for their inability to lose weight performs a much needed service" (Yanovski, 1993). This attitude needs to be conveyed for positive patient outcomes to help achieve weight loss.

Professionalism in medicine involves respect for all patients. Providers with a positive and more respectful attitude toward patients have a greater impact during direct patient encounters in comparison to those who do not show a respectful attitude. General biases with regard to obesity will continue to exist; however, it is those who lead by positive example who will make a greater impact (Huizinga, Cooper, Bleich, Clark, & Beach, 2009).

Huizinga et al. (2009) found that an increased body mass index (BMI) led to lower physician respect. "A ten-unit higher BMI was associated with a 14% higher prevalence of low physician respect" (n.p.). This study correlates to previous studies that also show negative attitudes toward obesity. This study also found that a higher BMI, independent of other patient and provider characteristics, led to lower physician respect. This distinction provides insight that patient care may be compromised by the negative attitudes toward obesity (Huizinga et al., 2009). Future research should focus on the impact of negative attitudes toward overweight and obese patients and the result of these outcomes.

WEIGHT DISCRIMINATION—PATIENT

Patient perceptions of weight bias concur with the perceptions stated earlier. Puhl and Brownell (2001) found that as many as 52% of women (overweight and obese) reported an occurrence with weight-related bias from a physician. This same study reported physicians as the most common source of weight bias.

Another study that surveyed obese patients after treatment found that patients were pleased with the general care received, but they were less satisfied with the care and treatment of their obesity. That same study found that nearly 50% of patients did not receive any weight-loss advice, whereas another 75% looked to the physicians for only a "slight amount" of weight-loss advice (Wadden et al., 2000).

Olson, Schumaker, and Yawn (1994) found that overweight and obese patients often had delayed care. Many times, this was due to delayed appointments or cancellations that were secondary to fear of weight. BMI was found to be significant with regard to appointment cancellations or missed appointments. As many as 12% of women had concerns with weight and therefore delayed an appointment. This study also found that 32% of women with a BMI greater than 27 kg/m² and 55% of women with a BMI greater than 35 kg/m² either delayed or cancelled appointments for fear of being weighed (Olson et al., 1994). A similar study also found that women delayed care and/or avoided breast and gynecological examinations, papanicolaou smears, and other preventive services (Fontaine, Faith, Allison, & Cheskin, 1998).

Wadden et al. (2000) found that nearly 80% of the patients (women) surveyed reported no concerns with physicians with regard to their weight. Also, "approximately 80% indicated that they rarely or never (a) had 'been very upset by comments that doctors have made about my weight,' (b) had physicians say 'critical or insulting things to me about my weight,' or (c) had 'doctors criticize me for not trying harder' when patients lost weight and regained it" (n.p.). However, in contrast to the earlier findings with this study, nearly two-thirds of patients indicated a lack of understanding in difficulty with being overweight. Another one-third of patients responded that they did not feel that doctors believed them when reporting what was eaten. Also, a majority of female patients felt that they were not disrespected with regard to their weight. This finding is welcomed, as the general picture paints practitioners as hostile and belittling patients who are unsuccessful with weight loss.

This study also found that most female patients blame themselves for their weight and view the excess weight as a personal failing. This being said, the study found that more than two-thirds of physicians never or rarely approached the topic of weight control and almost half of the physicians did not prescribe or suggest any weight-loss methods. In general, this study found that female patients have few expectations for assistance with weight loss from their physicians (Wadden et al., 2000).

Prior studies show that providers admit to negative attitudes toward obese patients; therefore, the anti-fat attitudes still exist. Numerous studies suggest that providers prefer not to treat obese patients or obesity, finding it unrewarding or ungratifying. These studies coincide with patient perceptions; however, no evidence has been found that shows overweight or obese patients receive less than the recommended care in comparison to those patients with a normal weight (Chang et al., 2010). The hope is that care for the obese patient will improve as bias decreases (Puhl & Brownell, 2001).

Several methods were used by doctors in which weight-loss guidance was provided. Counseling, offering dietary sheets, and providing handouts on healthy eating were the most common at 98%, 93%, and 89%, respectively. Group counseling and counseling with the family or significant others was less common at 17% and 32%. Treatment advice consisted of recommending eating less (78%), exercise (77%), or attending a "slimmers group" (54%). As per patient report, these types of advice were not found as helpful as group or family counseling; hence, they were commonly less used (Cade & O'Connell, 1991). This study proves that providers need to listen to patient needs and provide advice based on patient learning.

THE PROVIDER–PATIENT RELATIONSHIP

Encouraging wellness, preventing illness, and providing care are the provider's responsibility. Many times, the "chief complaint" for the visit is not the real or actual problem. Careful listening as well as providing a warm and open environment is essential. Rendering support for the patient and family as well as providing education is what providers have done capably for hundreds of years. "Patients need to feel connected to their provider and know that each infirmity and each anxiety is heard with compassion" (Buttaro, Trybulski, Bailey, & Sandberg-Cook, 2003, p. 10). Providers must advocate for patients and ensure that their well-being is acknowledged.

Provider attributes such as attentiveness, respect, humility, and fortitude promote positive provider–patient relationships. Attentiveness is noted when the provider listens or observes with open body language. Respect for the patient is demonstrated by listening and being nonjudgmental. Humility is listening to the patient and focusing on the strengths as well as improving the weaknesses. Fortitude is the ability or courage used to deal with a situation.

Efficiency as well as time management is important during each patient's visit. The focus must be on the patient, and distractions should be kept to a minimum. A quiet setting and an examination room are essential. Confidentiality must also be ensured. This part of the provider–patient bond is needed for growth and mutual respect. Several strategies can be used to enhance provider–patient interactions. One of the first strategies is to introduce oneself to the patient and proceed with a handshake. Allowing the patient to remain in street clothes for the initial contact may help the patient feel more at ease or comfortable. Sitting at the patient's level can also promote a safe environment. The health care provider should listen to the patient to promote his or her commitment to the patient. Also, the provider should not allow his or her personal feelings or prejudices to alter the conversation or relationship. It is critical to allow the patient to participate in the future plan, as this helps the patient feel more accountable for his or her actions. The provider should schedule follow-up with the patient to establish a timeline to complete goals. Finally, the provider should address further questions or concerns that the patient may have before ending the visit (Buttaro et al., 2003).

QUICK TIPS—STEPS FOR PATIENT COMMUNICATION

- Maintain confidentiality
- Ensure privacy
- Offer introduction/handshake
- Convey compassion/attentiveness/respect
- Promote efficiency/time management
- Evaluate weight/vitals
- Perform physical examination
- Listen
- Establish goals with timeline
- Schedule follow-up
- Address further questions/concerns

Obesity is a difficult topic to address with a patient. Biased attitudes are an issue, as negative attitudes about overweight and obese individuals exist among many health care professionals and the general public. These overweight and obese individuals can be reluctant to seek medical care, due to fear of humiliation. That is why quality care is not only necessary but also a careful approach of the subject (Puhl & Brownell, 2001).

In general, obese patients have more medical problems in comparison to someone of a normal weight, thus increasing the complexity of care. With the increase in clinical complexity, there is an increase in frequency of office visits, thereby increasing the likelihood of recommended care (Higashi et al., 2007; Werner & Chang, 2008). Again, Chang et al. (2010) found no evidence of lower quality of patient care in overweight or obese patients; in fact, those with a higher BMI had higher success rates in many of the performance measures. These results were found in large samples of Medicare and Veterans Health Administration (VHA) populations with an additional eight performance measures present. This study found that overweight and obese individuals with diabetes mellitus (DM) had increased laboratory testing, including lipids and hemoglobin A1C (HgA1c). Both populations also had increased vaccinations. Overweight and obese Medicare populations also had increased odds of mammography, whereas the VHA population had higher odds of colorectal cancer (CRC) and cervical cancer screening (Chang et al., 2010).

Respect, trust, and caring should be elicited in the provider–patient relationship. Those who approach patient relationships from this perspective as well as using therapeutic communication will have increased patient quality and interactions (Buttaro et al., 2003).

THERAPEUTIC COMMUNICATION

Trust, mutual respect, and communication are required for effective care of the obese patient (Wee et al., 2002). Communication is a vital part of each provider–patient relationship. One such type of communication is called therapeutic communication.

Therapeutic communication is defined as actively listening to the patient. Being an "active" listener involves listening to and paying attention to what is being said first, and then restating what was said to make sure everyone is on the same page. Verbal conversation is important as well as proper use of nonverbals. Pullen and Mathias (2010, p. 4) define a *therapeutic nurse–patient relationship* as, "a helping relationship that's based on mutual trust and respect, the nurturing of faith and hope, being sensitive to self and others, and assisting with the gratification of your patient's physical, emotional, and spiritual needs through your knowledge and skill." Simple steps can be done to reassure one's patient that an equal partnership exists. The first step is introduction. This can be done with a simple handshake and stating one's name. Using the patient's name throughout the conversation also provides additional patient comfort. Providing privacy is the next step. This allows the patient to feel safe and comfortable. Using active listening skills also relays attentiveness to the patient. One could restate what the patient has said, but should not use this too much, as this technique could indicate a lack of listening. One should be genuine and maintain eye contact. Use of nonverbals, such as head nodding and smiling, also allows for inviting, engaging conversation. Professional boundaries should also be maintained at all times. This includes respect for different cultures.

Providing wellness of the mind, body, and spirit is an important aspect of achieving therapeutic communication. Caring behavior is portrayed in effective therapeutic communication. Growth is achieved with continued conversation and patient progression (Pullen & Mathias, 2010).

Along with therapeutic communication, a team approach, counseling, and flexibility are also key aspects in establishing a successful weight-loss clinic (Frezza & Wachtel, 2008; Fujioka & Bakhru, 2010). A positive attitude is also essential when treating obese patients, as many patients feel providers are discriminatory about weight and pass prior judgment when treating obesity (Chang et al., 2010; Ferrante et al., 2009; Wadden et al., 2000). Clinics providing education, evaluation, assessment, and treatment of obesity need to be aware of the challenges with preventative treatment; however, success has been shown through promotion of a safe and friendly environment as well as patient trust.

QUICK TIPS—HOW TO APPROACH A PATIENT'S WEIGHT (PROVIDER-LED DISCUSSIONS)

- In reviewing your chart, I see you have _____ (health conditions/diseases); this/these put you at a higher risk for the development of cardiovascular disease (CVD). One of the ways I can help reduce your risk is to discuss your weight and start to think about ways you can work on weight loss.
- What are your thoughts/feelings on your weight today?
- I see that this visit was scheduled to discuss your weight. What are your thoughts on this?
- How can I best help you work on weight loss?
- How can I best help you work on weight maintenance?
- Today you weigh _____ pounds. What would you like to weigh? Is this a realistic goal? How are we going to work to accomplish this?
- I see that your weight is up _____ pounds from your last visit (this usually opens up for the patient to discuss thoughts, feelings, etc.).

QUICK TIPS—PATIENT STATEMENTS/QUESTIONS WITH PROVIDER RESPONSES

Patient: "I'm embarrassed to bring up my weight, but know I need to do something."

Provider: "I'm here to help. I want you to feel comfortable talking about this. What do you think has led to your current weight?"

Patient: "I know that a lot of my problems are from my weight. . . . "

Provider: "Losing weight will help reduce your current health conditions as well as reduce your risk factors for CVD. Let's look at how we can get started with weight loss."

Patient: "I know I need to lose weight, but right now, I just can't do that."

Provider: "Tell me more about that."

Patient: "But I'm eating right and exercising; why am I not losing weight?"

Provider: "Let's take a look at what you're doing each day and see if we can come up with some answers."

Patient: "I only eat about 1,500 calories daily. I don't understand this weight."

Provider: "Let's take a look at your journal. Or,
Let's have you start keeping a journal so we can figure this out."

ETHICAL PRINCIPLES

With the increased role responsibilities, advanced practice nurses (APNs) may need to handle clinical situations that involve ethical conflicts. Many times, ethical dilemmas occur when the patient and provider have different views on the same clinical problem. The way these situations are viewed is often due to one's own personal experience and health status. Several ethical principles exist, such as autonomy, beneficence, nonmaleficence, justice, veracity, and fidelity. For a review of these terms, please refer to Chapter 2.

The code of ethics of the American Nurses Association (ANA) is one way to remind APNs of the professional adherence in such situations. Additional perspectives are provided for "adherence to principles grounded in nursing's long tradition and commitment to ethical practice" (Buttaro et al., 2003, p. 11). Patients' privacy as well as their worth and dignity are also emphasized. Patient protection, including the provider's responsibility to defend against negligent practice, is also included in the code. Finally, the APN should promote professional competency through continued research, public health initiatives, and policies that support social change and access to health care (Buttaro et al., 2003).

ADDRESSING LEGAL ISSUES—MALPRACTICE

As health care continues to change rapidly, so does access to quality health care. That is why the following areas, such as The Patient's Bill of Rights, informed consent, and privacy and confidentiality, should be addressed by the office staff and/or provider. The Patient's Bill of Rights, adopted in 1973, has two basic tenets. The first is respect for the patient in decision making, whereas the second is "sensitivity to racial, cultural, linguistic, religious, and gender differences, as well as to the needs of the persons with disabilities" (Buttaro et al., 2003, p. 13). Informed consent should be addressed while the patient is checked in as a new patient and covers the "sharing" of information. This includes interaction and the provider–patient relationship. Goals, as well as different approaches to the subject, should also be addressed. This is where alternative approaches to the management of a health issue—or, in this case, weight loss or weight management—exist and should be properly addressed. The procedure or medication should be explained to the patient as well as the risks, benefits, and/or alternatives to treatment. The ANA considers confidentiality to be one of the basic provisions of health care. Personal and psychological issues are kept between the provider and patient and should not be disseminated (Buttaro et al., 2003).

Malpractice is not something APNs should have to worry about; however, cases do occur. Most malpractice cases usually result from a lack of communication and/or poor or no follow-up of patients. Most malpractice lawsuits against APNs usually include the supervising physician as well, because most supervising physicians sign off or are liable for reviewing the overall treatment plan. In order for a malpractice suit to exist, the patient must show evidence of duty, breach of duty, proximate cause, and damages (Buttaro et al., 2003). Box 5.1 includes ideas that may help reduce the risk of malpractice.

BOX 5.1 REDUCING MALPRACTICE RISK

1. Use direct patient quotes, especially under chief complaint and in the subjective part of the note.
2. In sensitive examinations or situations, have a medical assistant or nurse accompany you. Document, with name, that the additional medical professional was present with you and for what parts he or she was there.
3. If the possibility of differential diagnoses exists, document with exact thoughts.
4. Document risks, benefits, or alternatives to the treatment or procedure. Document patient's acceptance or refusal to treatment and plan.
5. Document goals and treatment plan. Document that the patient was agreeable or disagreeable.
6. Document new medications with the exact dose and frequency that you are prescribing. Document patient instructions on the medication.

It is important to have a healthy provider–patient relationship. This allows for the patient to open up about issues relating to obesity. The provider should deliver a caring environment. Therapeutic communication is an essential piece of the relationship, as this allows open lines of communication.

REFERENCES

Buttaro, T. M., Trybulski, J., Bailey, P. P., & Sandberg-Cook, J. (2003). *Primary care: A collaborative practice* (2nd ed.). St. Louis, MO: Mosby.

Cade, J., & O'Connell, S. (1991). Management of weight problems and obesity: Knowledge, attitudes and current practice of general practitioners. *British Journal of General Practice, 41*, 147–150.

Chang, V. W., Asch, D. A., & Werner, R. M. (2010). Quality of care among obese patients. *JAMA, 303*(13), 1274–1281. doi:10.1001/jama.2010.339

Christou, N., & Efthimiou, E. (2009). Five-year outcomes of laparoscopic adjustable gastric banding and laparoscopic Roux-en-Y gastric bypass in a comprehensive bariatric surgery program in Canada. *Canadian Journal of Surgery, 52*(6), E249–E258. Retrieved from http://www.ncbi.nlm.nih.gov/pmc/articles/PMC2792387/

Ferrante, J. M., Piasecki, A. K., Ohman-Strickland, P. A., & Crabtree, B. F. (2009). Family physicians' practices and attitudes regarding care of extremely obese patients. *Obesity, 17*, 1710–1716. doi:10.1038/oby.2009.62

Fontaine, K. R., Faith, M. S., Allison, D. B., & Cheskin, L. J. (1998). Body weight and health care among women in the general population. *Archives of Family Medicine, 7*, 381–384.

Frezza, E. E., & Wachtel, M. S. (2008). A successful model of setting up a bariatric practice. *Obesity Surgery, 18*, 877–881. doi:10.1007/s1169-007-9377-7

Fujioka, D., & Bakhru, N. (2010). Office-based management of obesity. *Mount Sinai Journal of Medicine, 77*, 466–471. doi:10.1002/msj.20201

Higashi, T., Wenger, N. S., Adams, J. L., Fung, C., Roland, M., McGlynn, E. A., . . . Shekelle, P. G. (2007). Relationship between number of medical conditions and quality of care. *New England Journal of Medicine, 356*(24), 2496–2504.

Hoppe, R., & Ogden, J. (1997). Practice nurses' beliefs about obesity and weight related interventions in primary care. *International Journal of Obesity Related Metabolic Disorders, 21*, 141–146.

Huizinga, M. M., Cooper, L. A., Bleich, S. N., Clark, J. M., & Beach, M. C. (2009). Physician respect for patients with obesity. *Journal of General Internal Medicine, 24*(11), 1236–1239. doi:10.1007/s11606-009-1104-8

Klein, D., Najman, J., Kohrman, A. F., & Munro, C. (1982). Patient characteristics that elicit negative responses from family physicians. *Journal of Family Practice, 14*, 881–888.

Maddox, G. L., & Liederman, V. (1969). Overweight as a social disability with medical implications. *Journal of Medical Education, 44*, 214–220.

Maroney, D., & Golub, S. (1992). Nurses' attitudes toward obese persons and certain ethnic groups. *Perceptual and Motor Skills, 75*, 387–391.

Olson, C. L., Schumaker, H. D., & Yawn, B. P. (1994). Overweight women delay medical care. *Archives of Family Medicine, 3*, 888–892.

Price, J. H., Desmond, S. M., Krol, R. A., Snyder, F. F., & O'Connell, J. K. (1987). Family practice physicians' beliefs, attitudes, and practices regarding obesity. *American Journal of Preventive Medicine, 3*(6), 339–345.

Puhl, R., & Brownell, K. D. (2001). Bias, discrimination, and obesity. *Obesity Research, 9*(12), 788–805.

Pullen, R. L., & Mathias, T. (2010). Fostering therapeutic nurse-patient relationships. *Nursing Made Incredibly Easy!, 8*(3), 4. doi:10.1097/01.NME.0000371036.87494.11

Wadden, T. A., Anderson, D. W., Foster, G. D., Bennett, A., Steinberg, C., & Sarwer, D. B. (2000). Obese women's perceptions of their physicians' weight management attitudes and practices. *Archives of Family Medicine, 9*, 854–860.

Wee, C. C., Phillips, R. S., Cook, E. F., Haas, J. S., Puopolo, A. L., Brennan, T. A., & Burstin, H. R. (2002). Influence of body weight on patients' satisfaction with ambulatory care. *Journal of General Internal Medicine, 17*(2), 155–159. doi:10.1046/j.1525-1497.2002.00825.x

Werner, R. M., & Chang, V. W. (2008). The relationship between measured performance and satisfaction with care among clinically complex patients. *Journal of General Internal Medicine*, 23(11), 1729–1735.

Yanovski, S. Z. (1993). A practical approach to treatment of the obese patient. *Archives of Family Medicine*, 2, 309–316.

Patients' Stories

Communication is essential in patient care and treatment. As previously mentioned, initiation of the topic of weight or obesity can be difficult. Positive avenues of this discussion are preferred for better patient–provider relationships. Important issues are addressed in every visit. Also imperative is the thorough documentation that conveys the timeline of this communication throughout the visit.

The following are excerpts from actual patient charts. Patient names and ages have been changed to protect patient privacy. The purpose of these excerpts is to provide a sample of patient visit flow and content with regard to his or her struggles with obesity, weight loss, and weight maintenance. The office notes from a nurse practitioner (NP), registered dietitian (RD), and exercise specialist detail each patient's clinical course through a SOAP (subjective, objective, assessment, plan), which consists of samples that can be used in clinical practice. There are two separate notes on each patient, including a first patient appointment summary and a second note done just prior to publication. A comparison of the patient's progress is documented as well as an actual patient testimony. This is a sample that has proved successful; however, it is meant to be used, changed, and interpreted by advanced practice nurses (APNs) for his or her own patient population.

The following are four actual patients who have participated in weight loss and have agreed to share their journeys and success.

Patient #1

Total Amount of Weight Lost: 42.6 pounds (according to chart review)
Total Percentage of Weight Lost: 12.12

First Patient Appointment Summary

CENTER FOR LIFESTYLE MEDICINE (CLM) CLINIC

CHIEF COMPLAINT: Obesity-related medical illness, osteoarthritis, gastroesophageal reflux disease (GERD), hyperlipidemia, hypertension (HTN), prediabetes, vitamin deficiency, and shortness of breath.

HISTORY: Mrs. JP is a pleasant 65-year-old woman referred by her primary care provider for risk factor modification aimed at weight loss. She has significant comorbid conditions and is prediabetic. The patient herself states that she is not sure why she is gaining weight and that she had tried several times in the past to lose weight. She had tried Dexatrim on and off over the past several years. She also tried liquid diets, including maple syrup, vinegar, and cayenne pepper. She reports that she tried some type of grapefruit diet and some type of beef and vegetable diet. She states that she tried numerous cleanses but they only work for approximately 2 to 3 days. She reports that she has gained about 40 pounds since she has moved to town. She snacks late at night anywhere from 11 p.m. to 1 a.m. She craves meats, especially hot dogs, and says it is not uncommon for her to eat an entire package of hot dogs in one sitting. She reports that her daughters cook and do the shopping. She says that they do stick to using a grocery list. The patient herself denies any current complaints of chest pain, pressure, or heaviness, but does notice significant shortness of breath. She does not complain of paroxysmal nocturnal dyspnea (PND) or orthopnea. Her shortness of breath is clearly related to any activity or exertion. She reports that it seems to be getting worse. She also has a significant family history of coronary artery disease (CAD). She denies any palpitations, dizziness, lightheadedness, fevers or chills, or syncope. She has lower-extremity edema. She also reports significant arthritic pain when she gets up and moves around and because of this is not too active.

Allergies

Bactrim
Purified protein derivative of tuberculosis (PPD)

Current Medications

Cyclobenzaprine HCl 10 mg PO (by mouth) daily prn (as needed)
Famotidine 40 mg PO daily
Flaxseed oil 1,000 mg PO daily
Klor-Con 10 mEQ PO daily
Loratadine 10 mg PO prn
Multivitamin one tablet PO daily
Triamterene–hydrochlorothiazide (HCTZ) 37.5 to 25 mg PO daily
Omega-3 capsule one tablet PO daily
Meloxicam 7.5 mg PO BID (twice a day)
Vitamin D_3 50,000 units once weekly
Metformin HCl 500 mg PO daily
Atorvastatin 10 mg PO daily HS (at bedtime)

Past Medical History

Arthritis
Chronic allergic rhinitis
Chronic reflux esophagitis
Diabetes mellitus (DM)
Gout
Hyperlipidemia
HTN
Hypokalemia

Gynecological History

Age of first menstrual cycle: 11
Age of menopause: 44, hysterectomy
Number of pregnancies: 5
Number of births: 3
Any history of abnormal vaginal bleeding? Yes

Past Surgical History

Dental surgery
Dilation and curettage
Hysterectomy
Sinus surgery
Tonsillectomy

Psychiatric History

Patient denies any depression signs or symptoms. No suicidal thoughts or ideations.
Beck Depression Inventory score: Not applicable
Depression: No
Anxiety: No
Adjustment disorder: No
Stress: No
Stress level: None
Stress frequency: Almost never
Binge eating disorder: No
Bulimia: No
Purging patterns: No
Anorexia nervosa: No

Previous Weight-Loss Attempts

What have you tried in the past? Dexatrim on and off for the past 20 years, liquid diets (maple syrup, vinegar, cayenne pepper), grapefruit diet.
What has worked best for you? Why? 2 to 3 days body cleanse and then cut back portions. Not sure why it has worked.
What has not worked? Why? Appetite suppressants. Not sure why it has not worked.
What are your current expectations? Learn to change dietary habits for a lifetime, increase mobility.

Anorectic Use

Which drugs have you used in the past? Dexatrim
When did you take it? Late 20s to early 30s
What was the effect? Increased heart rate (HR)
Are there any problems with medications in the past? Not applicable
What do you expect from the use of medication now? Not applicable

History of Weight Gain

Gradual onset: Yes
Onset: Childhood
Lifestyle changes: None, but gained about 40 pounds after moving back to town.
Stress: Yes, due to husband's health.
Why do you think you have gained weight? When distracted/too busy and loses focus on eating.

Dietary History

Is there a tough time of day? Bedtime (11 p.m.–1 a.m.)
Are there problem foods? Meats
Is volume an issue? No
Are cravings an issue? Yes, meats and hot dogs
Are there certain triggers? No
Who shops and cooks? Daughters
Do you use a shopping list? Yes, and stick to it
Do you eat out? How often? Yes, about 2×/week
What are your snack habits? Crackers
Do you have any food dislikes? No
Are you a nighttime eater? Yes
Are you a stress eater? No
Are you a volume eater? No

Exercise History

Current level of activity? None, supposed to start physical therapy in May.
  Type:
  Frequency:
  Duration:
Past activity level? Has always been sedentary
Favorite activity? None
Barriers to exercise? Bilateral knee and back pain

Family History

Family history of cancer
Family history of DM
Family history of epilepsy
Family history of HTN
Family history of rheumatoid arthritis
Family history of transient ischemic attack (TIA)

Personal History

Caffeine use
Smoking status: Never a smoker

Review of Systems (ROS)

She has weight gain, shortness of breath, daytime somnolence, and tiredness/
  fatigue. All other reviews of systems are negative.

Vital Signs

Neck circumference: 18 inches
Chest circumference: 68 inches
Waist circumference: 62 inches
Hip circumference: 70 inches
Waist-to-hip ratio: 0.89
Height: 63 inches, **Weight:** 351.3 pounds, Body mass index (**BMI**): 62.25 kg/m^2,
  Body surface area (**BSA**): 2.46

Blood pressure (BP): 128/80 mmHg left upper extremity (LUE) sitting
HR: 56 beats per minute, apical, pulse quality regular
Respiratory rate: 20 respirations per minute

Physical Examination

Head, Eyes, Ears, Nose, Throat (HEENT): PERRLA, extraocular muscles were
   intact. Conjunctiva normal, anicteric
Neck: Supple, no jugular vein distension (JVD). No thyromegaly or masses
Skin: Warm and moist
Mucosa: No cyanosis
Cardiovascular: Normal palpation, percussion. Normal S1 and S2. 1/6 systolic
   murmur. No clicks or gallops
Lungs: Normal palpation, percussion. Good bilateral air entry. No rales, rhonchi,
   or crepitation
Abdomen: Soft, nontender. Normal bowel sounds. No rebound or rigidity
Extremities: 1+ edema, no cyanosis or clubbing
Neurological: Alert and oriented ×3. No motor or sensory deficit

Health Management Plan

Lifestyle Modification Note: Today, the patient and her husband present themselves for an initial visit in the CLM Clinic. Our weight-loss program was explained,
body composition report was reviewed, and short- and long-term goals were set.
The patient's daughter is also present today and appears to take on a caretaker
role. She and her sister go grocery shopping and cook for the patient. The patient
reports trying many weight-loss/diet plans in the past; most of these were very
restrictive and were only meant to be followed for a few days. The patient states
that she does not know why she is overweight, as she does not eat large volumes
of food or snack throughout the day. She appears to understand but is hesitant
to admit that it is her food choices. She states that meats are a problem food and
that she often craves hot dogs. She has chronic pain in her back and lower body
with any weight-bearing activity; she ambulates with a cane but is severely sedentary. She is scheduled to begin physical therapy for her pain on May 7th. I believe
dietary changes will be the most beneficial at this time, but the next time I meet her,
I would also like to introduce exercises she can complete while sitting down. She is
scheduled to see the RD at her next appointment in 2 weeks. —Exercise Specialist.

Goals

- Keep dietary and exercise journal daily
- Lose weight of 1 to 2 pounds per week
- Aim for 1,500 to 1,600 calories daily
- Consume three to five servings of fruits and vegetables daily
- Consume 64 ounces of fluid daily

Impression/Plan

1. Obesity-related medical illness: Her weight and BMI are elevated today at
   351 pounds and a BMI of 62. She met me and the exercise specialist today.
   She had several questions throughout today's visit. Much of the time was spent
   gathering and collecting information as well as setting goals. Her goals were
   set as earlier to include beginning a dietary and activity journal and aiming

for 1,500 to 1,600 calories per day. I think that she will require a lot of education because she has several questions with regard to food consumption as well as exercise. At today's visit, more than 60 minutes of total patient time was spent. Out of the more than 60 minutes, at least 50 minutes was spent with one-on-one weight counseling and health coaching. During that time, I addressed the 5As—asking, advising, assessing, assisting, and arranging—for weight-loss follow-up. I clearly think that she needs risk factor modification as well as a cardiac workup prior to her baseline. I will order at least a resting EKG prior to her next appointment. I will review and determine if she needs further cardiac follow-up prior to exercise recommendations.

2. HTN: Fairly well controlled.
3. Hyperlipidemia: On statin therapy. I will obtain a copy of her lipid/liver panel.
4. Anemia.
5. GERD.
6. Osteoarthritis.
7. Prediabetes: I will obtain a copy of a fasting glucose as well as the previous glycated hemoglobin (HgA1c).
8. Vitamin D deficiency: I will obtain a copy of her previous vitamin D level.
9. Shortness of breath and lower-extremity edema: I think this is multifactorial in nature and related to her weight, deconditioning, and multiple underlying comorbid conditions. I will order an EKG to further rule out any EKG changes as well as any underlying cardiac condition.
10. Fatigue: She has some complaints of underlying obstructive sleep apnea (OSA). I will screen her for an Epworth score at her next appointment. I discussed the possibility of a sleep study, but she does not wish to consider it at this time. I explained the risk associated with possible undertreated OSA.
11. Beck Depression Inventory score: She did not complete a Beck Depression Inventory score due to the length of her appointment. I will assess this at her next appointment and rule out any underlying depression. She has no current complaints of any suicidal thoughts or ideations.
12. Laboratories: At this time, I would like to obtain a copy of her baseline laboratories. If she has not had laboratories drawn in the past 3 months, I would recommend the following: complete blood count (CBC), comprehensive metabolic panel (CMP), thyroid-stimulating hormone (TSH), Free T3, Free T4, lipid level, vitamin D level, and HgA1c.

Again, I clearly think she needs further workup, including baseline EKG, if not a stress test and echocardiogram along with screening for sleep apnea and depression. I will assess these at her next visit prior to any recommendations for exercise therapy.

Follow-Up Appointment Summary: (9 months after initial appointment)

CLM CLINIC

CHIEF COMPLAINT: Shortness of breath

HISTORY: Mrs. JP is a pleasant 66-year-old woman who I last saw on December 31. She is down by almost 7 pounds since she was last seen. She reports that she is eating better. She is eating three meals a day. She has been more consistent with her portion control. She feels like she has "cheated," because she had a piece of cake for her husband's birthday. She reports that when she has something like a sweet treat or snack, she goes right back to eating how she should. She "does not overeat." She feels she has changed her taste for certain foods and does not crave the sweets as she used to. She is not going to the Wellness Center, but reports being much more active throughout the day. She reports it has been too cold for her to be outside, but she has been tolerating the weather by doing more activities and more work around the house. She has no current complaints of any chest pain, heaviness, or pressure; no radiation of any pain to the arm, neck, jaw, or back. She complains of shortness of breath noticeable with activity. She has no PND, orthopnea, or palpitations. She denies any dizziness, lightheadedness, or syncope. There is no evidence of any lower-extremity edema, no fevers or chills. She reports having a pending appointment to see an orthopedic doctor for bilateral knee pain tomorrow.

Allergies

Bactrim TABS
PPD

Current Medicines

Cyclobenzaprine HCl 10 mg PO daily prn
Famotidine 40 mg PO daily
Flaxseed oil 1,000 mg PO daily
Klor-Con 10 mEQ PO daily
Loratadine 10 mg PO prn
Multivitamin one tablet PO daily
Triamterene–HCTZ 37.5 to 25 mg PO daily
Vitamin D_3 50,000 units once weekly

Vital Signs

Neck circumference: 15.4 inches
Chest circumference: 58 inches
Waist circumference: 56 inches
Hip circumference: 64.25 inches
Waist-to-hip ratio: 0.87
Height: 63 inches, Weight: 308.7 pounds, BMI: 54.7 kg/m², BSA: 2.33
BP: 120/84 mmHg LUE sitting
HR: 78 beats per minute, apical, pulse quality regular
Respiratory rate: 16 respirations per minute

Physical Examination

General: Looks stated age, appropriate conversation, in no acute distress
HEENT: PERRLA, extraocular muscles were intact. Conjunctiva normal, anicteric
Neck: Supple, no JVD
Skin: Moist, dry
Mucosa: No cyanosis, moist
Cardiovascular: Normal S1 and S2. 1/6 systolic murmur
Lungs: Good bilateral air entry

Abdomen: Obese, round, soft, and nontender. Normal bowel sounds. No rebound pain or rigidity

Extremities: Trace edema, no cyanosis or clubbing

Neurological: Alert and oriented ×3. No motor or sensory deficit

Health Management Plan

Mrs. JP presents for a follow-up regarding her weight and need for weight loss related to her health. She has lost nearly 45 pounds since April 2013. She reports that she has not had to make drastic changes to lose weight. Over time, she has made several small changes, which have now become a part of her regular routine. She no longer eats high-calorie desserts on a regular basis and has increased the amount of fruits, vegetables, and lean meat in her diet. She reports feeling as though she is "cheating" when eating cake or other goodies as she is still losing weight. Her daughter, who was present, stated that when she does have a higher-calorie food item, she recognizes it, chooses a small portion, and then consumes low-calorie foods the remainder of the day. She reports drinking water all day long and feels she is getting an adequate amount for her needs. She has been eating more fruits, vegetables, and nonfat yogurt in the past 2 weeks. Her activity level has consisted of chasing after and playing with grandchildren. She plans to start back at the Wellness Center 3 days weekly this next month. It has been hard to go due to the extreme cold temperatures we have been experiencing. I will continue to give the encouragement, education, and counseling needed to lose the desired weight successfully and healthily. —Registered Dietitian

Goals

- Keep a dietary and exercise journal daily
- Lose weight of 1 to 2 pounds per week
- Consume three to five servings of fruits and vegetables daily
- Continue to choose small portions
- Engage in physical activity for 15 minutes or more daily

Met Previous Goals

- 1 to 2 pounds of weight loss per week
- Cardiovascular exercise
- Dietary goals

Impression/Plan

1. Abnormal EKG: She had a previous EKG done showing anterior T-wave changes. She reported mild shortness of breath, but reports improved symptoms. I offered further testing, but she wished to hold off. Certainly, if she decided to have any type of orthopedic surgery done, I would have recommended further testing at that time due to her numerous risk factors.
2. HTN: Well controlled.
3. Hyperlipidemia: She was taken off her cholesterol medication secondary to fatty liver disease (FLD).
4. Pre–type 2 diabetes mellitus (T2DM): Her metformin had previously been stopped. She reports that her blood sugars are under good control. I will obtain a copy of her most recent laboratories for review.

5. FLD: She had recent laboratory work, but does not have the results available to her. I recommended continued efforts for weight loss.
6. Anemia.
7. GERD.
8. Osteoarthritis.
9. Vitamin D deficiency.
10. Shortness of breath: She reports improving symptoms. She has been more active and has not noticed any chest heaviness, pain, or pressure. I recommended stress testing in the near future.
11. Right-sided abdominal pain: This has resolved.
12. Obesity-related medical illness: Her weight is down by nearly 7 pounds since she was last seen. I commended her on this. I encouraged her continued efforts. She is consuming three meals a day, which appear to be very well balanced. I encouraged her to continue with her activity. She has been inconsistent in going to the Wellness Center, but reports that she feels more mobile because she is able to get up and move around with less effort. She met me and the RD. New goals were revised as earlier. The Health Management Plan could be also referred to. I will continue to follow her routinely and, per her request, will follow her on a consistent basis. In the meantime, I recommended continuing to monitor her portions as well as to reduce her sweets. I recommended increased activity, as tolerated.

Comparison

With weight loss, she is no longer on the following medications:
Omega-3 capsule one tablet PO daily
Meloxicam 7.5 mg PO BID
Metformin HCl 500 mg PO daily
Atorvastatin 10 mg PO daily HS

Patient Testimony

I started with the CLM Clinic in April 2013. Since that time, I have lost 43 pounds. Never before have I lost this much (weight). I started at 351 pounds and now am 308 pounds. I changed my eating habits and I don't feel like I am dieting at all. I eat what I want, I changed how and what I eat and learned a better way to lose weight without surgery or medication. I thank the team for working with me. Thank you!

Patient #2

> **Total Amount of Weight Lost:** 49.1 pounds (according to chart review)
> **Total Percentage of Weight Lost:** 17%

First Patient Appointment Summary

CLM CLINIC

CHIEF COMPLAINT: "I need help with weight loss."

HISTORY: Mr. SM is a pleasant 73-year-old gentleman who presents to the CLM Clinic for his first appointment today. He is accompanied by his wife. He reports that he is here because this was a doctor-recommended program. He reports that weight loss is very important to him at this time. His weight makes it harder for him to bend over, and he also complains of lower back pain after prolonged periods of standing and walking. He needs support, individual counseling, and accountability. He would like to lose weight to feel better about himself and have more energy. He reports that he is currently active and tries to ride 3 miles a day on his stationary bike. He usually stops because his "behind" hurts from sitting on the seat too long. He could go farther and reports that he could tolerate the activity easily. He denies any current complaints of any chest pain or discomfort; no radiation to the arm, neck, jaw, or back. He does complain of shortness of breath, especially with overexertion. He denies any palpitations, PND, orthopnea, dizziness, lightheadedness, or syncope. He had mild lower-extremity edema due to being on his feet all day but had no fevers or chills.

Allergies

No known drug allergies

Current Medicines

Actos 30 mg PO daily
Metformin HCl 1,000 mg PO BID
Simvastatin 20 mg PO daily HS
Alprazolam 0.25 mg PO one tablet TID prn
Lisinopril–HCTZ 20 to 25 mg PO BID
Aspirin 81 mg PO daily
Glimepiride 2 mg PO BID
Fish oil 1,000 mg PO 2 capsules daily
Metoprolol succinate ER 100 mg PO one tablet TID

Past Medical History

Anxiety
DM
Hypercholesterolemia
HTN
OSA
Rhythm disorder
Supraventricular tachycardia

Past Surgical History

Orthopedic surgery; broken leg
Tonsillectomy

Psychiatric History

Patient denies any depression signs or symptoms. No suicidal thoughts or ideations
Beck Depression Inventory score: 1
Depression: No
Anxiety: Yes

Adjustment disorder: No
Stress: No
Stress level: None
Stress frequency: Almost never
Binge-eating disorder: No
Bulimia: No
Purging patterns: No
Anorexia nervosa: No

Previous Weight-Loss Attempts

What have you tried in the past? Nothing really
What has worked best for you? Why? Not applicable
What has not worked? Why? Not applicable
What are your current expectations? Patient does not have a goal in mind, but
    would just really like to lose something. He would like to lose as much as
    possible.
Anorectic use: Not applicable
Which drugs have you used in the past? Not applicable
When did you take them? Not applicable
What was the effect? Not applicable
Were there any problems with medications in the past? Not applicable
What do you expect now from the use of medication? Not applicable

History of Weight Gain

Gradual onset: Yes
Onset: Adult life
Lifestyle changes: Nothing significant. Life in general.
Stress: No
Why do you think you have gained weight? Patient is unsure why he has put on
    weight.

Dietary History

Is there a tough time of day? Not a particular time in the day when he eats a lot.
    If patient wants a snack, he will have one.
Are there problem foods? Patient is not a picky eater. Patient drinks three cans
    of diet pop daily. Patient does not drink coffee or alcohol.
Is volume an issue? Yes
Are cravings an issue? No
Are there certain triggers? No
Who shops and cooks? Patient and wife do both
Do you use a shopping list? Yes, but frequently buys items that are not on the list
Do you eat out? How often? Yes, couple of times/week
What are your snack habits? Sugar-free candy, fruit
Do you have any food dislikes? Yes, eggs, oranges, cereals high in sugar, coffee,
    ham, chicken, turkey, soup, and rice
Are you a nighttime eater? Yes, patient does have a snack before bed
Are you a stress eater? No
Are you a volume eater? Yes

Exercise History

Current level of activity? Yes
   Type: Stationary bike
   Frequency: 3 miles/day
   Duration: 15 to 20 minutes daily
Past activity level? Walking, golfing
Favorite activity? No favorite exercise
Barriers to exercise? Patient is unsure why he does not exercise more. Patient says
   that he always thought 3 miles daily is adequate. Also, the seat on his station-
   ary bike gets uncomfortable. Patient also had lateral meniscus tear and ended
   up having surgery.

Family History

Maternal history of acute myocardial infarction; died at 78 years
Maternal history of HTN
Paternal history of pneumonia; died at 78 years

Personal History

Denied alcohol use; asked on November 9, 2011
Caffeine use; four cans of soda per day
Living independently with spouse
Marital history—currently married
Smoking Status: Former smoker; smoked pipe 30 years ago
Denied tobacco use; asked on November 9, 2011

Review of Systems (ROS)

He has weight gain, shortness of breath, and tiredness/fatigue.
All other review of systems is negative.

Vital Signs

Neck circumference: 18.75 inches
Waist circumference: 50 inches
Hip circumference: 49 inches
Waist-to-hip ratio: 1.02
Height: 70 inches, Weight: 265.4 pounds, BMI: 38.1 kg/m^2, BSA: 2.36
BP: 134.70 mmHg left upper extremity (LUE) sitting
HR: 64 beats per minute, apical, pulse quality regular
Respiratory rate: 16 respirations per minute

Physical Examination

HEENT: PERRLA, extraocular muscles were intact. Conjunctiva normal, anicteric
Neck: Supple, no JVD. No thyromegaly or masses
Skin: Warm and moist
Mucosa: No cyanosis
Cardiovascular: Normal palpation, percussion. Normal S1 and S2. 1/6 Systolic
   murmur. No clicks or gallops
Lungs: Normal palpation, percussion. Good bilateral air entry. No rales, rhonchi,
   or crepitation

Abdomen: Soft, nontender. Normal bowel sounds. No rebound or rigidity
Extremities: No edema, cyanosis, or clubbing
Neurological: Alert and oriented ×3. No motor or sensory deficit

Health Management History

Dietary Note: Mr. SM is here for his first visit today for weight-loss assistance. He has already lost 5 pounds in the past 2 months according to his wife. He has done this by cutting back on portions and high-calorie snacks. He would like to lose 15 pounds in the next 3 months. We set a 10% weight-loss goal of 26 pounds in 6 months. His wife brought a typed journal of the past 5 days, which was very helpful. He has regular meals and snacks. His portions currently are on the large side for his supper meal. He enjoys cookies every other day. We discussed cutting back on the serving sizes at meals and switching cookies for fruit most of the time. He agreed with this plan, as he likes fruit a lot. He drinks diet soda and only one bottle of water daily. We discussed the importance of increased water to aid with weight loss and help with hydration. As for activity, he has been riding his bike 3 days per week, for the past few years, according to his wife. He used to walk daily, but has not done so in the past year due to hurting his knee and having knee surgery. We set goals today. We will continue to assist with meeting them in future appointments. —Registered Dietitian

Goals

- Keep a dietary and exercise journal daily
- Lose weight of 1 to 2 pounds per week
- Cut back portion
- Switch cookies for fruit
- Consume three to five servings of fruits and vegetables daily
- Consume 64 ounces of fluid daily
- Continue biking 3 days per week; introduce walking, as tolerated

Impression/Plan

1. Obesity-related medical illness: Again, he is here for his initial appointment today. He met me and the RD. New goals were discussed as earlier. He is here and is willing to lose weight. I followed the 5As of asking, advising, assessing, assisting, and arranging. Specific goals were suggested and discussed as earlier for his weight-loss plan. I think it is really important for him to continue to follow this routinely with the RD and exercise specialist for more specific goals. At today's appointment, approximately 60 minutes of total patient time was spent. Of that 60 minutes, at least 50 minutes were spent with one-on-one weight counseling and health coaching. I think this will benefit his overall health as well as reduce his number of comorbidities.
2. History of atrial arrhythmia: He does appear irregular today. I got an EKG that showed a normal sinus rhythm with premature atrial contractions (PACs). He is asymptomatic with this. I advised him to continue with his aspirin and beta-blocker therapy.
3. Normal left ventricular (LV) function
4. Shortness of breath: According to his cardiac note, this is chronic and stable. I think this would be improved by weight loss, as he carries a lot of abdominal/central obesity.

5. Negative stress test
6. Anxiety
7. Diabetes: This is oral controlled. I would like to obtain a copy of his previous HgA1c for further review.
8. Hyperlipidemia: He remains on statin therapy. His cholesterol has been further followed by his primary care provider. I will obtain a copy of his previous lipid and liver panel.
9. HTN: Well controlled today
10. Severe OSA: He remains on BiPAP therapy. He is further followed in the sleep apnea clinic.
11. Cardiolite stress test showing scar versus artifact in inferior wall: Again followed in cardiac clinic
12. Pulmonary HTN with a right ventricular systolic pressure (RVSP) of 62: I think this is more in relation to his weight as well as his sleep apnea. I clearly think we could also help with this. We discussed this in great detail today.
13. Beck Depression Inventory score: His Beck Depression Inventory score is stable and within normal limits at 1. No current suicidal thoughts or ideations
14. Laboratories: At this time, I would like to obtain a copy of baseline laboratories. If he has not had baseline laboratories drawn within the past 3 months, I would recommend the following: CBC, CMP, TSH, Free T3, Free T4, lipid panel, and vitamin D level

I look forward to working with this patient and helping him achieve his weight-loss needs.

Follow-Up Appointment Summary:
(12 months after initial appointment)

CLM CLINIC

CHIEF COMPLAINT: Follow-up weight-loss and risk factors

HISTORY OF PRESENTING ILLNESS: Mr. SM is a pleasant 74-year-old gentleman who returns to the clinic for a follow-up today. He was last seen in September by our RD. Since that time, he is down by 3 pounds. He is still working on losing weight and also wonders what a good goal weight would be for him. He recently had skin cancer removed off his left ear. He reports that his activity has been somewhat more limited; however, he is still riding the bike at least 6.5 miles daily. He has now split this up into 2.5 miles in the morning, 2 miles at noon, and 2 miles in the afternoon. He has also increased his resistance with his weights and is doing continued resistance therapy. He reports that when he had ear surgery, he was unable to use his seat belt for about 12 days, but has resumed this. Overall, he feels good. He is down by more than 50 pounds in the previous year. He is off Actos and Glucophage. He has lowered his cholesterol and BP medications. He reports pending laboratory work from Monday. There are no current complaints of any chest pain, heaviness, or pressure; no radiation of any pain to the arm, neck, jaw, or back; minimal mild shortness of breath; no PND, orthopnea, and palpitations; no episodes of any dizziness, lightheadedness, or syncope; no evidence of any lower-extremity edema; and no fevers or chills.

Allergies

No known drug allergies

Current Medications

Metformin HCl 1,000 mg PO BID
Simvastatin 20 mg half tablet PO daily HS
Alprazolam 0.25 mg PO one tablet TID prn
Lisinopril–HCTZ 20 to 25 mg PO BID
Aspirin 81 mg PO daily
Fish oil 1,000 mg PO 2 capsules daily
Metoprolol succinate ER 100 mg PO one tablet TID
ZYRTEC allergy 10 mg PO daily

Vital Signs

Neck circumference: 18 inches
Waist circumference: 44 inches
Hip circumference: 44 inches
Waist-to-hip ratio: 1.0
Height: 69.5 inches, **Weight:** 226.6 pounds, **BMI:** 33 kg/m^2, **BSA:** 2.19
BP: 150/66 mmHg LUE sitting
HR: 54 beats per minute, apical, pulse quality regular
Respiratory rate: 20 respirations per minute

Physical Examination

General: Looks stated age, appropriate conversation, in no acute distress
HEENT: PERRLA, extraocular muscles were intact. Conjunctiva normal, anicteric
Neck: Supple, no JVD
Skin: Warm, pink, and dry
Mucosa: No cyanosis, moist
Cardiovascular: Normal S1 and S2. 1/6 systolic murmur
Lungs: Good bilateral air entry
Abdomen: Soft and nontender. Normal bowel sounds. No rebound pain or
    rigidity
Extremities: No edema, cyanosis, or clubbing
Neurological: Alert and oriented ×3. No motor or sensory deficit

Health Management Plan

Dietary Note: Mr. SM presents for a follow-up appointment for weight loss today.
His weight is down by 3 pounds since I last visited him in September. He is pleasant and happy with his weight loss today. According to his journal, he continues
with the same exercise routine, is typically eating the same type of food, and practicing portion control. He reports that he would like to continue what he is currently doing and does not want to add any more exercises at this time. His wife
would like him to try to add more, but seemed to understand his preference of
maintaining what he is currently doing. His wife continues to keep track of his
intakes and activity using a form of her own. She is quite detailed with this, which
helps in understanding what he is doing on a daily basis. His intakes appear to be
very similar to the last time we met. His wife stated that they had made the slight

recommendations I had given them the previous time concerning the types of meat at his lunch meal. He had been consuming bologna and sausage sandwiches. He does not like turkey or chicken in his sandwiches, but has switched to lean ham or roast beef. He continues to consume at least five servings of fruits and vegetables every day, three meals and two snacks, and appropriate portions at meals and snacks. Overall, he has made several positive changes toward healthy weight loss. All questions were answered. I will continue to assist as needed and will see him again in 3 months. —Registered Dietitian

Goals

- No longer keep a journal
- Lose weight of 1 to 2 pounds per week
- Continue with current dietary routine—small servings, five servings of fruits and vegetables, lean meats, and low-fat dairy
- Continue with current activity routine

Met Previous Goals

- Kept a food and activity journal
- Cardiovascular exercise
- Strengthening exercises
- Stress management
- Dietary goals

Impression/Plan

1. History of atrial arrhythmia with atrial runs: He has a pending Holter monitor for February to assess for any underlying atrial arrhythmia. He was advised to keep this. No concerning palpitations. He remains on beta-blockade therapy and aspirin. I will continue to follow him routinely.
2. Normal LV function per echocardiogram in October 2012.
3. History of cardiolite showing a scar versus artifact: No concerning angina-type symptoms. On aspirin and beta-blockade therapy.
4. Anxiety.
5. T2DM: He is only on metformin therapy. He has significantly reduced his HgA1c and has got off Actos and Glucophage. He has pending laboratory work on Monday. I will await these results.
6. Hyperlipidemia: With his known risk factors, especially diabetes, I would recommend an LDL less than 100. He is further followed up by his primary NP. He is on statin therapy.
7. HTN: Slightly elevated, but he reports it is usually better controlled.
8. OSA: He remains on BiPAP therapy. He is further followed up in the sleep apnea clinic.
9. History of pulmonary HTN: He has pending testing. I advised him to keep this. No new or change in symptoms.
10. Recent squamous cell carcinoma: Status postsurgery on his left ear: Further followed up by ear, nose, and throat (ENT) services.
11. Beck Depression Inventory score: Stable. No current suicidal thoughts or ideations.
12. Obesity-related medical illness: His weight is down by 3 pounds from his previous appointment with our RD in February. He met me as well as our

RD today. His wife is keeping a detailed journal with regard to his weight and of exactly what he is eating. He has been keeping his journal for more than a year and is very meticulous in measuring and calculating his food consumption. I did talk with him about foregoing the journal and at this time, per patient request and after further discussion with the patient and his wife, I feel comfortable with this recommendation and will be doing so. Certainly, if they would notice weight gain they would resume the journal. In the meantime, I also encouraged continued activity with his biking and resistance band therapy. I will continue to follow him routinely. I advised him to contact me with any questions and/or concerns.

I will schedule him for a return visit in the next 4 months.

Comparison

With weight loss, no longer on the following medications:
Actos 30 mg PO daily
Glimepiride 2 mg PO BID
He has also reduced his cholesterol medication by half tablet.

Patient Testimony

I made a commitment to lose weight in response to my heart doctor recommending weight loss.

In 1 year, I have lost nearly 50 pounds and am maintaining this weight loss. I feel better plus I am healthier. My high BP, cholesterol levels, and blood glucose reading have been reduced as a result of my weight loss. All of these reductions have resulted in my doctor taking me off my two or three diabetic medications plus reducing both my BP and cholesterol medications by half.

I have learned better self-control, portion control, and am making healthy choices with regard to the food I eat. After incorporating these healthier ways of eating plus daily exercise/fitness exercises, I found doing all of this got easier over time. I became used to this healthier way of eating, which has now become for me my everyday eating habit, which is a "lifestyle" change that has really worked for me.

The CLM Clinic has a great support team (Accredited Registered Nurse Practitioner [ARNP], RD, and Exercise/Fitness Specialist) who guide and support one along the way with lots of good advice, positive encouragement, and information. They helped me regain control of my weight, my health, and the quality of my life. My energy today is great. Thank you, CLM Clinic! I could not have done this without you!

Patient #3

> **Total Amount of Weight Lost:** 101.8 pounds (according to his chart)
> **Total Percentage of Weight Lost:** 33%

First Patient Appointment Summary

CLM CLINIC

CHIEF COMPLAINT: Shortness of breath secondary to weight

HISTORY: Mr. BA is a pleasant 52-year-old gentleman who presents to the CLM clinic today for the first time. He was referred by his cardiologist for further workup and weight management. The patient has a significant history of atrial fibrillation, diabetes, HTN, hyperlipidemia, and possible sleep apnea. He has tried exercise in the past and reports that this has kept his weight down; however, this is not helping as much anymore. He reports he would like to lose at least 50 pounds. He has not tried any medications in the past. He reports that the tough time of day for him is during the evening hours. He likes a lot of meat, potatoes, and carbohydrates. He is currently followed up in a cardiac clinic for his history of atrial fibrillation. He denies any current complaints of chest pain or discomfort. He experiences no radiation to the arm, neck, jaw, or back. He does have significant shortness of breath. This is clearly with exertion. He has no PND or orthopnea; no palpitations; no dizziness, lightheadedness, or syncope; mild lower-extremity edema; and no fevers or chills.

Allergies

No known drug allergies

Current Medicines

Aspirin 325 mg PO daily
Benazepril–HCTZ 20-12.5 mg PO daily
Amlodipine besylate 10 mg PO daily
Simvastatin 20 mg PO daily HS
Bystolic 10 mg PO daily
Actoplus Met 15-500 PO TID
Onglyza 5 mg PO daily
Warfarin PO daily as directed

Past Medical History

Atrial fibrillation
Diabetes mellitus (DM)—type 2
Hyperlipidemia
HTN
Male erectile disorder

Past Surgical History

Complete colonoscopy
Foot surgery; ingrown toe nail

Psychiatric History

Patient denies any depression signs or symptoms. No suicidal thoughts or ideations
Beck Depression Inventory score: 0
Depression: No
Anxiety: No
Adjustment disorder: No
Stress: Yes, at times
Binge-eating disorder: Yes

Bulimia: No
Purging patterns: No
Anorexia nervosa: No

Previous Weight-Loss Attempts

What have you tried in the past? Exercise
What has worked best for you? Why? The exercise does help.
What has not worked? Why? N/A
What are your current expectations? Goal would be to lose at least 50 pounds
  or more.
Anorectic use: No
Which drugs have you used in the past? N/A
When did you take them? N/A
What was the effect? N/A
Are there any problems with medications in the past? N/A
What do you expect now from the use of medication? N/A

History of Weight Gain

Gradual onset: Yes
Onset: After he graduated high school
Lifestyle changes: N/A
Stress: Job-related stress may have contributed to weight gain.
Why do you think you have gained weight? Stress. Patient takes relief from stress
  by eating.

Dietary History

Is there a tough time of day? Evening hours
Are there problem foods? Meats, potatoes, salty foods, sweets, and carbohydrates
Is volume an issue? Yes
Are cravings an issue? Yes, at times
Are there certain triggers? No
Who shops and cooks? Patient and patient's wife
Do you use a shopping list? Yes, but buys items not on the list as well
Do you eat out? How often? Once/week
What are your snack habits? Chocolate, candy
Do you have any food dislikes? No
Are you a nighttime eater? No
Are you a stress eater? Yes
Are you a volume eater? Yes

Exercise History

Current level of activity? Yes
  Type: Walking
  Frequency: Daily
  Duration: 50 minutes (about 2 miles)
Past activity level? Football
Favorite activity? Walking
Barriers to exercise? Time

Family History

Weight gain or loss: Yes, relation: Brother and sister are overweight
Anorexia: No
Bulimia: No
Binge eating: No
High BP: Yes, relation: Majority of family
High cholesterol: Unsure
Diabetes: No
Coronary disease: No
Metabolic syndrome: No
Mental illness: No
Sororal history of breast cancer
Maternal history of colon cancer; passed at age 56
Sororal history of HTN

Personal History

Alcohol use; two drinks on the weekends
Marital history—currently married
No tobacco use; lifetime nonsmoker
Working full time

Review of Systems (ROS)

He has weight gain, shortness of breath, palpitations, and daytime somnolence.
All other review of systems is negative.

Vital Signs

Neck circumference: 17.5 inches
Waist circumference: 52.75 inches
Hip circumference: 50 inches
Waist-to-hip ratio: 1.06
Height: 70 inches, **Weight:** 308 pounds, **BMI:** 44.2 kg/m^2
BP: 140/86 mmHg LUE sitting
HR: 84 beats per minute, apical, pulse quality regular
Respiratory rate: 16 respirations per minute

Physical Examination

HEENT: PERRLA, extraocular muscles were intact. Conjunctiva normal, anicteric
Neck: Supple, no JVD. No thyromegaly or masses
Skin: Warm and moist
Mucosa: No cyanosis
Cardiovascular: Normal palpation, percussion. Irregular S1 and S2. 1/6 murmur. No clicks or gallops
Lungs: Normal palpation, percussion. Good bilateral air entry. No rales, rhonchi, or crepitation
Abdomen: Soft, nontender. Normal bowel sounds. No rebound or rigidity
Extremities: 1+ edema, no cyanosis or clubbing
Neurological: Alert and oriented ×3. No motor or sensory deficit

Health Management Plan

Physical Activity Note: This is the patient's first appointment in the CLM Clinic for weight loss. Due to a discussion with his cardiologist in the beginning of September, the patient now walks approximately 2 miles daily and has seen weight loss. He reports low back pain while walking and therefore takes breaks during exercise. I commended him for his efforts and encouraged him to continue; I believe he will be a compliant patient to work with. I explained the exercise component of our program and the baseline fitness assessment he will complete the next time I meet him. He has a sedentary job and reports working through his morning and afternoon 15-minute breaks. Therefore, he was encouraged to at least get up and walk around 2× each day. —Exercise Specialist

Goals

- Keep a dietary and exercise journal daily
- Lose weight of 1 to 2 pounds per week
- Monitor and limit portions
- Aim for 2,200 calories per day
- Continue to cut down on regular soda
- Continue to walk ~2 miles daily with breaks as needed
- Walk around 2× each day at work

Impression/Plan

1. Obesity: His BMI is elevated at 44.0, which places him in the Class III or morbid obesity category. Counseling was provided regarding the importance of good dietary and exercise choices. At this time, he met me, the RD, and the exercise specialist. I counseled him regarding the importance of good dietary and exercise choices. I helped him set goals as stated earlier. This included beginning a dietary and exercise journal along with a weight loss of 1 to 2 pounds per week. He was instructed to aim for around 2,200 calories per day and to walk at least 2 miles daily with breaks as needed. At today's visit, I spent approximately 60 minutes of total patient time. Of that total patient time, at least 50 minutes was spent with one-on-one weight counseling and health coaching. I will schedule him for a return visit in the next 2 weeks. At that time, he will complete his baseline physical assessment.
2. Atrial fibrillation: He is anticoagulated on Coumadin therapy. His rate seems well controlled. He has a pending cardioversion. He is followed closely in the cardiac clinic.
3. Shortness of breath: This is clearly with exertion. He has multiple risk factors for coronary disease and is pending further cardiac workup. Most likely, this is multifactorial and also due to his weight.
4. T2DM: Oral controlled. I will obtain a copy of his previous HgA1c.
5. HTN: Slightly elevated today. I will continue to monitor this.
6. Hypercholesterolemia: On simvastatin therapy. I will obtain a copy of his previous lipid and liver panel.
7. Possible OSA: He has a pending sleep study.
8. Beck Depression Inventory score: His Beck Depression Inventory score is within normal limits at 0. He denies any current suicidal thoughts or ideation.

9. Laboratories: At this time, I will obtain a copy of his baseline laboratories. If he has not had laboratories drawn in the past 3 months, I will order the following: CBC, CMP, TSH, Free T3, Free T4, vitamin D level, lipid level, and HgA1c.

I will schedule him for a return visit in the next 2 weeks.

Follow-Up Appointment Summary: (26 months after initial appointment)

CLM CLINIC

CHIEF COMPLAINT: Continued weight maintenance management

HISTORY: Mr. BA is a pleasant 64-year-old gentleman who returns to the clinic for a follow-up today. He is doing well and is down by 3 pounds since his last appointment with our exercise specialist in June. I have not seen him since November 2012. He is down by more than 102 pounds since beginning this program in September 2011. He reports that he has had many events over the summer and has even gone on vacation for a period of 10 days and maintained his weight loss. He still eats reasonably. He eats when he is hungry and is eating three meals a day. He continues to exercise in the mornings for at least an hour at the gymnasium. He is participating in the "SLED program." He reports this is a series of exercises, which he changes every couple of months. He reports that he had run six different 5Ks this summer. He feels good and reports that he can usually tolerate at least 30 minutes running on the treadmill. He denies any problems or current complaints of any chest pain, heaviness, or pressure. There is no radiation of any pain to the arm, neck, jaw, or back. He has minimal mild shortness of breath. There is no PND or orthopnea. He denies any palpitations. There are no episodes of dizziness, lightheadedness, or syncope; no evidence of any lower-extremity edema; and no fevers or chills.

Allergies

No known drug allergies

Current Medicines

Aspirin 325 mg PO daily
Benazepril–HCTZ 20-12.5 mg PO two tablets daily
Amlodipine besylate 10 mg PO daily
Propafenone HCl 150 mg PO TID

Vital Signs

Neck circumference: 15 inches
Waist circumference: 39.5 inches
Hip circumference: 41 inches
Waist-to-hip ratio: 0.96
Height: 71 inches, Weight: 206.2 pounds, BMI: 28.8 kg/m²
BP: 158/80 mmHg LUE sitting
HR: 52 beats per minute, apical, pulse quality regular
Respiratory rate: 16 respirations per minute

Physical Examination

General: Looks stated age, appropriate conversation, in no acute distress
HEENT: PERRLA, extraocular muscles were intact. Conjunctiva normal, anicteric
Neck: Supple, no JVD
Skin: Warm, pink, and dry
Mucosa: No cyanosis, moist
Cardiovascular: Normal S1 and S2. 1/6 systolic murmur. No clicks. No gallops
Lungs: Good bilateral air entry
Abdomen: Soft and nontender. Normal bowel sounds. No rebound pain or rigidity
Extremities: No edema, no cyanosis, or clubbing
Neurological: Alert and oriented ×3. No motor or sensory deficit

Health Management Plan

Dietary Note: Mr. BA presents himself to the clinic today. His weight is down by another 3 pounds from his previous visit in June. Since his first cardiac appointment here in September 2011, he has lost 102 pounds! His goal is to maintain his current weight, as he feels comfortable here. He continues to exercise on his own for approximately 60 minutes every day. He has been exercising in the morning before work. He does not meet with a trainer twice weekly as he had in the past, but has been given instructions of different exercises and weights to do on his own. He has been compliant with these and determined to keep the weight off. He typically eats breakfast after his workout and before starting his workday. He will stop for lunch most days at the local convenience store, but typically chooses small portions of one slice of pizza or a 6-inch submarine sandwich with lean meat. We talked about having a healthy high-protein snack before exercising to help with satiety and to prevent overeating afterward. It was also recommended that he continue to pay close attention to the serving sizes and increase his vegetable intake at this time to prevent eating too many calories in one sitting. He has been trying to eat more vegetables and would like to work on this goal. He plans to return in 5 months. He was commended on all of his efforts and encouraged to continue. —Registered Dietitian

Goals

- Keep a dietary and exercise journal daily
- Lose weight of 1 to 2 pounds per week
- Continue with current exercise routine (60 or more minutes each day)
- Continue to choose small portions and consume three meals daily

Met Previous Goals

- Kept food and activity journal
- 1 to 2 pounds of weight loss per week
- Cardiovascular exercise
- Strengthening exercises
- Stress management
- Dietary goals

Impression/Plan

1. Atrial fibrillation: He remains on propafenone therapy. He is tolerating this well. He is on a full-strength aspirin. There are no recent breakthroughs or any palpitations.
2. Shortness of breath: He is able to now tolerate 30 minutes of running on the treadmill with no problems.
3. No ischemia by cardiolite as of September 2011.
4. Cardiomyopathy with reduced LV function: His echocardiogram in September 2012 showed a normalized LV function with an ejection fraction of 50% to 55%. There were absolutely no acute signs or symptoms of any decompensation.
5. Diabetes: He is no longer on any oral diabetes medication therapy. This is managed with diet and exercise. He had laboratories drawn on Saturday and has a pending appointment with his primary care provider.
6. HTN: His BP is elevated today. He remains on benazepril–HCTZ therapy and amlodipine. Upon recheck, it was essentially the same at 150/80. I recommended follow-up with his primary care provider.
7. Hypercholesterolemia: He is no longer on any medication therapy.
8. OSA: He remains on BiPAP therapy. There are no current problems. He is tolerating this well.
9. Beck Depression Inventory score: Stable. There are no current suicidal thoughts or ideations.
10. Obesity-related medical illness: His weight is down by an additional 3 pounds since his appointment in June. He is down by 102 pounds. He is off all his diabetic medication and is feeling great. He continues to make good dietary choices as well as has consistent exercise. I encouraged him to continue with his efforts for weight loss and risk factor modification. I will continue to follow him routinely and see him on an as-needed basis. I commended his efforts and am very happy with his overall progress. Today, he met me and the RD. New goals were revised as earlier. During that time, I addressed the 5As—asking, advising, assessing, assisting, and arranging for weight-loss follow-up and risk factor modification.

I will follow him on an as-needed basis.

Comparison

With weight loss, no longer on the following medications:
Simvastatin 20 mg PO daily HS
Bystolic 10 mg PO daily
Actoplus Met 15-500 PO TID
Onglyza 5 mg PO daily
Warfarin PO daily as directed
His combination of benazepril–HCTZ was increased to two tablets daily
He was also put on propafenone HCl 150 mg PO TID

Patient Testimony

After being diagnosed with type 2 diabetes at least 10 years ago and continually gaining weight since graduating high school along with countless warnings from my family doctor, I weighed in for a physical at 318 pounds. Then, about 1 year later, I was diagnosed with atrial fibrillation. My family doctor referred me to a cardiologist. After meeting with the cardiologist, he suggested weight loss through a monitor program at his office. Around that same time, I also joined a gym (thanks to my son). After meeting with the NP, RD, and exercise specialist, I started watching what I ate, worked with a personal trainer, and started daily cardiovascular exercise. I started to lose weight! After going through a few plateaus, I have lost a total of 110 pounds and I feel great!

I realize this is a lifetime change. I have to work daily at this change! Monitoring what and how much I eat as well as my daily workouts is what I have to do.

I have now been "cleared" of diabetes completely! This means no more medications for diabetes, although I change my HgbA1c level every 6 months.

I would like to thank the talented staff at the clinic as well as my cardiologist for helping change my life! It's good to go there and see all the smiles and encouragement! I get very emotional for a 55-year-old.

I would also like to say that nothing comes easy, but with determination—you can do it!

My favorite piece of exercise equipment at the gym is the treadmill. I find that I can burn the most calories by running. I have run six 5Ks in 2013 alone!

My (new) hobbies are

- Working out
- Motorcycling
- Horseback riding
- Running 5Ks

Patient #4

Total Amount of Weight Lost: 120.1 pounds (according to chart review)
Total Percentage of Weight Lost: 34.99%

First Patient Appointment Summary

CLM CLINIC

CHIEF COMPLAINT: Shortness of breath; struggles with weight

HISTORY: Ms. CK is a pleasant 53-year-old woman who presents to the CLM Clinic as a new patient today. She reports that she wants to lose weight, because a doctor had recommended this. She also reports that she is desperate to lose weight and has hit rock bottom. She reports that she needs help. She has a history of lap-banding surgery and has gained weight back after this. She reports that her biggest obstacles in losing weight include lack of motivation, poor dietary choices, late night snacking, lack of physical activity, and pain with physical activity. She reports that she also has no support at home and that she is a workaholic. She is currently working two jobs. She reports that her efforts, which influence her to lose weight, include her health, job, family, and grandchildren. She reports that she has no time to plan meals and has poor food choices. She reports that she has pain and limited time to exercise. She currently weighs in at 343.2 pounds. Her highest weight was 376 pounds, and she would consider around 130 pounds to be a good target weight for herself. She reports weighing this approximately

12 years ago. One of her jobs is very sedentary, as she is a polysomnogram technician monitoring overnight sleep studies. She reports that she gets up and down to help patients, but for the most part sits a lot during this time. She currently denies any complaints of any chest pain or discomfort. There is no radiation to the arm, neck, jaw, or back. She does have shortness of breath. There is no PND or orthopnea. She denies any palpitations. There is no dizziness, lightheadedness, or syncope. She has some lower-extremity edema. There are no fevers or chills. All other review of systems is negative.

Allergies

Iodine

Current Medicines

Norvasc 10 mg PO daily
HCTZ 12.5 mg PO daily
Furosemide 20 mg PO daily
Ventolin HFA (90 base) MCG/ACT aerosol solution; inhale two puffs prn

Past Medical History

HTN
Type 2 diabetes; diet controlled

Gynecological History

Age of first menstrual cycle: 13
Age of menopause: N/A
Number of pregnancies: 1
Number of births: 1
Any history of abnormal vaginal bleeding? Yes

Past Surgical History

Cholecystectomy
Lap band surgery

Psychiatric History

Patient denies any depression signs or symptoms. No suicidal thoughts or ideations
Beck Depression Inventory score: 22
Depression: Yes, only with her weight
Anxiety: No
Adjustment disorder: No
Stress: No
Stress level: Fairly light
Stress frequency: Occasionally
Binge-eating disorder: Yes
Bulimia: No
Purging patterns: No
Anorexia nervosa: No
Previous weight-loss attempts: Yes

Previous Weight-Loss Attempts

What have you tried in the past? Weight watchers, human chorionic gonado-
tropin (HCG), fen-phen, lap band surgery, fasting
What has worked best for you? Why? HCG patient lost 46 pounds
What has not worked? Why? "Almost everything I have tried."
What are your current expectations? Patient would really like to be 150 pounds.
Patient just wants to be healthier.

Anorectic Use

Which drugs have you used in the past? Fen-phen, Lipozene. Patient has taken
others, but does not remember the names.
When did you take them? In the 1990s
What was the effect? Patient lost 46 pounds.
Were there any problems with medications in the past? N/A
What do you now expect from the use of medication? N/A

History of Weight Gain

Gradual onset: Yes
Onset: Childhood
Lifestyle changes: Patient thinks weight gain stems from some stressful events
during her childhood.
Stress: Yes, family and financial stressors.
Why do you think you have gained weight? "Food is comforting." "Almost like
a friend."

Dietary History

Is there a tough time of day? Patient is a third-shift worker and notices that she
eats mostly during these hours.
Are there problem foods? Loves junk food.
Is volume an issue? Yes
Are cravings an issue? Yes, chicken wings from KFC, chips
Are there certain triggers? Yes, emotional eater
Who shops and cooks? Patient's mother
Do you use a shopping list? No
Do you eat out? How often? Yes, three times per month. These are usually fast
food restaurants.
What are your snack habits? Chips, Snickers (during menstrual cycle), ice cream
Do you have any food dislikes? Vegetables give her gas. She does not like cot-
tage cheese. Patient does not eat much red meat.
Are you a nighttime eater? Patient is a third-shift worker. Majority of eating
habits are during the night when she is awake.
Are you a stress eater? Yes
Are you a volume eater? Yes

Exercise History

Current level of activity? No
  Type: N/A
  Frequency: N/A
  Duration: N/A

Past activity level? Walking, had gymnasium membership, weight lifting, active in sports

Favorite activity? Walking

Barriers to exercise? Pain in her knees. Plantar fasciitis. Also, lack of motivation

Family History

Weight gain or loss: Yes. Relation: Daughter
Anorexia: No
Bulimia: No
Binge eating: No
High BP: Relation: Majority of family
High cholesterol: Yes. Relation: Mother
Diabetes: Yes. Relation: Mother, brothers, and daughter
Coronary disease: Yes. Relation: Parents
Metabolic syndrome: Unsure
Mental illness: Yes. Relation: Mother has depression.

Personal History

Single
Working
Nonsmoker

Review of Symptoms (ROS)

She has weight gain, shortness of breath, and tiredness/fatigue.
All other review of systems is negative.

Vital Signs

Neck circumference: 15 inches
Chest circumference: 48.5 inches
Waist circumference: 51 inches
Hip circumference: 62 inches
Waist-to-hip ratio: 0.82
Height: 63 inches, **Weight:** 343.2 pounds, **BMI:** 60.8 kg/m^2
BP: 126/80 mmHg LUE sitting
HR: 70 beats per minute, apical, pulse quality regular
Respiratory rate: 16 respirations per minute

Physical Examination

HEENT: PERRLA, extraocular muscles were intact. Conjunctiva normal, anicteric
Neck: Supple, no JVD. No thyromegaly or masses
Skin: Warm and moist
Mucosa: No cyanosis
Cardiovascular: Normal palpation, percussion. Normal S1 and S2. No murmur. No clicks or gallops
Lungs: Normal palpation, percussion. Good bilateral air entry. No rales, rhonchi, or crepitation
Abdomen: Soft, nontender. Normal bowel sounds. No rebound or rigidity
Extremities: 1+ edema, no cyanosis or clubbing
Neurological: Alert and oriented ×3. No motor or sensory deficit

Health Management Plan

Dietary Note: Patient presents for her first visit for weight loss today. Her current weight is 343.2 pounds. Her personal weight goal is to be 130 pounds. We discussed setting short-term goals to reach her long-term goal. A minimum of 34 to 35 pounds in 6 months was recommended by the doctor of nursing practice (DNP). We discussed a healthy weight loss of 1 to 2 pounds per week. She seemed agreeable with this number. Her current barriers to weight loss include her work schedule and her mother's shopping and cooking. Her mother tends to fry foods at many meals and will get upset if she does not eat them. She reported that she recently talked with her mother about the importance of weight loss and has been buying some of her own foods. She works third shift at Allen and tends to snack on foods during working hours. We discussed a healthy eating plan consisting of eating three meals and two snacks at consistent times during the day. Her caloric needs for weight loss were discussed, and a calorie guide was given to help her get started. A list of healthy snacks that are less than 100 calories was given as well. On her next visit, she will meet with the exercise specialist for further activity goals. —Registered Dietitian

Goals

- Keep a dietary and exercise journal daily
- Lose weight of 1 to 2 pounds per week
- Aim for 1,800 calories daily
- Consume no more than 100 to 150 calories per snack 1 to 2 times daily
- Walk 5 minutes daily

Impression/Plan

1. Obesity: Status post-lap banding surgery: Her weight and BMI are elevated at 343.2 pounds with a BMI of 60.8. This places her in the Class III category for morbid obesity. Counseling was provided regarding the importance of good dietary and exercise choices. Today, she met me and an RD. Goals were set as earlier. She was instructed to begin keeping a dietary and exercise journal and encouraged to aim for a weight loss of 1 to 2 pounds per week. She was also encouraged to walk 5 minutes daily, which will be an increase from her current activity level. She was also encouraged to aim for 1,800 calories per day and to not eat more than 100 to 150 calories per snack. At today's visit, approximately 60 minutes of total patient time was spent. Of that 60 minutes, at least 50 minutes was spent with one-on-one weight counseling and health coaching. She rescheduled for a return visit in the next 2 weeks. At that appointment, she will meet with the exercise specialist to further complete a baseline physical assessment. This will help determine further exercise prescription.
2. HTN: Her BP is well controlled today.
3. Unknown cholesterol levels: I will obtain a copy of her previous lipid/liver panel.
4. T2DM: She reports this is controlled by diet. I will obtain a copy of her previous fasting glucose and her HgA1c.
5. Shortness of breath: Most likely, this is multifactorial in nature and largely due to her weight and deconditioning.
6. History of lap band surgery.

7. Beck Depression Inventory score: Her Beck Depression Inventory score is elevated at 22, which places her in the moderate depression category. She states that this is purely due to her weight. She denies any suicidal thoughts or ideations.
8. Laboratories: At this time, I will obtain a copy of baseline laboratories. She has not had laboratories drawn within the previous 3 months. I would recommend the following: CBC, CMP, TSH, Free T3, Free T4, lipid panel, and vitamin D level.

She will be scheduled for a return visit in 2 weeks.

Follow-Up Appointment Summary (23 months after initial appointment):

CLM CLINIC

HISTORY: Mrs. CK is a pleasant 55-year-old woman who returns to the clinic for a follow-up today. She is down by an additional 6 pounds since she was last seen on November 26. She has recently joined Planet Fitness and will be going a couple of days a week. She reports that she is tolerating water a lot better and drinking more of this. She has been tolerating activity well and reports she has been trying to challenge herself by doing the elliptical. Otherwise, she is doing her normal things and is eating three meals. When she has a snack, she reports this is healthy. She feels good about herself. She has good self-esteem. There are no current complaints of any chest pain, heaviness, or pressure; no radiation of any pain to the arm, neck, jaw, or back. There is minimal mild shortness of breath with activity, but she reports that each day she is tolerating this a little better. There is no PND or orthopnea; no palpitations; no episodes of dizziness, lightheadedness, or syncope; no evidence of any lower-extremity edema; and no fevers or chills. She reports that this is the lowest weight she has been since before her daughter was born more than 30 years ago. All other review of systems is negative.

Allergies

Iodine
Shellfish

Current Medicines

Norvasc 5 mg PO daily
Ventolin HFA (90 base) MCG/ACT aerosol solution; inhale 2 puffs prn
Aspirin 81 mg PO daily
Prilosec OTC 20 mg PO daily
Biotin 1,000 mcg five tablets daily

Vital Signs

Neck circumference: 13 inches
Chest circumference: 39 inches
Waist circumference: 37.5 inches
Hip circumference: 48 inches

Waist-to-hip ratio: 0.78
Height: 63 inches, **Weight:** 223.1 pounds, **BMI:** 39.5 kg/m², **BSA:** 2.03
BP: 110/72 mmHg LUE sitting
HR: 70 beats per minute, apical, pulse quality regular
Respiratory rate: 16 respirations per minute

Physical Examination

General: Looks stated age, appropriate conversation, in no acute distress
HEENT: PERRLA, extraocular muscles were intact. Conjunctiva normal, anicteric
Neck: Supple, no JVD
Skin: Warm. Dry
Mucosa: No cyanosis, moist
Cardiovascular: Normal S1 and S2, 1/6 systolic murmur
Lungs: Good bilateral air entry
Abdomen: Soft and nontender. Normal bowel sounds. No rebound pain or
    rigidity
Extremities: No edema, no cyanosis, or clubbing
Neurological: Alert and oriented ×3. No motor or sensory deficit

Health Management Plan

Dietary Note: Mrs. CK presents for a follow-up visit for weight-loss assistance today. Since her last appointment on November 26, her weight is down by 6 pounds. The team commended her on her success and the efforts she has made in reaching her goals. She reports having increased energy and less shortness of breath. She recently joined Planet Fitness and plans to go there at least twice weekly. She continues to practice portion control by reading labels, measuring, and weighing food. She reported that she continues to choose small portions. She continues to avoid high-fat meat and desserts. She is proud to report that she has been able to resist sweet treats that are offered to her and resisted eating any of the high-calorie/high-fat food items at Christmas time, with the exception of a piece of pie. She plans to come back next week for the support group. She remains with a positive outgoing attitude about her weight loss and attempts at it. She plans to continue to lose weight of 1 to 2 pounds per week in a healthy manner. She continues to also follow up with her bariatric surgeon. Goals were set for the next month. —Registered Dietitian

Goals

- Keep a dietary and exercise journal daily
- Lose weight of 1 to 2 pounds per week
- Continue to practice portion control
- Continue to limit/avoid sweet treats
- Consume 64 ounces of water daily
- Cardio activity for 20 or more minutes daily

Met Previous Goals

- 1 to 2 pounds of weight loss per week
- Stress management
- Dietary goals

Impression/Plan

1. Status post-Roux-en-Y gastric bypass surgery in November 2012
2. History of lap band surgery
3. History of HCG and fen-phen use
4. HTN: Well controlled today
5. T2DM
6. Shortness of breath: This is relatively stable at this time. I will continue to watch this.
7. No EKG evidence of ischemia per treadmill stress test in July 2012
8. Normal LV function per ECG in July 2012
9. Mild mitral and tricuspid regurgitation: Stable. No acute signs or symptoms of any decompensation
10. Beck Depression Inventory score: Stable
11. Obesity-related medical illness status post-Roux-en-Y gastric bypass surgery and history of lap band surgery: She is doing well. She is down by an additional 5 pounds. She is at the lowest weight since before she gave birth to her child more than 30 years ago. She is very excited about this. She is very motivated to keep up her current lifestyle means, including exercise and monitoring what she is eating. She met me and the RD today. New goals were revised as earlier. I commended her on her progress and encouraged continued follow-up. She wishes for further accountability. I will follow up routinely. I am very happy with her progress.

Comparison

With weight loss, no longer on the following medications:
Furosemide 20 mg PO daily
HCTZ 12.5 mg PO daily
Her Norvasc has been cut in half, and she now takes 5 mg PO daily
The following medications have been added to her medication regimen:
Aspirin 81 mg PO daily
Prilosec OTC 20 mg PO daily
Biotin 1,000 mcg five tablets daily

Patient Testimony

First, I would like to say "Thank You" to the staff at the CLM Clinic and support group for guiding me and teaching me this past year. I am also thankful that my primary health care provider recommended this program.

The staff has been with me through the death of both parents and my personal struggles this past year. They have taught me to how to take care of "me." I feel very comfortable sharing my life history with them.

I also thank you for allowing me to participate in such a good program that addresses issues that will change lives if that person is willing to allow information that will enhance or, shall I say, improve their lives.

To the support group: Thanks for your support. The sessions that are held each month are very helpful, informative, and most of all fun.

Keep up the good work! We need more people, programs, and caring establishments such as this. Those of you who know me personally always hear me say, "I'm not going 'nowhere,' I'm here to stay!"

Case Study 2

This case study builds upon information acquired in Chapters 4 to 6 dealing with communication:

- *Chapter 4: Addressing Pediatric Obesity*
- *Chapter 5: How to Initiate the Weight Conversation With Patients*
- *Chapter 6: Patients' Stories*

Ryan is an 11-year-old Black boy who comes in for his school physical. He is getting ready again for school in the fall. He is accompanied by his mother. He says that he is excited about starting the fifth grade.

His vitals are as follows:

Blood pressure: 116/76
Pulse: 80 bpm
Respirations: 16
Height: 55 inches (slightly greater than 25th percentile)
Weight: 150 pounds (greater than 95th percentile)
Body mass index (BMI): 34.85 kg/m^2
Pulse oximetry: 98% on room air

He reports that he was active playing baseball over the summer. He enjoys playing video games with his friends. He also loves watching television. He says that he watches at least 4 hours of television per day. When asked to recall what he ate the previous day, he says the following:

- Breakfast: two cherry pop tarts, one banana, one glass of orange juice, and one glass of milk
- Morning snack: one package of nutty bars
- Lunch: two hot dogs, chips, and four chocolate chip cookies
- Afternoon snack: yogurt, two chocolate chip cookies
- Supper: one hamburger, one baked potato (with butter and cheese), and a fruit cup
- Nighttime snack: two scoops of chocolate ice cream

His physical examination shows the following:

General: Looks stated age, appropriate conversation, in no acute distress
Head, Eyes, Ears, Nose, Throat (HEENT): PERRLA, extraocular muscles intact.
   Conjunctiva normal, anicteric
Neck: Supple, no jugular vein distension (JVD). Acanthosis nigricans
Skin: Warm and dry
Mucosa: No cyanosis, moist
Cardiovascular: Normal S1 and S2. No murmur
Lungs: Good bilateral air entry
Abdomen: Obese, soft, and nontender. Normal bowel sounds. No rebound pain
   or rigidity
Extremities: No edema, no cyanosis, or clubbing
Neurological: Alert and oriented ×3. No motor or sensory deficit

In reviewing his family history, one could see that his mother is obese. She reports she has hypertension (HTN) and type 2 diabetes mellitus (T2DM). Her husband, the child's father, has high cholesterol. The child's maternal grandmother has HTN, T2DM, and coronary artery disease (CAD). The child's paternal grandfather has a history of stroke and CAD. The child has an 8-year-old sister with no reported health problems.

Is he overweight or obese? What category does his BMI fall into? Would you use BMI in an 11-year-old?

How would you address his weight?

What has led to his obesity?

Is he a candidate for weight loss?

How would you present him with a plan for weight loss? What would this include?

Would you make any additional referrals?

Would you order any testing? If yes, what testing and why?

What dietary advice would you provide?

What lifestyle changes would you suggest?

Would you recommend any family lifestyle counseling?

You also draw fasting blood work on him and find the following:

Thyroid-stimulating hormone (TSH): 3.5

Fasting lipid panel:

Total cholesterol: 215
Triglycerides: 550
High-density lipoprotein (HDL): 30
Low-density lipoprotein (LDL): 150

Would you consider any medications? If yes, what?

When would you repeat laboratory work?

When would you schedule his next follow-up appointment?

Would you involve any other advanced practice nurses (APNs) in his care?

What additional education, if any, would you provide?

Assessment

Overview of Genetics and Pathophysiology of Obesity

This chapter focuses on the pathophysiology of obesity. There are many components to this, although this chapter explains only the basics. There have been entire books written on these complex issues and subjects alone. The explanation of the pathophysiology is not easy, as there are numerous diseases and comorbidities associated with obesity, thus the complexity. The disease of obesity has a direct correlation with numerous comorbid conditions.

ENERGY BALANCE

It is important to understand the concept of energy balance with obesity. Energy storage is part of the physiological process that is needed for survival. If energy is not used secondary to more intake than output, this energy is stored as triglycerides found in adipose tissue. "The release of fatty acids by the hydrolysis of white adipose tissue triglyceride stores allows us to face periods of food shortage or increased energy expenses" (Clement & Ferre, 2003, p. 722).

The distribution of adipose tissue is different in women and men. Women usually carry subcutaneous adipose tissue in the lower areas of the trunk, whereas men commonly have more in the upper trunk and intra-abdominal areas. Adipose tissue may vary throughout one's life span. This is because white adipocytes may take an entire life span to progress through the differentiation process.

It is not only important to know that adipocytes change throughout life but also important to understand the function of adipocytes. Much of this function involves secretion that is important for the energy balance as well as carbohydrate metabolism. These key factors can include the following: angiogenic factors, angiotensinogen, immunorelated factors, prostaglandins, and protein (Clement & Ferre, 2003).

The discovery of the human obese (OB) gene, and its product, leptin, has led to a better understanding of energy storage regulation, as it has been found to inhibit hunger (Clement & Ferre, 2003; Klok, Jakobsdottir, & Drent, 2006). This effect has been demonstrated in many rodent studies. Leptin has a large role in many biological mechanisms:

- Angiogenesis
- Bone formation
- Hematopoiesis

- Immune response
- Inflammatory response
- Wound healing

Leptin influences both orexigenic and anorexigenic peptides. The following are orexigenic peptides:

- Neuropeptide Y (NPY)
- Melanin-concentrating hormone (MCH)
- Agouti-related protein (AgRP)
- Galanin
- Orexin
- Galanin-like peptide (GALP)

The following are anorexigenic peptides influenced by leptin:

- Proopiomelanocortin (POMC)
- Cocaine-regulated transcript
- Amphetamine-regulated transcript
- Neurotensin
- Corticotropin-releasing hormone (CRH)
- Brain-derived neurotrophic factor

These neuropeptides can be found in several of the hypothalamic regions (arcuate nucleus [ARC], paraventricular nucleus, or lateral or perifornical hypothalamus) (Klok et al., 2006).

Leptin has been found primarily in the adipocytes of white adipose tissue. Leptin, a cytokine-like polypeptide, produced through hypothalamic receptors by activation, is proportionate to the adipose mass, thus providing signals to the brain about the fat stores. Leptin can affect both the lateral and medial hypothalamus to inhibit hunger and induce satiety. NPY is counteracted by leptin in the lateral hypothalamus. Along with this, leptin impedes AgRP. The combination of leptin and both peptides inhibits hunger. Leptin combines and secretes alpha-Melanocyte-stimulating hormone (α-MSH) from POMC. This process occurs in the medial hypothalamus, more specifically in the hypothalamic ARC. After this process, α-MSH then binds to the melanocortin 4 receptor (MC4R), deterring hunger (Clement & Ferre, 2003).

Ghrelin also has an important role in energy balance. The ghrelin peptide was originally found in the stomach. Other forms of the protein ghrelin and the ghrelin-producing neurons have been found in several other areas of the body, including the brain and gastrointestinal tract. Secreted by the stomach, ghrelin is affected by age, gender, growth hormone (GH), weight or body mass index (BMI), glucose, and insulin, as well as one's nutritional state. Ghrelin also increases preprandial and decreases postprandial. Ghrelin and leptin have been hypothesized to work together for satiety (Klok et al., 2006).

ENVIRONMENTAL AND GENETIC FACTORS

Parental obesity has been found to be the strongest risk factor associated with obesity, more so if both parents are obese. Some studies have associated maternal obesity as a stronger predictor than paternal obesity; some have thought this to be because of pregnancy weight gain. Pregnancy weight gain is directly related to the child, as well as the adult's weight and BMI.

There has long been the battle about weight gain—is it genetic or environmental? Twin, family, and adoption studies have led the way to prove a high value with regard to genetic studies. Both twin and adoption studies have shown a 60% to 90% correlation of BMI and genetics.

Weight has also been found to correlate with the intrauterine environment. Numerous studies have been done with twins, including monozygotic (MZ) twins. One study with more than 3,500 twin sets found a positive correlation with genetics, progressing BMI, and childhood. This study showed a larger genetic influence on increasing age. Another study showed heritability of increased BMI later in childhood. One should be reminded to review twin studies cautiously. This is because twin studies can overestimate dominant genetics as well as underestimate environmental factors.

Genetic determination has been seen with intake and physical activity levels. Eating behaviors have also shown heritability. Having said this, obesity is a complex disease that is complicated by both pathophysiology and behavior; therefore, further research is warranted (Hinney, Vogel, & Hebebrand, 2010).

GENETIC SYNDROMES

Numerous genetic syndromes—perhaps at least 25—exist in combination with obesity (Clement & Ferre, 2003). According to Goldstone and Beales (2008), some of the common disorders include the following:

- Prader–Willi
- Bardet–Biedl syndrome (BBS)
- Alstrom syndrome
- Cohen syndrome
- Albright's hereditary osteodystrophy (pseudohypoparathyroidism)
- Carpenter syndrome
- MOMO syndrome
- Rubinstein–Taybi syndrome
- Fragile X syndrome
- Borjeson–Forssman–Lehmann syndrome

Challenges lie ahead to determine responsible genes and their susceptible roles in accompanying disease (Clement & Ferre, 2003).

GENE AND PROTEIN FUNCTION

Obesity, a complex disorder, has continued to advance in gene research and mapping, which is an important part of investigation and treatment. Caused by genetic and nongenetic factors, the advancement in obesity research has changed over the past 100 years. Biological, psychological, and psychosocial developments have occurred, thus leading to the current research and theories of thought. Historically, the early 1900s saw pituitary and/or hypothalamic dysfunction as the cause of obesity. Psychological theories emerged and continued from the 1940s through 1970s along with the first syndromal form of obesity. Body weight regulation was studied through twins and adoption in the 1980s and 1990s, thus leading the way to the cloning of the leptin gene in 1994. This was a major breakthrough in obesity studies and was instrumental in further biomedical research—large-scale, molecular genetic studies and pediatric treatment of leptin deficiency. This paved the way for thought that a single gene mutation could enhance and lead to an increase in hunger and/or obesity. The latest research focuses on the neuroendocrine disorder of obesity, genetic predispositions, environmental risk factors, and polygenetic variants (Hinney et al., 2010).

> Environmental changes affecting both energy intake and expenditure are assumed to underlie the recent obesity epidemic, as the gene pool of a population is unlikely to have changed substantially within the past generation. This is in accordance with the "thrifty genotype hypothesis." This hypothesis implies that gene variants, which result in an increased energy deposition as fat, have accumulated over time to maintain the reproductive function as long as possible and to enhance survival during famines. (Hinney et al., 2010, p. 298)

Gene studies in the obese can prove helpful; however, it is still unclear whether predictive genetics will be incorporated into obesity prevention.

PATHOPHYSIOLOGY

The human body is smart. It is made for survival. One of the body's natural reactions is to store extra fat as fuel for survival in case of starvation. If the body repeatedly gets too much food or fat, its natural process is to store the extra as fat. This, over a period of time, causes obesity. Enhanced lipolysis, secondary to the sympathetic state of obesity, leads to the release of excessive fatty acids that stimulate lipotoxicity. Lipid accumulation in the nonadipose tissues generates oxidant stress to the endoplasmic reticulum and mitochondria. This inhibits lipogenesis, stimulates lipotoxicity, increases hyperglycemia and hepatic glucose production, decreases secretion of pancreatic beta-cell insulin, and results in beta-cell exhaustion.

Normal adiposity is exaggerated in obesity because of the excess secretion of adipokines. In each disease associated with obesity, the body's immune response stimulates inflammation, causing tissue dysfunction primarily in adipose tissue. However, since obesity affects the entire body, it can also be seen in muscle, organ, or vascular endothelium (Redinger, 2007).

As previously seen, adipocytes not only store triacylglycerol but also regulate secretagogues, which, in turn, regulate body fat mass. The release of secretagogues by the adipocytes includes lectin, adiponectin, and visfatin. Cytokines, growth factors, and complement proteins are also involved with adipocyte adipokines. Inflammatory adipokines are found throughout the body in muscle and surrounding organs (visceral fat). Those responsible are the following: tumor necrosis factor-alpha (TNF-α), interleukin (IL)-1, and IL-6.

Adipokines have different roles within the body. Endothelial function may be enhanced when adipokines encourage the secretion of renin, angiotensinogen, and angiotensin II, thus increasing hypertension (HTN). The secretion of TNF-α increases fatty liver inflammation as well as the inflammation in the gut, pancreas, mesentery, and bronchial trees. Along with TNF-α and IL-6, C-reactive protein (CRP), alpha-1 acid glycoprotein, and specific amyloid antigen are also seen, especially in those with fatty liver disease (FLD). CRP, alpha-1 acid glycoprotein, and specific amyloid antigen are considered acute-phase reactants that are also more commonly seen in those with type 2 diabetes mellitus (T2DM).

Adipocytes also play a role in insulin sensitivity. They are responsible for the stimulation of monocyte chemoattractant protein 1 (MCP-1), macrophage migration inhibiting factor (MM1F), and resistin. Along with stimulation and secretion, fat-associated macrophages enhance the body's inflammatory state. The specific macrophages that are responsible are the mitogen-activated protein kinase family, which consists of C-Jun N-terminal Kinase, inhibitor of nuclear factor kappa beta (NF-KB) Kinase b, and phosphatidylinositol 3-Kinase (Redinger, 2007). The enhanced mitogen-activated family of protein kinases induces "[T]he transcription factor NF-KB that allows dephosphorylation of the IRS-1 and IRS-2 docking proteins. The latter inhibits the GLUT4 transporter of glucose, resulting in insulin resistance" (Redinger, 2007, p. 858).

The systemic inflammation in obesity has been found to produce atherogenesis throughout development. This is seen in early endothelial fatty streaks, later progressing into thrombosis through plaque formation and rupture. White fat cells secrete vasoactive endothelial growth factor, plasminogen activator inhibitor-1, angiotensinogen, renin, and angiotensin II, which form foam cells, thus enhancing endothelial uptake of lipids and free fatty acids. IL-6 inhibits lipolysis, thus increasing hypertriglyceridemia.

Secretion of cytokines MCP-1, MMIF, and endothelin-1 enhances the progress of atherosclerosis and the inflammatory process, thus increasing plaque located in the vascular wall. The rupture of plaque and thrombosis are caused by plasminogen activator inhibitor-1, IL-6, tumor growth factor-β, and TNF-α. Matrix metalloproteinases also cause increased progression of plaque formation, thus leading to atheroma cap thinning and further plaque rupture (Redinger, 2007).

Adipose cells also secrete anti-inflammatory hormones as somewhat of a protective mechanism. These hormones include the following: adiponectin, visfatin, and complement-related acylation-stimulating protein. Improvement of insulin sensitivity as well as vascular endothelium dysfunction is seen. This is most apparent when the levels of anti-inflammatory adipokines are reduced, as the weight continues to climb. "In summary, inflammatory, insulin-resistant, hypertensive, and thrombotic-promoting adipokines that are atherogenic are counterbalanced by anti-inflammatory and anti-atherogenic adipocyte hormones, such as adiponectin, visfatin, and acylation-stimulating protein, whereas certain actions of leptin and resistin are pro-atherogenic" (Redinger, 2007, p. 859).

The disease of obesity deals directly with the accumulation of fat, thus leading to an increase in cardiovascular risk factors as well as systemic diseases. Physical symptoms

QUICK TIPS—ROLES OF ADIPOCYTES

1. Store triacylglycerol
2. Regulate secretagogues that regulate body fat mass
3. Enhance endothelial function
4. Stimulate fat-associated macrophages
5. Secrete anti-inflammatory hormones

associated with obesity and its comorbid conditions can include arthritis, back pain, breathlessness, cellulitis, edema, sweating, stress incontinence, and/or sweating. Surgical hazards, social or psychological issues, and metabolic or endocrine issues are also seen in overweight or obese individuals. Problems related to surgery or anesthesia can include poor wound healing or dehiscence, hernia, chest infection, or problems related to sleep apnea. Social or psychological issues can include isolation, agoraphobia, discrimination, family or marital stress, unemployment, tiredness, low self-esteem, depression, self-deception, or thought distortion. Metabolic diseases can include HTN, hyperlipidemia, stroke, hypercoagulation, or diabetes. Hirsutism, oligomenorrhea, infertility, menorrhagia, or estrogen-dependent cancers (breast, endometrium, and prostate) fall under the category of endocrine disease (Lean, 2000).

Metabolic and organ dysfunction is seen with obesity. Adiponectin, exclusively produced and secreted by adipocytes, regulates the metabolism of glucose and lipids as well as influences the body's response to insulin (Redinger, 2007).

Obesity directly causes cardiac pathology, including atheroma, thrombosis, left ventricular hypertrophy (LVH), and arrhythmia. The compounding effect of obesity and any of the following risk factors or diseases greatly increases the risk of cardiovascular disease (CVD). These can include, but are not limited to, smoking, noninsulin-dependent diabetes mellitus (NIDDM), hyperlipidemia, and/or HTN (Lean, 2000).

Although it would seem simple to focus only on obesity and weight loss with regard to caloric intake versus caloric energy expenditure, a physiological and metabolic fulcrum can help in better understanding fat storage and release. Certainly, lifestyle factors may upset the balance; once this is off, it is difficult to rebalance. Durstine and Moore (2003) discuss the complexity of the altered physiological fulcrum:

"The altered physiological fulcrum in obesity includes the following:

- Increased fasting insulin
- Increased insulin response to glucose
- Decreased insulin sensitivity
- Decreased GH
- Decreased GH response to insulin stimulation
- Increased adrenocortical hormones
- Increased cholesterol synthesis and excretion
- Decreased hormone-sensitive lipase" (p. 149)

As the prevalence of obesity continues to rise, so does the importance of understanding not only the genetic components involved but also the pathophysiology. This disease is complicated by its numerous comorbid conditions, therefore adding to the complexity. It is essential to educate patients, families, and providers on this multifaceted disease.

REFERENCES

Clement, K., & Ferre, P. (2003). Genetics and the pathophysiology of obesity. *Pediatric Research, 53*(5), 721–725. Retrieved from http://www.nature.com/pr/journal/v53/n5/pdf/pr2003291a.pdf

Durstine, J. L., & Moore, G. E. (2003). *ACSM's exercise management for persons with chronic disease and disabilities* (2nd ed.). Champaign, IL: Human Kinetics.

Goldstone, A. P., & Beales, P. L. (2008). Genetic obesity syndromes. *Frontiers of Hormonal Research, 36*, 37–60. doi:10.1159/0000115336

Hinney, A., Vogel, C. I. G., & Hebebrand, J. (2010). From monogenic to polygenic obesity: Recent advances. *European Child and Adolescent Psychiatry, 19*(3), 297–310. Retrieved from http://www.ncbi.nlm.nih.gov/pmc/articles/PMC2839509

Klok, M. D., Jakobsdottir, S., & Drent, M. L. (2006). Appetite regulatory peptides: The role of leptin and ghrelin in the regulation of good intake and body weight in humans: A review. *Obesity Reviews, 8*, 21–34.

Lean, M. E. J. (2000). Pathophysiology of obesity. *Proceedings of the Nutrition Society, 59*, 331–336. Retrieved from http://journals.cambridge.org/download.php?file=%2FPNS%2FPNS59_03%2FS0029665100000379a.pdf&code=c21dc022c3943ead6cb278dbfe6e39fd

Redinger, R. N. (2007). The pathophysiology of obesity and its clinical manifestations. *Journal of Gastroenterology and Hepatology, 3*(11), 856–863. Retrieved from http://www.ncbi.nlm.nih.gov/pmc/articles/PMC3104148

Behaviors, Addiction, and Eating Disorders

This chapter focuses on behaviors, addiction, and eating disorders. These conditions play a major role in the recognition and treatment of obesity. The following sections focus on and identify specific diseases in relation to the understanding of this complex issue.

BEHAVIORS AND ADDICTION

Prior to understanding the complexities of eating disorders, it is important to define *behavior*. Defining this helps identify why the behavior is done and what can be done to treat it. According to Bicard and Bicard (2013), *behavior* is defined as actions that are observed and can be measured. This refers specifically to the actions and does not involve any type of personal motivation or feelings. Data collection allows for optimization of the behavior and for design and implementation of their intervention (Bicard & Bicard, 2013).

Behavior can be established at ages as early as toddlers or preschool age. This includes basic eating patterns. In children, these are seen as learned or observed behaviors from parents. Research has shown that leading by example promotes more positive eating habits. Therefore, adults who encourage children for "less fat" or "more fruits and vegetables," without positive demonstration, actually hinder good eating habits. Development of good eating habits is further promoted by adult influence. Providing a variety of healthy options falls on parental or adult responsibility, whereas the amount and type of food falls on the child. Appetite fluctuations throughout childhood are normal. The child or patient should never be "pushed" or "forced" to eat, as this may cause aversions to certain foods, overeating, or acting out.

The advanced practice nurse (APN) should provide education and encourage the patient and/or family to engage in the eating experience. This includes the following:

- Positive examples of eating
- Education about sugars
- Food preparation
- Structured mealtimes
- A relaxed mealtime environment

- Age-appropriate snacks
- Opportunities to prepare and serve meals
- Adequate exercise
- Adequate sleep

The APN is responsible for providing adequate education for proper growth and development. This includes patient and family education with regard to food behaviors (Buttaro, Trybulski, Bailey, & Sandberg-Cook, 2003).

Considered a disease that causes loss of control compared with eating certain types of foods, food addiction is founded on the theoretical basis that palatable food is regulated by the same regions of the brain as that of highly abused drugs (Institute for Natural Resources [INR], 2014). *Palatable foods* are defined as "1. agreeable to the palate or taste or 2. agreeable or acceptable to the mind" (Merriam-Webster, 2014). Palatable foods and highly abused drugs share the same pathways to the mesolimbic system that is used in behavior motivation. A "rewiring" of the brain can take place, as repeated exposure to large amounts of the palatable foods promotes almost a "loss of control." Dr. Nora Volkow, director of the National Institute on Drug Abuse at the National Institutes of Health (NIH), states, "It's more difficult for people to control their eating habits than narcotics" (INR, 2014, n.p.).

Although palatable food initially serves as positive and negative reinforcing, as food consumption repeats more frequently with palatable food choices, the brain stress circuitry and reward pathways expect these foods more often. If this does not occur, a negative emotional state ensues; thus, food serves as an escape or a way to relieve stress or comfort (INR, 2014). "Neurotransmitters that are implicated in drug-seeking behaviors are also implicated in food intake" (INR, 2014). This includes dopamine, especially its release in the nucleus accumbens (NAcc). Repeated overconsumption of food leads to decreased sensitivity and again causes the person to overeat or eat compulsively to gain the sense of reward or satisfaction. The satisfaction is only temporary; thus, the cycle of overeating continues. "It is clear that modern-day foods have reinforcing abilities similar to alcohol or other drugs of abuse" (Avena, 2012, as cited in INR, 2014). Distorted thinking occurs over time and the person may want to, but cannot, stop these cravings.

Addiction can be referred to as an illness, one that encompasses physical and mental aspects. Personality, especially of those with doubt, insecurity, or even negativity, can lead to further destructive behavior. Dr. David Kessler, the former commissioner of the U.S. Food and Drug Administration (FDA), estimates that as many as 20% of people who are considered a healthy weight are addicted to specific foods, a combination of foods, or even the volume or amount of food. Many times, these patients will eat more food than the body needs or eat even when they know it is not good for them (Food Addiction Institute [FAI], 2014).

A number of questionnaires exist to determine if someone is addicted to food; however, these are best administered by an APN with further education in mental health or counseling. Not all people who have a food addiction are obese, but many times one, if not all three, of the following can be seen: obesity, eating disorders, and/or chemical dependency. Research on food addiction has been ongoing since 1995. Current research is focused on chemical dependency of food, human genetic research, animal studies, brain imaging of dopamine receptors, and biochemical studies of the digestive processes (INR, 2014). Further treatment of obesity can be understood, as more research is done on food addiction.

Food Addicts (FA) in Recovery Anonymous is an organization formed out of the organization Overeaters Anonymous (OA). FA is based on the 12 steps of Alcoholics Anonymous (AA) and encompasses all types of persons struggling with eating disorders. Meetings are available nationwide (Box 8.1).

> **BOX 8.1 ADDICTION RESOURCES**
>
> **FA in Recovery Anonymous**
> www.foodaddicts.org
>
> **Food Addiction Institute**
> www.foodaddictioninstitute.org
>
> **Food Addiction Research Foundation**
> www.foodaddictionresearch.org

EATING DISORDERS

Obesity is defined as "a situation where the time spent eating (or not eating) in response to an external stimulus is greater than the time spent eating in response to internal hunger cues" (Hahn, 1998 as cited in Burns, Dunn, Brady, Barber Starr, & Blosser, 2004, p. 245). Some authors refer to obesity itself as an eating disorder, as it appears to fit the definition given earlier. Eating disorders can be seen in both the pediatric and adult populations. If the APN suspects an eating disorder, proper referral to a psychiatric mental health nurse practitioner (PMHNP), psychologist and/or psychiatrist, and/or treatment center can be considered.

The exact cause of eating disorders is not known, although there are several theories that exist. In addition, several types of eating disorders exist. Many of these diseases include issues surrounding food; they can also involve emotional issues and lead to physical issues. These disorders affect both genders and can lead to life-threatening consequences if not treated (National Eating Disorders Association [NEDA], 2014).

Anorexia Nervosa

Anorexia nervosa most often is a disorder found in adolescent girls. Although most commonly seen in girls, this disorder can also occur in adolescent boys (approximately 10%). The peak age of this disease is from 14.5 years through 18 years of age. It is a disease where individuals are fearful of becoming obese and feel that they are fat even when they are thin, underweight, or even emaciated. Anorexia nervosa is defined as a body weight that is 15% less than what is considered an ideal body weight. In girls, this disease causes the absence of three consecutive menstrual cycles, when no known physical illness is present (Burns et al., 2004).

Anorexia nervosa is also seen as a result when food intake is inadequate. Fear or weight gain, or an obsession with weight gain, is also seen. Low self-esteem and poor body image are also seen, as well as the inability to appreciate the severity of the weight loss (NEDA, 2014).

Although the exact cause of this disorder is unknown, several theories are suggested: psychological, biological, behavioral, sociocultural, and family systems theories. Young women can also suffer from anorexia secondary to insecurity, low self-esteem, poor attachment, and fear of abandonment.

The patient should be assessed for a history of any of the following: amenorrhea, dizziness, lightheadedness or syncope, lack of hunger, a very rigid structure, and inflexibility to change. These patients also use statements such as "I feel fat";

display moods of irritability, hostility, and unhappiness; and express suicidal ideations.

Physical examination findings of an anorexic patient may include any of the following:

- Abdominal pain
- Abdominal distension
- Decreased bowel sounds
- Dry, cracked, yellowish, or grayish skin color
- Dry mucous membranes
- Thin, brittle, or dull hair
- Alopecia
- Lanugo
- Weak muscles
- Decreased muscle mass
- Drowsiness
- Confusion
- Irritable mood

Changes in vital signs, such as changes in temperature, blood pressure (BP), pulse, or respirations, can also be seen (Burns et al., 2004).

Bulimia

Bulimia is characterized by repeated episodes of binging and purging, with self-induced vomiting to compensate for the guilt and overeating. Another characteristic of bulimia is a sense of feeling out of control. Warning signs of bulimia can be seen in the disappearance of large amounts of food. Frequent trips to the bathroom after meals, as well as laxative or diuretic use, are also signs of bulimia. Exercise programs, especially those that are extremely rigid, can also be a sign. Staining of the teeth, swelling of the cheeks or jaw, and calluses on the knuckles or hands can also be seen. Other signs include being withdrawn from friends, family, or activities. The person with bulimia can also be seen as focused on dieting, weight loss, or food control (NEDA, 2014).

Bulimia is seen in approximately 1% to 2% of adolescents and peaks between 18 and 19 years of age (Burns et al., 2004; NEDA, 2014). A majority of bulimia patients, as great as 80%, are women (NEDA, 2014). Many times, the onset of binge eating is seen approximately 2 years before the onset of purging. As with anorexia, the cause of the onset of bulimia is often unknown. Numerous theories also exist and can include biological, behavioral, sociocultural, psychodynamic, and family systems. Bulimia is often seen as a learned behavior, typically from peers.

A clinical assessment can be used to gain insight on the disease and current findings. The patient with bulimia may identify excessive concern about weight. He or she may express specific plans of dieting, purging, or binge eating. Many times, the patient also expresses guilt about eating and uses overeating as a form of stress management. The patient may discuss self-induced vomiting after eating or binging or complain of frequent constipation or diarrhea. The patient may display mood swings, but more often depression. Bulimia may also coexist with other destructive behaviors such as substance abuse or shoplifting. Finally, the patient may have a family history of abuse, such as sexual abuse.

Physical examination findings of a bulimic patient may include any of the following:

- Abnormal weight gain or weight loss
- Tooth decay
- Loss of enamel
- Enlarged parotid glands
- Dry, rough, or cracked skin
- Sores of the mucous membranes
- Sores around fingernails
- Broken blood vessels in the face
- Muscle weakness
- Fatigue
- Arrhythmias
- Edema

Changes in vital signs, including decreased BP, can also be seen (Burns et al., 2004).

Differential diagnoses for both anorexia nervosa and bulimia should also be considered along with the patient assessment and treatment plan. These diagnoses include, but are not limited to, the following:

- Hyperthyroidism
- Diabetes mellitus (DM)
- Inflammatory bowel disease (IBS)
- AIDS
- Malignancy
- Central nervous system neoplasm
- Systemic lupus erythematosus
- Pregnancy
- Depression
- Substance abuse

Long-term complications of anorexia nervosa and/or bulimia should also be discussed with the patient. These complications range from mild in nature to severe. All should be considered and discussed in depth. These complications include, but again are not limited to, the following:

- Growth retardation
- Dehydration
- Hypokalemia
- Alcohol addiction
- Drug addiction
- Osteoporosis
- Gynecological problems—amenorrhea
- Fertility problems
- Gastrointestinal problems
- Cardiac arrhythmia
- Congestive heart failure (CHF)
- Suicide
- Death

Eating Disorder Not Otherwise Specified

An eating disorder not otherwise specified is defined as a disorder that causes impairment or distress on the body, but does not meet the criteria for anorexia nervosa, binge-eating disorder, or bulimia. There are five examples of an eating disorder not otherwise specified by the *DSM-IV* criteria: atypical anorexia nervosa, bulimia nervosa (with less frequent occurrences), binge-eating disorder (with less frequent occurrences), purging disorder, and night eating syndrome. In contrast to anorexia, where the weight is less than normal, in patients with atypical anorexia nervosa, the person's weight is not below normal. The *purging disorder* is defined as purging without the binging of food present prior to the purge. Finally, *night eating syndrome* is defined as an excessive consumption of food at night (INR, 2014).

Additional Eating or Feeding Disorders

The following are additional eating or feeding disorders that should also be considered when working with overweight or obese patients: avoidant/restrictive food intake disorder, Pica, rumination disorder, and unspecified feeding or eating disorder. Avoidant/restrictive food intake disorder is similar to anorexia nervosa, but does not have the psychological features. It is the lack of consumption of an adequate amount of food, and thus, the risk of serious nutritional deficiencies. Reasons for food avoidance or restriction can include food dislike, dislike of textures, or fear of vomiting. *Pica* is defined as eating nonfood items (e.g., wood). Rumination disorder is the regurgitation of food that has already been consumed and swallowed. This food is then reswallowed or sometimes spat out. An unspecified feeding or eating disorder is when the behaviors portrayed do not meet any of the other eating disorder criteria, but the person still portrays eating disorder-like problems (INR, 2014).

> **QUICK TIPS—EATING DISORDERS**
>
> **Anorexia**—inadequate food intake
>
> **Bulimia**—binging and purging
>
> **Eating Disorder Not Otherwise Specified**
> - Atypical anorexia nervosa
> - Bulimia nervosa
> - Binge-eating disorders
> - Purging disorders
> - Night eating syndrome
>
> **Additional Eating/Feeding Disorders**
> - Avoidant/restrictive food intake disorder
> - Pica
> - Rumination disorder
> - Unspecified feeding or eating disorders

UNINTENTIONAL WEIGHT LOSS

A good APN uses differentials in diagnoses and treatment of weight gain. However, one must also be aware that there are some cases where weight loss is unintentional. The following are provided as a reference for differential diagnoses for weight loss. These are found more commonly in the older adult and may range from a broad spectrum of physiological and/or psychosocial disorders (Buttaro et al., 2003).

Decreased Caloric Intake

- Malignancies
- Gastrointestinal/bowel distress
- Depression/anxiety/stress/hypomania
- Anorexia nervosa/bulimia
- Poor nutrition
- Alcoholism
- CHF
- Chronic respiratory disease
- HIV/AIDS/infectious diseases
- Poor dentition
- Decreased smell/taste
- Functional obstacles or eating
- Decreased access to food
- Dementia
- Social isolation
- Drug side effects

Decreased Caloric Absorption

- Uncontrolled DM
- Renal disease
- Small bowel disease
- AIDS wasting syndrome
- Post-gastrectomy surgery
- Alcoholism/liver disease
- Repeated vomiting or diarrhea from illness/chemotherapy
- Gallbladder disease
- Open skin wounds

Increased Metabolic Demands

- Hyperthyroidism
- Malignancies
- Fever
- Mania
- Chronic respiratory disease or
- Cocaine abuse

Behaviors and addiction are important while addressing the overweight or obese patient. Eating disorders are also essential to address and treat. If left untreated, they can cause serious injury or death. Collaboration and patient referrals to other specialists are always appropriate and should be considered with any of these diseases due to the pure complexity and need for ongoing and lifelong treatment.

REFERENCES

Bicard, S. C., & Bicard, D. F. (2013). *The Iris center case study: Defining behavior.* Vanderbilt. Retrieved from http://iris.peabody.vanderbilt.edu/wp-content/uploads/2013/05/ICS-015.pdf

Burns, C. E., Dunn, A. M., Brady, M. A., Barber Starr, N., & Blosser, C. G. (2004). *Pediatric primary care: A handbook for nurse practitioners* (3rd ed.). St. Louis, MO: Saunders.

Buttaro, T. M., Trybulski, J., Bailey, P. P., & Sandberg-Cook, J. (2003). *Primary care: A collaborative practice* (2nd ed.). St. Louis, MO: Mosby.

Food Addiction Institute. (2014). Retrieved from http://foodaddictioninstitute.org

Institute for Natural Resources. (2014). *Food addiction, obesity, & diabetes*. Concord, CA: INR Seminars.

Merriam-Webster. (2014). *Palatable*. Retrieved from http://www.merriam-webster.com/dictionary/palatable

National Eating Disorders Association. (2014). Retrieved from https://www.nationaleatingdisorders.org

Which "Way" Is the Right "Weigh?"

Many theories exist about how to determine the proper measurement, weight, and body composition and which type of scale provides the most accurate answer. This chapter addresses different methods to weigh and measure body fat. Appropriate assessment of the patient's weight is critical for further treatment of the overweight and/or obese patient.

Evaluating and understanding the distribution of body fat is also an important factor in determining overall health risk. Higher levels of abdominal fat also place the patient at higher risk for metabolic syndrome and other comorbid diseases. A generalized representation of body composition may also be seen by measuring the circumference. A cloth tape measure, which is flexible; duplicate measurements; and a rotational order are most accurate, as they provide consistency in measuring. It is thought that a rotational order is best, as it allows the skin to regain its natural texture. The tape measure should be applied directly on the skin and over as few layers as possible. The measurements should also be taken while the patient is standing. The average of the two measurements should be taken. If measurements differ by more than 5 mm, the measurements should be retaken (Pescatello, Arena, Riebe, & Thompson, 2014). The American College of Sports Medicine (ACSM) describes the recommended method for measuring the circumference (Box 9.1).

The waist-to-hip ratio (WHR) identifies those individuals with a higher amount of abdominal fat and those at increased health risk (Pescatello et al., 2014). Although the waist circumference (WC) is helpful to measure in normal and overweight patients, it is not necessarily recommended for those with a body mass index (BMI) greater than 35 kg/m². WCs above 40 inches in a man and/or above 35 inches in a woman are considered at high risk for comorbid conditions (National Institutes of Health [NIH], National Heart, Lung, and Blood Institute [NHLBI], & North American Association for the Study of Obesity, 2000).

MEASURING BODY FAT

BMI, which takes into account the patient's weight and height, has been referred to as the "fifth vital sign." This measurement is used as a quick way to determine the classifications of weight. BMI gives a generalized idea of obesity; however, it is not always seen as accurate in some body types. In the elderly population and muscular people, this may give an inaccurate indication of classification of weight due to variations in lean body mass. Three terms are commonly used to identify

BOX 9.1 HOW TO MEASURE CIRCUMFERENCE

Abdomen
With the subject standing upright and relaxed, a horizontal measure is taken at the height of the iliac crest, usually at the level of the umbilicus.

Arm
With the subject standing erect and arms hanging freely at the sides with hands facing the thigh, a horizontal measure is taken midway between the acromion and olecranon processes.

Buttocks/Hips
With the subject standing erect and feet together, a horizontal measure is taken at the maximal circumference of the buttocks. This measure is used for the hip measure in a waist/hip measure.

Calf
With the subject standing erect (feet apart ~20 cm), a horizontal measure is taken at the level of the maximum circumference between the knee and the ankle, perpendicular to the long axis.

Forearm
With the subject standing, arms hanging downward but slightly away from the trunk and palms facing anteriorly, a measure is taken perpendicular to the long axis at the maximal circumference.

Hips/Thigh
With the subject standing, legs slightly apart (~10 cm), a horizontal measure is taken at the maximal circumference of the hip/proximal thigh, just below the gluteal fold.

Mid-Thigh
With the subject standing and one foot on a bench so the knee is flexed at 90°, a measure is taken midway between the inguinal crease and the proximal border of the patella, perpendicular to the long axis.

Waist
With the subject standing, arms at the sides, feet together, and abdomen relaxed, a horizontal measure is taken at the narrowest part of the torso (above the umbilicus and below the xiphoid process). The National Obesity Task Force (NOTF) suggests obtaining a horizontal measure directly above the iliac crest as a method to enhance standardization. Unfortunately, current formulae are not predicated on the NOTF suggested site (Pescatello et al., 2014, n.p.).

three categories of obesity: *sarcopenic obese, normal obese*, and *hypermuscular obese* (Bessesen & Kushner, 2002). *Sarcopenic obesity* is defined as a disease of aging where fat mass increases as lean body mass or muscle decreases. This is associated with decreased muscle mass as well as with loss of strength. It can lead to a reduction in the quality of life or early death (Benton, Whyte, & Dyal, 2011). It is thought to have resulted from numerous medications, inactivity, or diseases. Corticosteroid use, inactivity, or prolonged bed rest are thought to be some of the causes, whereas diseases such as hypogonadism, age-related hypogonadism, hypopituitarism, neuromuscular diseases, and menopause can also increase the patient's risk for sarcopenic obesity. Certain genetic influences could also increase one's risk. *Normal obesity* is defined as increased body fat with reduced lean body mass. *Hypermuscular obesity* is defined as both increased body fat and lean mass. This is common in those who participate in heavy resistance training (Bessesen & Kushner, 2002).

Scales can be bought anywhere. They come in a wide variety of prices. However, they provide only one piece of information—weight. Weight can determine overweight or obesity, but cannot provide the makeup details of the body. Several methods exist to determine body composition as follows: anthropometry and the use of calipers, near-infrared interactance (NIR), hydrostatic weighing, air displacement, dual-energy X-ray absorptiometry (DEXA), and bioelectrical impedance (BIA).

Calipers are a way to provide skinfold measurements. These measurements are determined by handheld calipers that exert a standardized pressure (Bessesen & Kushner, 2002). Calipers are widely used because of their inexpensiveness, ease, and simplicity. They are used to determine the amount of fatness and distribution of subcutaneous adipose tissue. Well over 100 articles have been published on the skinfold method technique, with more than 100 equations used to figure skinfold measurements for a range of patients, from children to elderly, athletic to sedentary. Skinfold measurements are also dependent on the patient's age, genetics, nutritional status, and activity (Brodie, Moscrip, & Hutcheon, 1998).

Anywhere from three to seven sites are used to determine skinfold thickness. There are two common three-site methods used in determining the percentage of body fat in male and female patients. Measurements in the male patient should include the chest, abdomen, and thigh, or include the chest, subscapular, and triceps. Measurements in the female patient should include the triceps, suprailiac, and thigh, or include the abdomen, suprailiac, and triceps. The seven sites used in both men and women in determining the percentage of body fat are the chest, midaxillary, triceps, subscapular, abdomen, suprailiac, and thigh (Barreira, Renfrow, Tseh, & Kang, 2013; Pescatello et al., 2014). There are different equations used to determine the percentage of body density; however, the Jackson and Pollock equation and the Durnin and Womersley equation are two of the most recognized. Vertical folds are used to measure the abdominal site, triceps, biceps, medial calf, midaxillary, and thigh. Diagonal folds are used to measure the chest/pectoral site, subscapular, and suprailiac skinfold sites. The following describes the ACSM's skinfold sites and how to measure them (Box 9.2).

Measurements are done by grasping the skin and tissue in a pinching motion, shaking the muscle loose, and "measuring" with the jaw of the calipers. This method raises concerns with regard to the accuracy of the findings (Bessesen & Kushner, 2002). One concern with the use of calipers is that it does not measure visceral fat (Cannon, 2011). The quality of the calipers as well as the skill of the person making the measurement also plays an important role. This method is also more difficult in the obese patient, as the "pinch" may require a larger skinfold and a more qualified person.

NIR uses a digital analyzer that measures the tissue makeup of the body (Bessesen & Kushner, 2002). This is done with a fiber optic probe connection that emits infrared light that passes through muscle and fat. Body composition is then estimated by using the patient's age and activity level (Cannon, 2011). This method, commonly used in the 1960s, is liked for its fast and noninvasive approach, although it is neither widely used nor recommended, secondary to the lack of research on validity and accuracy (Bessesen & Kushner, 2002). Research suggests that NIR may overestimate a lean person's body fat, whereas it may underestimate body fat in those who are overweight (Cannon, 2011).

BOX 9.2 SKINFOLD MEASUREMENTS

Abdominal
Vertical fold; 2 cm to the right side of the umbilicus

Triceps
Vertical fold; on the posterior midline of the upper arm, halfway between the acromion and olecranon processes, with the arm held freely to the side of the body

Biceps
Vertical fold; on the anterior aspect of the arm over the belly of the biceps muscle, 1 cm above the level used to mark the triceps site

Chest/Pectoral
Diagonal fold; one-half the distance between the anterior axillary line and the nipple (men) or one-third of the distance between the anterior axillary line and the nipple (women)

Medial calf
Vertical fold; at the maximum circumference of the calf on the midline of its medial border

Midaxillary
Vertical fold; on the midaxillary line at the level of the xiphoid process of the sternum. An alternate method is a horizontal fold taken at the level of the xiphoid/sternal border in the midaxillary line

Subscapular
Diagonal fold (at a 45° angle); 1 to 2 cm below the inferior angle of the scapula

Suprailiac
Diagonal fold; in line with the natural angle of the iliac crest taken in the anterior axillary line immediately superior to the iliac crest

Thigh
Vertical fold; on the anterior midline of the thigh, midway between the proximal border of the patella and the inguinal crease (hip; Pescatello et al., 2014, n.p.)

Hydrostatic or underwater weighing is considered an accurate method to determine weight; however, it is not ideal for everyone. It uses the Archimedes principle of fluid displacement (Cannon, 2011). A stainless steel tank with a cot or chair is mounted on an underwater scale and is suspended from a diving board over a body of water (usually a pool or tub). For accurate results, the individual is weighed outside the tank and then fully immersed underwater. Underwater weighing allows calculation of body fat percentage by determining the volume of the body and the patient's body density. Bone and muscle are more dense, and fat is less dense; therefore, an obese patient would have a higher proportion of body fat and a lower proportion of body density (Bessesen & Kushner, 2002). Although considered the "gold standard" by the ACSM for weighing due to its accuracy, certain population groups may have skewed data (Cannon, 2011). Athletes and the elderly are two such populations. Athletes may have an underestimated body fat percentage with hydrostatic weighing due to their denser bones. The elderly suffering from osteoporosis may have the opposite problem—an overestimation of body fat. Finally, the residual lung volume of the patient should be considered. Ideally, this volume should be directly measured; however, residual lung volume should be estimated as well, although this will not be as accurate. This method is costly, requires specialized equipment and space, and is also intimidating to many, as it is usually performed while the patient is in a bathing suit (Bessesen & Kushner, 2002; Cannon, 2011).

Measurement with the BOD POD uses air displacement instead of water displacement. The BOD POD takes only seconds and has accuracy results similar to those of underwater weighing (Cannon, 2011; McCoy, 2012). The BOD POD is a two-chambered fiberglass "pod" that contains a reference chamber and a chamber for a test subject (Fields, Higgins, & Hunter, 2004). It uses a fiberglass plethysmograph, which measures body volume. This is done in a closed chamber using computerized sensors to measure how much air is displaced while the patient is sitting. Body density is computed, and body fat is estimated. This chamber is widely used, as it accommodates many body types. One downfall to the BOD POD is that the patients must wear tight-fitting clothing and a swim cap. Uncovered or loose hair can underestimate body fat by more than 2%, whereas loose-fitting clothing may underestimate body fat by more than 5% (Bessesen & Kushner, 2002). The high cost is another limitation in using the BOD POD (Bessesen & Kushner, 2002; Cannon, 2011).

DEXA is another method used to measure body composition. Total body mineral, fat-free lean mass, and fat tissue mass are measured by a scanner that uses low-dose X-rays. An entire body scan takes anywhere from 10 to 20 minutes and is done while the individual lies still. DEXA is considered reliable, as it shows the distribution of fat tissue. This method of body composition is considered accurate in the obese patient.

BIA is also readily used to determine body composition due to its simplicity and accuracy. Low-intensity electric current is passed throughout the body and determines fat mass, percentage of total body weight, lean body mass, basal metabolic rate, and target weight. These numbers are determined as the muscle conducts the electricity, whereas the fat does not, thus producing the measure of electrical impedance (Bessesen & Kushner, 2002). The ACSM recommends the following for an accurate BIA analysis: no eating or drinking for 30 minutes prior to weighing, no exercise for at least 12 prior hours, and no alcohol for 48 prior hours. In addition to an empty stomach, it is also recommended that the patient should have an empty bladder and void at least 30 minutes prior to weighing (Cannon, 2011).

It is important that the advanced practice nurse (APN) learns and understands the differences between scales and measurements of body composition. The APN should also be able to determine which method is appropriate for each patient. Finally, it is important that the patient feel comfortable with whatever method is chosen.

REFERENCES

Barreira, T. V., Renfrow, M. S., Tseh, W., & Kang, M. (2013). The validity of 7-site skinfold measurements taken by exercise science students. *International Journal of Exercise Science, 6*(1), 20–28. Retrieved from http://digitalcommons.wku.edu/cgi/viewcontent.cgi?article=1413&context=ijes

Benton, M. J., Whyte, M. D., & Dyal, B. W. (2011). Sarcopenic obesity: Strategies for management. *American Journal of Nursing, 111*(12), 38–44. Retrieved from http://www.ncbi.nlm.nih.gov/pubmed/22082499 doi: 10.1097/01.NAJ.0000408184.21770.98

Bessesen, D. H., & Kushner, R. (2002). *Evaluation and management of obesity*. Philadelphia, PA: Hanley & Belfus, Inc.

Brodie, D., Moscrip, V., & Hutcheon, R. (1998). Body composition measurement: A review of hydrodensitometry, anthropometry, and impedance methods. *Nutrition, 14*(3), 296–310. Retrieved from http://www.uni.edu/dolgener/Fitness_Assessment/Body_Comp_Methods_Review.pdf

Cannon, J. (2011). Body fat measurement—A review of different methods. *Today's Dietitian, 13*(5), 66. Retrieved from http://www.todaysdietitian.com/newarchives/050311p66.shtml

Fields, D. A., Higgins, P. B., & Hunter, G. R. (2004). Assessment of body composition by air displacement plethysmography: Influence of body temperature and moisture. *Dynamic Medicine, 3*(3). Retrieved from http://www.dynamic-med.com/content/3/1/3

McCoy, K. (2012). *Your body fat percentage: What does it mean?* NYU Langone Medical Center. Retrieved from http://www.med.nyu.edu/content?ChunkIID=41373

National Institutes of Health, National Heart, Lung, and Blood Institute, & North American Association for the Study of Obesity. (2000). *The practical guide identification, evaluation, and treatment of overweight and obesity in adults*. Retrieved from http://www.nhlbi.nih.gov/files/docs/guidelines/prctgd_c.pdf

Pescatello, L. S., Arena, R., Riebe, D., & Thompson, P. D. (2014). *ACSM's guidelines for exercise testing and prescription* (9th ed.). Philadelphia, PA: Lippincott Williams & Wilkins.

Physical Assessment of the Adult Obese Patient

Critical thinking is required in performing an accurate physical assessment. Critical thinking encompasses analysis of data using the scientific knowledge base, experience, clinical competencies, attitude, and standard of care. These specific areas allow the advanced practice nurse (APN) to hone in on the health assessment and physical examination.

The scientific knowledge base allows one to understand and identify the normal findings for each body system through analysis of anatomy and physiology. It also allows for variations in the obese patient. Experience develops physical examination skills of inspection, palpation, percussion, and auscultation. Competency is used in collecting an accurate history, forming an accurate diagnosis, and evaluating nursing care through the reassessment of findings. Attitude allows for collaboration in uncertainty and thorough examination and review. Finally, two standards of care—intellectual and professional—allow the APN to apply appropriate diagnostic criteria for symptom analysis, as well as identify the characteristics, signs, and symptom abnormalities, and relay the results to the patient. This way of thinking allows for a thorough physical examination, especially in the obese patient (Potter & Weilitz, 2003).

Prior to the physical examination, a thorough health history needs to be taken. Biographic information is essential and can usually be filled out ahead of time either prior to the appointment or in the waiting room. This includes the patient's name; age; birth date; sex; race; ethnic origin; living arrangement; marital status; address; cell phone, home, and work number; employment status; occupation; emergency contact; and religious preference. The chief complaint identifies the reason for the visit, usually described in the patient's own words. The health history or history of present illness (HPI) provides the patient's reason for seeking out the APN and documents the chronological signs and symptoms of the problem from beginning to end. A past medical history (PMH) includes any medical conditions, allergies, current medications, and immunizations. Past surgical history (PSH) reviews any previous surgeries. Women should also be asked about obstetric and gynecological history. This includes pregnancies, births, menstrual history, mammogram, breast self-examination, and sexually transmitted diseases. A man's health history is also important. Inquiry of testicular self-examination, prostate-specific antigen (PSA) testing, and sexually transmitted diseases is also essential. A psychiatric history is also important to assess in the overweight and/or obese patient. Depression can be evaluated by asking about suicidal thoughts or ideations. Depression screening tools can also be used, such as the Beck Depression Inventory score. Asking the patient about anxiety, adjustment disorder, stress, binge-eating disorder, bulimia, purging patterns, and anorexia nervosa also reveals important data.

A nutritional assessment is also important, especially in the care and treatment of the overweight and/or obese patient. This might involve a 24-hour diet recall or a previously recorded 3-day food diary. Family history collects information of family members and their medical conditions, as well as if they have died; if they have died, a cause of death is noted. This history should also include questions about family members' weight history. Finally, the APN can inquire about the environmental history, such as living and working environments and exposure to pollutants, hazardous wastes, chemicals, and noise exposure.

Previous weight-loss attempts, anorectic use, history of weight gain, dietary history, and exercise history are other important categories to ask the overweight or obese patient about during the initial visit. This questioning helps the provider gain further insight into the patient's weight history.

Figure 10.1 is a sample of a health history list of questions.

Chief Complaint

HPI

Allergies

Current Medications

PMH

(Females) Gynecological History
Age of first menstrual cycle:
Age of menopause:
Number of pregnancies:
Number of births:
Any history of abnormal vaginal bleeding?
Last mammogram:
Breast self-examination:
Sexually transmitted diseases:

(Males) Health History
Testicular self-examination:
PSA testing:
Sexually transmitted diseases:

PSH

Psychiatric History
Beck Depression Inventory score:
Depression: Yes/No
Anxiety: Yes/No
Adjustment disorder: Yes/No
Stress: Yes/No
Binge-eating disorder: Yes/No
Bulimia: Yes/No
Purging patterns: Yes/No
Anorexia nervosa: Yes/No

FIGURE 10.1 Sample new patient health history questions.

HPI, history of present illness; PMH, past medical history; PSA, prostate-specific antigen; PSH, past surgical history.

Previous Weight-Loss Attempts
What have you tried in the past?
What has worked best for you? Why?
What has not worked? Why?
What are your current expectations?

Anorectic Use
Which drugs have you used in the past?
When did you take them?
What was the effect?
Are there any problems with medications in the past?
What do you expect from medication now?

History of Weight Gain
Gradual onset: Yes/No
Onset: Childhood/Adult
Lifestyle changes:
Stress: Yes/No
Why do you think you have gained weight?

Dietary History
Is there a tough time of day?
Are there problem foods?
Is volume an issue?
Are cravings an issue?
Are there certain triggers?
Who shops and cooks?
Do you use a shopping list?
Do you eat out? How often?
What are your snack habits?
Do you have any food dislikes?
Are you a nighttime eater?
Are you a stress eater?
Are you a volume eater?

Exercise History
Current level of activity:
　　Type:
　　Frequency:
　　Duration:
Past activity level:
Favorite activity:
Barriers to exercise?

Family History

Weight gain or weight loss: Yes/No	Relation:
Anorexia: Yes/No	Relation:
Bulimia: Yes/No	Relation:
Binge eating: Yes/No	Relation:
High blood pressure (BP): Yes/No	Relation:
High cholesterol: Yes/No	Relation:
Diabetes: Yes/No	Relation:
Coronary artery disease (CAD): Yes/No	Relation:
Metabolic syndrome: Yes/No	Relation:

FIGURE 10.1 (*continued*)

Mental illness: Yes/No   Relation:
Congestive heart failure (CHF): Yes/No   Relation:
Obstructive sleep apnea (OSA): Yes/No   Relation:
Liver cancer: Yes/No   Relation:

Personal History
Alcohol use:
Tobacco use:
Illegal drugs:
Caffeine use:
Current work status:
Marital status:

FIGURE 10.1 (continued)

This sample can be used on the initial visit to help gain a better understanding of the patient and his or her weight status prior to the present appointment. The sample may be tailored as needed for each patient and APN.

Another good method used for history taking is mailing patients a health questionnaire prior to their arrival at the first appointment (Figure 10.2). This should be filled out along with a 3-day food diary and brought to the initial visit. The questionnaire is a way to get the patient thinking about his or her goals prior to meeting with the APN. A sample questionnaire is given next.

Please complete and bring with you to your next office visit.

Name: _____   Date: _____

What brought you to the clinic/why do you want to lose weight? (e.g., doctor recommended, desire weight loss, health reasons, and mental health)

_____
_____
_____

What do you believe is your biggest obstacle in losing weight? (e.g., motivation, dietary choices, late night snacking, physical activity, and pain with physical activity)

_____
_____
_____

What factors influence your effort to lose weight? (e.g., kids/family, job, time management, social life—busy schedule with no time to exercise or plan meals and lack of resources)

_____
_____
_____

What do you expect from the program? (e.g., individual counseling, group educational classes, and support and accountability) The better we fit your needs, the more successful you will be in developing healthier lifestyles.

_____
_____
_____

FIGURE 10.2 First-visit questionnaire.

What is your long-term goal? (e.g., desired weight to achieve—ideal body weight; decrease/stop prescription used for health issues such as hypertension (HTN), hypercholesterolemia, diabetes; feel better about yourself; and have more energy)

_____

_____

_____

Are you currently exercising? Yes _____   No _____
If yes, what activity do you do and how often and for how long do you normally exercise?

_____

_____

_____

In the past, what had caused you to stop exercising? Circle all that apply
It caused too many aches and pains   It was boring
Illness   Lack of resources/place to be active
Lost motivation   Schedule became too busy
Did not see a benefit from exercising   Other _____

What do you consider a "good" weight for you? _____

When did you weigh this? _____

What is the most you have ever weighed? _____

When did you weigh this? _____

In the past 5 years, how often have you attempted to lose weight? _____

_____

What diets have you tried? _____

How many meals do you usually eat per day? _____

How many servings (1 shot, glass of wine, 12 oz beer) do you drink per week? _____

On average, how often do you eat the following foods per week?

_____ Cheese

_____ Fast food

_____ Meat

_____ Eggs (alone or in foods)

_____ Fried foods (nonfast food)

_____ Vegetables

_____ Fruit

_____ Regular pop (not diet)

What is your present occupation? _____

How would you describe the average physical demands of your job?
Light _____ Fairly light _____ Somewhat hard _____ Hard _____ Very hard _____

Approximately how much of your normal day is spent:
Sitting _____ Standing _____ Walking _____ Carrying objects _____ Lifting objects _____

FIGURE 10.2 (continued)

On average, how often do you feel stressed? Circle the most appropriate.

Almost never   Occasionally   Frequently   Very frequently   Constantly

How would you describe the stress? Circle the most appropriate.

Fairly light   Moderate   Severe   Very severe

Please record what you eat for at least 3 days prior to your first visit to the office. Be honest; only your health care provider will see it and we won't judge you! This will only be used to help us establish a starting point with your individualized program.

FIGURE 10.2 (*continued*)

Again, this too is a sample questionnaire. It may be adjusted to fit each patient and/or APN, as needed.

Upon arrival at the first visit, the patient should be checked in by a nurse or nursing assistant and asked a series of questions (Figure 10.1). A health history should be taken directly from the patient or from a family member, partner, or significant other. It is also important to use any previous medical records for a complete review (Potter & Weilitz, 2003). After this, he or she can be weighed. A variety of options exist for weighing, as addressed in Chapter 9. Blood pressure, heart rate (HR), respirations, and height (inches) should be recorded. Body measurements, including neck circumference (NC), waist circumference (WC), and hip circumference (HC), should also be measured in inches and recorded. Body mass index (BMI), basal metabolic rate (BMR), and the Harris–Benedict Formula can also be figured. Consideration can be taken to complete a baseline resting electrocardiogram (EKG) and to screen for depression or sleep apnea.

The APN should complete a head-to-toe physical assessment and review vitals and measurements. A complete physical examination for the obese patient should be similar to a normal physical examination with some slight variations. A head-to-toe physical examination includes four basic skills: inspection, palpation, percussion, and auscultation.

Inspection is based on observation. This includes knowledge of normal physical characteristics of each age group as well as the normal physical characteristics of the obese patient. Paying close attention to detail while learning to multitask in observing is a competency skill learned with practice and time. Another vital skill is comparing findings from one side of the body to the opposite side of the body. Finally, collaboration with a colleague is often used for confirmation of a finding.

Palpation is based on touch and performed after visual inspection. Any areas with suspected tenderness should be palpated last. Promoting a comfortable environment is the key, as it ensures that the patient is relaxed. "Use different parts of the hand to detect characteristics (e.g., texture, shape, temperature, perception of vibration, or movement and consistency)" (Potter & Weilitz, 2003, p. 36). However, one should remember that the fingertips are the most sensitive parts of the hands. Light, deep, and bimanual palpation are three different forms that can be used for examination.

Percussion is performed by tapping to determine the location, size, and density of the structure. Time and experience are key factors used to master the competency of percussion. Direct or indirect percussion is used to determine the sound heard. Sounds such as tympany (drumlike), resonance (hollow), hyperresonance (booming), dullness (thudlike), and flatness (flat) are produced by percussion. Practice, as well as using the appropriate amount of force, is essential for accurate comparison sounds.

Auscultation is based on listening through the stethoscope. As with percussion, auscultation takes practice. It is best done in a quiet environment so that the characteristics of sound can be best heard. Frequency, loudness, quality, and duration are characteristics of sound.

Having the room ready for the patient makes the examination easier. Patient positions are also essential for proper examination and patient comfort. Sitting, supine, dorsal recumbent, prone, and lateral recumbent are appropriate positions for the obese patient. The lithotomy, Sims, and knee–chest positions are usually not needed, as these are commonly used during a yearly health examination. The sitting position allows for the head, neck, back, posterior and anterior thorax, lungs, axillae, heart, breasts, and upper extremities to be properly examined. The supine position allows for examination of the head, neck, anterior thorax, lungs, breasts, axillae, heart, abdomen, extremities, and pulses. The dorsal recumbent is best for an abdominal assessment, but can also be used for further head and neck, anterior thorax, lungs, breasts, axillae, and heart. This position allows for abdominal relaxation and better abdominal assessment. The prone position is used for hip joint assessment and assessment of the musculoskeletal system. It is rarely used in the examination of the obese patient, but may be used to assess hip extension. The lateral recumbent position is useful in detecting heart murmurs and assessment of the heart. It is important to note that patients with respiratory illnesses may not tolerate this position well.

A physical examination should start with the head and progress down to the toe. A complete physical examination includes breast, genitourinary, and rectal examinations; however, these are not common in the assessment of the obese patient. A sample documentation of an obese patient's complete physical examination is seen in Figure 10.3.

Vital Signs

Neck circumference
Chest circumference
Waist circumference
Hip circumference
Waist-to-hip ratio
Height
Weight
Body mass index
Blood pressure
Heart rate
Respiratory rate

Physical Examination

General: Looks stated age, appropriate conversation, in no acute distress.
HEENT:
  Head: Normocephalic.
  Ears: Tympanic membranes and canals are clear bilaterally. Good light reflex.

FIGURE 10.3 Patient physical examination.

Eyes: PERRLA, extraocular muscles intact, conjunctiva normal, sclera anicteric.
Nose: No polyps.
Throat: Clear without exudate or drainage. Tonsils present.
Neck: Supple, no lymphadenopathy, no thyromegaly, and no jugular vein distension (JVD).
Skin: Warm, pink, dry. Good turgor.
Mucosa: No cyanosis, moist.
Cardiovascular: Point of maximal impulse (PMI) normal. Normal S1 and S2. No murmurs, rubs, or gallops. No carotid bruits present.
Lungs: Good bilateral air entry. Clear to auscultation and percussion.
Abdomen: Soft and nontender. Normal bowel sounds. No rebound pain or rigidity.
Extremities: No edema, cyanosis, or clubbing; range of motion (ROM) within normal limits (WNL). Pedal pulses 2+ bilaterally.
Neurological: Cranial nerves II through XII intact. Muscle strength 5/5. Romberg negative without pronator drift. Deep tendon reflex (DTR) 2+. Gait normal. Alert and oriented ×3.

FIGURE 10.3 (*continued*)

Variations in the obese patient's physical examination can be seen in multiple areas. The APN should assess for acne and/or hirsutism. This can correlate with polycystic ovary syndrome (PCOS). Physical findings observed in the obese patient might include acanthosis nigricans or striae. These findings could identify insulin resistance or Cushing's syndrome, respectively. Thyroid nodules or a goiter could indicate hypothyroidism. Elevation in BP or pulse can be seen as an abnormal finding that may indicate either hypertension (HTN) or simple deconditioning. Further attention to the cardiovascular system should be made to assess the cardiac rhythm and S3/S4 gallop. This could identify an arrhythmia or possibly congestive heart failure (CHF). A larger abdomen and WC indicate abdominal obesity, increasing the patient's risk for cardiovascular comorbidities. Peripheral edema could indicate venous stasis or pulmonary HTN. The presence of papilledema could indicate pseudotumor cerebri. Finally, muscular weakness, especially proximal muscle weakness, could indicate Cushing's syndrome, as well as identify osteoporosis (Tsai & Wadden, 2013).

QUICK TIPS: OBESITY EXAMINATION

Abnormal Finding	Disease
Acne	PCOS
Hirsutism	Insulin resistance
Acanthosis nigricans	Cushing's syndrome
Striae	Hypothyroidism
Thyroid nodule/goiter	HTN/deconditioned
Elevated BP	HTN/deconditioned
Elevated HR	Arrhythmia
Cardiac rhythm	CHF
S3/S4 gallop	Abdominal obesity
Larger abdomen	Venous statis/pulmonary HTN
Peripheral edema	Pseudotumor cerebri
Papilledema proximal muscle weakness	Cushing's syndrome/osteoporosis

The complete physical assessment should be thorough and will take time. The initial appointment may take at least 60 minutes. Any abnormality should be discussed with the patient and readdressed at the next visit. Any concern with a screening should also be discussed with the patient and referrals should be made as necessary. Most importantly, the APN should trust his or her instinct and place patient care at the forefront of the visit.

REFERENCES

Potter, P. A., & Weilitz, P. B. (2003). *Health assessment* (5th ed.). St. Louis, MO: Mosby.

Tsai, A. G., & Wadden, T. A. (2013). Obesity. *Annals of Internal Medicine, 159*(5). Retrieved from http://annals.org/article.aspx?articleid=1733379

Physical Assessment of the Pediatric Obese Patient

The physical assessment of the pediatric obese patient is similar, yet different, to that of an adult obese patient. It is important to include family in the interview and assessment, as the goal needs to be a collaborative effort for evaluation, assessment, and treatment. Similar to an adult assessment, key skills, including critical thinking, scientific knowledge bases, experience, clinical competencies, attitude, and standard of care, need to be utilized.

As with the adult patient, prior to the physical examination, a thorough health history needs to be taken. With a pediatric patient, some, if not all, of the questions may be answered by both the patient and family member. Please refer to Chapter 10 for further review of the health history, nutritional history, and previous attempts at weight loss, as well as conditions such as anorexia, bulimia, and binge eating. In pediatric patients, the history should also focus on the patterns of eating as well as on exercise for both the child and family unit. It would be beneficial to have a registered dietitian (RD) involved in the child/family interview process, as much of the focus includes dietary patterns. It is important to remember that the overweight or obese child may eat less in comparison to a normal weight child; however, the overweight or obese child tends to have less or lower exercise or energy output. Key questions should focus on dietary specifics: dietary intake, total caloric intake, fat and carbohydrate intake as percentages of total caloric intake, and nutrition of the intake. Exercise patterns for both the child and family should be assessed as well. Questions should also inquire about the weight and/or overweight or obese status of the family members as well as family medical conditions. The onset of obesity as well as any specifics about this period should be documented (trouble at school, in home situation, with friends, etc.). The child should also be asked about his or her peers, friendships, and any problems or difficulty at school. Finally, the readiness of family participation should be assessed in order to move forward with a treatment plan (Burns, Dunn, Brady, Starr, & Blosser, 2004).

Figure 11.1 shows a sample of a health history questionnaire. It is similar to the adult questionnaire with age-appropriate changes.

Chief Complaint

History of Present Illness

Allergies

Current Medications

Past Medical History

(Females) Gynecological History
Age of first menstrual cycle:
Number of pregnancies:
Number of births:
Any history of abnormal vaginal bleeding?
Breast self-examination:
Sexually transmitted diseases:

(Males) Health History
Testicular self-examination:
Sexually transmitted diseases:

Past Surgical History

Psychiatric History
Beck Depression Inventory score:
Depression: Yes/No
Anxiety: Yes/No
Adjustment disorder: Yes/No
Stress: Yes/No
Binge-eating disorder: Yes/No
Bulimia: Yes/No
Purging patterns: Yes/No
Anorexia nervosa: Yes/No

Previous Weight-Loss Attempts
What have you tried in the past?
What has worked best for you? Why?
What has not worked? Why?
What are your current expectations?

Anorectic Use
Which drugs have you used in the past?
When did you take them?
What was the effect?
Are there any problems with medications in the past?
What do you expect from medication now?

History of Weight Gain
Gradual onset: Yes/No
Onset:
Lifestyle changes:
Stress: Yes/No
Why do you think you have gained weight?

Dietary History
Is there a tough time of day?
Are there problem foods?

FIGURE 11.1 Sample pediatric new patient health history questions.

Is volume an issue?
Are cravings an issue?
Are there certain triggers?
Who shops and cooks?
Do you eat out? How often?
What are your snack habits?
Do you have any food dislikes?
Are you a nighttime eater?
Are you a volume eater?

Exercise History
Current level of activity:
    Type:
    Frequency:
    Duration:
Past activity level:
Favorite activity:
Barriers to exercise:

Family History

Weight gain or weight loss: Yes/No	Relation:
Anorexia: Yes/No	Relation:
Bulimia: Yes/No	Relation:
Binge eating: Yes/No	Relation:
High blood pressure (BP): Yes/No	Relation:
High cholesterol: Yes/No	Relation:
Diabetes: Yes/No	Relation:
Coronary artery disease (CAD): Yes/No	Relation:
Metabolic syndrome: Yes/No	Relation:
Mental illness: Yes/No	Relation:
Congestive heart failure (CHF): Yes/No	Relation:
Obstructive sleep apnea (OSA): Yes/No	Relation:
Liver cancer: Yes/No	Relation:

Personal History
Alcohol use:
Tobacco use:
Illegal drugs:
Caffeine use:

FIGURE 11.1 (*continued*)

This sample can be used on the initial visit to help gain a better understanding of the pediatric patient and family involved. Again, this sample may be tailored, as needed, for each patient and advanced practice nurse (APN).

Another good method used for history taking is mailing patients and family a health questionnaire prior to their arrival at the first appointment. This should be filled out, along with a 3-day food diary, and brought to the initial visit. It is helpful if the packet is filled out together by the pediatric patient and family. A sample questionnaire is seen in Chapter 10, Figure 10.2. Additional questions may be substituted to inquire about school. An example is shown in Figure 11.2.

What year in school are you? _____

How would you describe the average physical demands at school?
Light _____ Fairly light _____ Somewhat hard _____ Hard _____ Very hard _____

Approximately how much of your normal day is spent:
Sitting _____ Standing _____ Walking _____ Carrying objects _____ Lifting objects _____

FIGURE 11.2 Sample school questions.

Please refer to Chapter 10 for further review of the first appointment. The health history should be taken directly from the patient and a family member. It is also important to use any previous medical records for a complete review (Potter & Weilitz, 2003). After this, he or she can be weighed. Blood pressure (BP), heart rate (HR), respirations, and height (inches) should be recorded. Body measurements, including neck circumference (NC), waist circumference (WC), and hip circumference (HC), should also be measured in inches and recorded. Body mass index (BMI), basal metabolic rate (BMR), and the Harris–Benedict Formula can also be calculated. This would also be an opportune time to complete a baseline resting electrocardiogram (EKG), screen for depression, and/or test for sleep apnea.

A physical examination should start with the head and progress downward to the toe. A complete physical examination would include breast, genitourinary, and rectal examinations; however, these are not common in the assessment of the obese pediatric patient. The parent and/or family member may stay in the room; however, if it is an adolescent patient, he or she may prefer that the parent leave during the physical assessment. One should always have another medical professional (e.g., nurse) present in the room with one during the assessment. A sample documentation of a complete physical examination of an obese patient is shown in Figure 11.3.

Variations in the obese pediatric patient's physical examination can be seen in multiple areas. One should use the examination and documentation that best fit the situation and/or practice.

Pediatric variations also need to be considered in physical examination. The following are important pediatric considerations. Respirations should be counted for a full minute instead of 15 or 30 seconds and multiplied. BP should be taken at least 15 minutes after the child has come into the examination room. This allows possible anxieties to dissipate as well as ensures that the BP is not elevated due to activity while in the waiting room. Children who have been crying, sleeping, or have allergies may display evidence of periorbital edema. Facial acne may be seen as a developmental change. Hair growth amounts and distribution may change during adolescence. A child's HR is more variable than that for adults. Exercise may provoke a wider range of reactions (Potter & Weilitz, 2003).

Laboratory data can also be a useful tool in the assessment and treatment of pediatric obesity. A fasting lipid panel, fasting glucose, and thyroid screen, including thyroid-stimulating hormone (TSH) and T4, can be drawn. Other laboratories may be added and ordered, as the APN deems necessary.

Differential diagnoses should be considered with pediatric obesity. This includes hypothyroidism, Down syndrome, or Prader–Willi syndrome. If one suspects any of these conditions, further testing should be ordered and appropriate referrals should be made (Burns et al., 2004).

Vital Signs
Neck circumference
Chest circumference
Waist circumference
Hip circumference
Waist-to-hip ratio
Height
Weight
Body mass index
Blood pressure
Heart rate
Respiratory rate

Physical Examination
General: Looks stated age, appropriate conversation, in no acute distress
HEENT:
  Head: Normocephalic
  Ears: Tympanic membranes and canals are clear bilaterally. Good light reflex
  Eyes: PERRLA, Extraocular muscles intact, conjunctiva normal, sclera anicteric
  Nose: No polyps
  Throat: Clear without exudate or drainage. Tonsils present
Neck: Supple, no lymphadenopathy, no thyromegaly, and no jugular vein distension (JVD)
Skin: Warm, pink, dry. Good turgor
Mucosa: No cyanosis, moist
Cardiovascular: Point of maximal impulse (PMI) normal. Normal S1 and S2. No murmurs, rubs, or gallops. No carotid bruits present
Lungs: Good bilateral air entry. Clear to auscultation and percussion
Abdomen: Soft and nontender. Normal bowel sounds. No rebound pain or rigidity
Extremities: No edema, cyanosis, or clubbing. Range of motion (ROM) within normal limits (WNL). Pedal pulses 2+ bilaterally
Neurological: Cranial nerves II through XII intact. Muscle strength 5/5. Romberg negative without pronator drift. Deep tendon reflex (DTR) 2+. Gait normal. Alert and oriented ×3

FIGURE 11.3 Pediatric patient physical examination.

The complete physical assessment should be thorough and will take time. The initial appointment may take at least 60 minutes. Any abnormality should be discussed with the patient and readdressed at the next visit. Any concern with a screening should also be discussed with the patient and referrals should be made as necessary. Most importantly, the APN should trust his or her instinct and place patient care at the forefront of the visit.

REFERENCES

Burns, C. E., Dunn, A. M., Brady, M. A., Starr, N. B., & Blosser, C. G. (2004). *Pediatric primary care: A handbook for nurse practitioners* (3rd ed.). St. Louis, MO: Saunders.

Potter, P. A., & Weilitz, P. B. (2003). *Health assessment* (5th ed.). St. Louis, MO: Mosby.

Physical Activity, Exercise Assessment, and Patient Recommendations

Causes of obesity have been previously addressed to include genetic and comorbid conditions; two other primary causes include poor diet, physical inactivity, and lack of exercise. This chapter addresses physical activity and exercise with regard to overweight and obese patients.

HISTORY OF PHYSICAL ACTIVITY RECOMMENDATIONS

Public health recommendations for physical activity were first published in the United States in 1995. This was followed by additions and updated revisions in 1996, 2007, 2008, and the latest, 2013. The first federal guidelines were published in 2008. These guidelines included four major recommendations on activity. The first recommendation was that adults should not be sedentary or inactive. The second recommendation was about the amount, frequency, and duration of activity: One hundred fifty hours per week of moderate-intensity activity or 75 minutes per week of vigorous activity. Both these are recommended in more than or equal to 10-minute bouts of activity. The third recommendation was about increasing the amount of moderate-intensity activity to 300 minutes per week and vigorous-intensity activity to 150 minutes. The fourth and final recommendation was about the addition of strength training. This was recommended at more than or equal to 2 days per week and of moderate to high intensity (Strath et al., 2013).

The U.S. Department of Health and Human Services (HHS) and the World Health Organization (WHO) recommend that adults have at least 2.5 hours of moderate to vigorous activity per week, whereas it is recommended for children to get at least 1 hour daily (Harvard School of Public Health, 2014). The American Heart Association (AHA) recommends 30 to 60 minutes of physical activity 5 to 7 days per week. There is an ongoing debate about how much activity is enough for weight loss and weight maintenance. Although guidelines and recommendations exist, it is important for the advanced practice nurse (APN) to understand that physical activity should be something agreed upon by the patient and provider. What works for one patient may not for the next.

KEY CONCEPTS OF PHYSICAL ACTIVITY

The most popular definition of *physical activity* "was published by Caspersen and colleagues in 1985. Physical activity was defined as, 'any bodily movements produced by skeletal muscles that result in energy expenditure'" (Strath et al., 2013, p. 2). Structured and incidental are two types of physical activity. Structured physical activity is organized or planned, whereas incidental physical activity is that which occurs incidentally, usually throughout the day. This can be at home or at work and is done by completing the normal day-to-day activities.

Dimensions and Domains

Four types of dimensions are included under physical activity: type or mode, frequency, duration, and intensity. *Mode* is defined as the specific type of activity performed. *Frequency* is defined as how often the activity is done. *Duration* is defined as the amount of time (in minutes) spent on this activity. *Intensity* is defined as the amount of energy expended to complete the activity.

Four domains are also used to describe physical activity: occupational, domestic, transportation, and leisure time. *Occupational* is defined as work related to or involving work. *Domestic* is defined as any household or incidental chore or task. *Transportation* is best described as using the body as a means to get somewhere. This could include walking to work or riding a bike to the grocery store. *Leisure time* is defined as any recreational activity, sport, hobby, or additional work. Physical activity should encompass all domains of life. Historically, it was thought that physical activity could or should only be done during leisure time. The current method of thought highlights the importance of completing physical activity at any part of one's day (Strath et al., 2013).

Physical Activity Measurement

Physical activity intensity is measured in metabolic equivalents (METs). MET estimates are for healthy adults. One MET is the energy (or calories burned) required to sit quietly for 1 minute. MET values indicate intensity (Harvard School of Public Health, 2014). One MET is also "commonly defined as 3.5 mL $O_2 \cdot kg^{-1} \cdot min^{-1}$ or ~250 mL/min of oxygen consumed, which represents the average value for a standard 70-kg person" (Strath et al., 2013, p. 3).

Light MET levels are defined as less than three METs. *Moderate-intensity activity* is defined as three to six METs, whereas greater than six METs are required for vigorous-intensity activity. Light MET activities can include slow walking, light housework, sitting at the computer, fishing, or even playing a musical instrument. Moderate MET activities can include fast or brisk walking, light bicycling, heavy cleaning, push mowing the lawn, or even playing doubles tennis. Vigorous MET activities can include fast walking or hiking, jogging, fast bicycling, singles tennis, basketball, playing soccer, or shoveling snow (Harvard School of Public Health, 2014).

PATIENT EVALUATION

Patient evaluation of exercise can be as simple as having the patient assess activity prior to the appointment. This can be used in patient questionnaires or patient history forms similar to the ones seen in Chapter 10. The patient should be asked about activity and exercise history. This includes the current and past levels of activity—type, frequency, and duration. A thorough assessment will discuss the patient's favorite activities as well as barriers to activity. Barriers could be anything from weight, pain, shortness of breath, other medical conditions, or even embarrassment. The patient should also be asked what causes a cease in activity. These can include any of the following: aches and pains, illness, loss of motivation, no benefit seen, boredom, lack of exercise resources or place to be active, scheduling conflicts, time commitment, and friends or family.

Physical activity questionnaires (PAQ) can be divided into three categories: global, recall, and quantitative history. The following are examples of PAQ questionnaires:

- Global
  - Exercise Vital Sign
  - EPIC PAQ
  - Godin Leisure Time Exercise
  - Lipid Research Clinics
  - Minnesota Heart Health
  - Physical Activity Vital Sign
  - Rapid Assessment of Physical Activity
  - Stanford Usual PAQ
- Recall
  - ARIC-Baecke
  - Aerobic Center Longitudinal Study
  - BRFSS, 2001
  - CARDIA
  - CHAMPS
  - Global PAQ
  - International PAQ Short
  - International PAQ Long
  - Kaiser PAQ (KPAS)
  - LOPAR Pregnancy PAQ
  - Seven-Day PA Recall
  - Yale PAQ (YPAS)
- Quantitative
  - Freidenrich Lifetime Leisure
  - Minnesota Leisure-Time Physical Activity (LTPA) Questionnaire
  - Modifiable Activity Questionnaire
  - Tecumseh Self-Administered Occupational PAQ

These questionnaires allow the APN to get a better understanding of what the patient likes or dislikes and how to find and provide the patient's best option.

Another method is a patient activity diary or log. This allows patients to track their activities or lack thereof and allows the provider to get a better idea of activities. Diaries can be completed in the form of pencil and paper or online through a cell phone, computer, or any other electronic device. The Bouchard Physical Activity Record is another way that patients can keep track of activity. This well-known tool allows patients to track the type of activity performed in 15-minute increments. There are behaviors identified by numbers 1 to 9 that correspond with an MET level of 1.0 to 7.8. Again, each patient is different and should use the best tool for him or her (Strath et al., 2013).

OBJECTIVE METHODS TO ASSESS PHYSICAL ACTIVITY

There are many available methods by which to assess physical activity. The APN should be aware of these methods; however, referral may be made to an exercise specialist at any time. Four different objective groups can be summarized in the following categories: measures of energy expenditure, physiological measures, motion sensors, and more than one sensor.

Measures of energy expenditure include indirect calorimetry, the doubly labeled water (DLW) method, and direct observation. Indirect calorimetry is often performed in a laboratory setting. It measures the amount of inhaled oxygen and exhaled carbon dioxide. Whole-body room calorimeters as well as computerized metabolic cart systems are available. First used in the 1980s, the DLW method measures total energy expenditure in a period of 1 to 3 weeks. This method is based on two isotopes, oxygen-18 (^{18}O) and deuterium (^{2}H), and used to estimate carbon dioxide production. Direct observation is self-explanatory; it is any situation in which the observer either physically watches the person performing the activity or monitors him or her through video. This method is more utilized in children than adults.

Physiological measures are also used as an objective method to assess physical activity. Heart rate monitoring is a physiological measure assessed through a wrist-worn monitor. A receiver is strapped to the chest with electrodes that then transmit heart rate data. This type of data may be monitored for specific activities or even for longer periods of time.

Motion sensors are another objective method to assess physical activity. Accelerometers and pedometers are the most common types of motion sensors. Accelerometers measure both acceleration and movement, whereas pedometers measure the total number of steps and the distance walked. Commonly used accelerometers are Actical, ActiGraph, ActivPAL, GENEActiv, Lifecorder Plus, and RT3. Another new and popular accelerometer is the FitBit Tracker. Again, this is not an exhaustive list; however, it does denote commonly used devices. Pedometers are also a great way to monitor activity. Some commonly used pedometers include StepWatch, Omron, New Lifestyles, and Yamax. Again, this is not an exhaustive list, but it does provide different patient options.

The fourth objective method to assess physical activity is multisensing assessment methods. Investigations are ongoing to determine whether physical activity assessment could benefit from multiple methods of observation. This could consist of heart rate monitoring with an additional accelerometer or different places to apply heart rate monitors with the use of an accelerometer (Strath et al., 2013).

EFFECTS OF EXERCISE RESPONSE AND TRAINING

With regard to the obese and exercise, straightforward answers are not always present. Exercise testing may be difficult because of the excess body weight and low physical work capacity. Exercise testing should be done with caution and awareness to the simple fact that these individuals may have numerous underlying comorbidities that may not only affect exercise tolerance or testing but also produce abnormal test results. One example would be increased heart rate or blood pressure response or an abnormal electrocardiogram (EKG) with stress testing.

Exercise training is helpful with any body weight, although it may not be as effective in those with morbid or severe obesity. Exercise through aerobic or cardiovascular activity promotes the reduction in not only body weight but also body fat. This, in turn, maintains or increases lean body weight. Body fat distribution is affected through physical activity (Durstine & Moore, 2003).

Physical activity is also important in weight maintenance or to prevent weight gain. The more activity people engage in, the more likely they are to keep weight steady. Long periods of exercise or high-intensity activity provide the best chance for weight loss. Researchers have shown that physical activity prevents overweight or obesity in many ways. Physical activity decreases total body fat, especially fat around the abdomen and waist. Physical activity increases total energy expenditure. This can lead to a neutral weight or weight loss in correlation with the number of calories consumed. Strength training to build muscle mass also increases the total calories burned, thus helping with weight control. Physical activity is also good for the overall health. It can help reduce anxiety and depression and increase the natural endorphins, which enhance that "feel good" feeling (Harvard School of Public Health, 2014).

Although the effects of exercise training are not well established, "metabolic rate, including the caloric cost of physical activity, does decline with weight reduction via caloric restriction. In the starvation state, however, the maintenance of metabolic rate through exercise may not always counteract the reduction mediated by food restriction" (Durstine & Moore, 2003, p. 151). Exercise has been proven to have a profound effect on the body's regulation of glucose. This includes decreasing fasting glucose, fasting insulin, and insulin resistance. Exercise also increases glucose tolerance (Durstine & Moore, 2003).

EXERCISE TESTING

Exercise testing may be used in overweight and/or obese patients; however, it is not always necessary. Again, this is patient specific and should be determined by group decision involving the APN, exercise specialist, and patient. Exercise testing can be measured in three main areas: aerobic, flexibility, and neuromuscular. Other areas can be measured by testing agility and strength. Aerobic testing may include using the treadmill or bike. It can also be done with the 6-minute walk test. Flexibility can be measured using goniometry to test range of motion (ROM). Neuromuscular testing can include gait analysis and balance (Durstine & Moore, 2003).

Figure 12.1 is an example that is currently used in the Center for Lifestyle Medicine (CLM) Clinic.

Center for Lifestyle Medicine

Patient Name: _____ Date: _____

Age: _____ Sex: _____ DOB: _____ Height: _____ Weight: _____

BMI: _____ Neck Circumference: _____

Waist Circumference: _____ Hip Circumference: _____

Waist-to-Hip Ratio: _____ WHR Classification: _____

Pre-Vitals

BP: _____ HR: _____ R: _____ SpO_2: _____

Cardiorespiratory Endurance

Protocol Used: _____ Score (m/# marched) _____

Reason for Termination: _____ Classification: _____

BORG Score: Prefatigue _____ Shortness of breath _____

　　　　　　　　Postfatigue _____ Shortness of breath _____

Muscular Endurance

Wall Push-ups: _____ # Completed/Classification: _____

Seated Crunch: _____ # Completed/Classification: _____

Muscular Strength

Bicep Curl: _____ Classification: _____

Chair to Stand: _____ Classification: _____

Flexibility

Sit and Reach Distance (inches): Right _____ Classification: _____

　　　　　　　　　　　　　　　　　　Left _____ Classification: _____

Agility

Timed Up and Go Test: _____ Classification: _____

Post-Vitals

BP: _____ HR: _____ R: _____ SpO_2: _____

FIGURE 12.1 Baseline assessment.

BMI, body mass index; BP, blood pressure; DOB, date of birth; HR, heart rate; R, respirations.

Again, this is a sample that could be used or modified when assessing over-weight or obese patients.

EXERCISE PROGRAMMING

Exercise programming is aimed at promoting energy expenditure as well as at reducing possible injury risk. Exercise programming should consist of and include a combination of aerobic activity, flexibility, and functionality. Strength training can also be added as the patient progresses. Recommendations are to be patient and facility specific. Aerobic activity should be aimed at working large muscle groups. Activities can include walking, biking, or water aerobics. Caution should be taken with those complaining of arthritic or weight-related joint or muscle complaints. Resistance training or strength training can be done with various methods as well. Free weights, machines, bands, or even the patient's body weight can be used. Stretching is also important to increase the patient's flexibility and ROM. Functional activities should be aimed at activity-specific exercises and used to increase activities of daily living (ADLs). Functional activities can also be used to increase vocational potential as well as patient self-confidence in completing normal activities.

Figures 12.2 and 12.3 show examples of stretches and strengthening activities, respectively, similar to a handout given at the CLM Clinic. For the purpose of this book, there are two examples of each stretch and exercise. The first example under each stretch and strengthening exercise is the correct form and technique and is what each patient should strive for. The second example under each is an actual patient who has participated in the CLM program. With overweight or obese patients, modifications may be needed as demonstrated next. Bands and/or free weights can be used for these exercises. All stretches should be held for 10 to 30 seconds. Each strengthening exercise should start with 3 sets of 10 repetitions, working up to 3 sets of 12 repetitions, and then 3 sets of 15 repetitions before advancing either the bands or weights.

Triceps Stretch

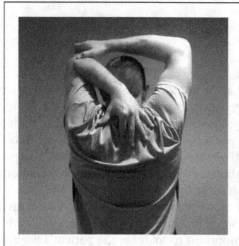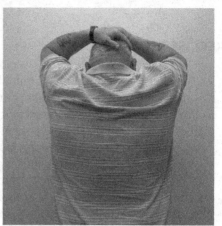

- Bring left arm up and place the palm of your hand down the center of your back with your elbow in the air.
- Place your right hand on your elbow and gently hold in place (may gently push if no stretch is felt) as you stretch your first arm.
- Hold for 10 to 30 seconds.
- Switch arms, repeat.

FIGURE 12.2 Stretches.

Bicep Stretch

This can be done while sitting or standing. When standing, make sure your feet are shoulder-width apart.

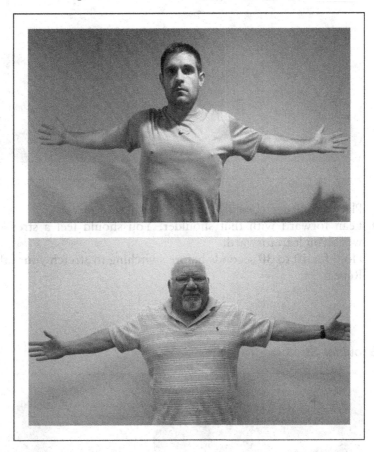

- Hold your arms out to the side, parallel with the ground with the palms of your hands facing forward.
- Stretch your arms back as far as possible.
- Hold for 10 to 30 seconds.
- A variation may be done with the thumbs pointing down.

FIGURE 12.2 (*continued*)

Chest Stretch

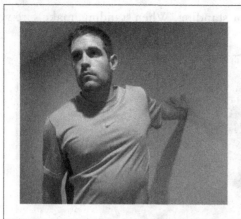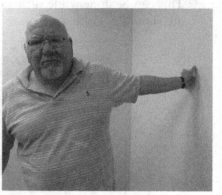

- Place an outstretched arm against a wall or doorway.
- Lean forward with that shoulder. You should feel a stretch in your chest when you lean forward.
- Hold for 10 to 30 seconds before switching to stretch your other arm.
- Repeat.

Shoulder Stretch

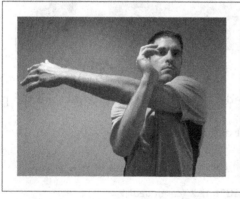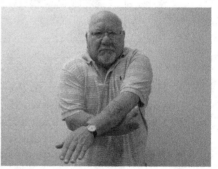

- Place one arm straight across your chest.
- Place the other arm on your elbow and pull your arm toward your chest.
- Hold for 10 to 30 seconds.
- Switch arms, repeat.

FIGURE 12.2 (continued)

Side Stretch

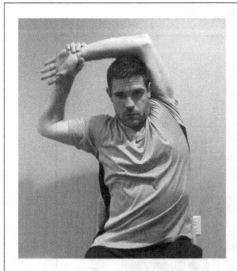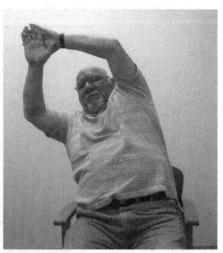

- Sitting in a chair with both feet flat on the floor, reach your arms above your head.
- Press your arms as far back as you can and hold for 10 to 30 seconds.
- Then, slowly lean to one side and hold for 10 to 30 seconds before returning to the upright, starting position.
- Repeat on the other side.

FIGURE 12.2 *(continued)*

Hamstring Stretch

You may hold onto a wall or a chair for balance.

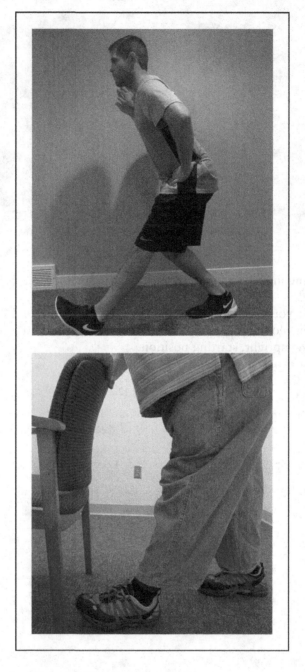

- Stand with one leg just in front of the other.
- Bend the back knee and rest your weight on the bent knee.
- Keeping your back straight, push your hips out behind you and lean forward.
- Hold for 10 to 30 seconds.
- Repeat with other leg.

FIGURE 12.2 (continued)

Quadriceps Stretch

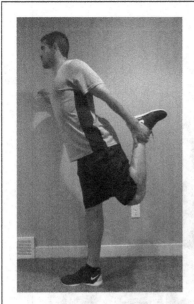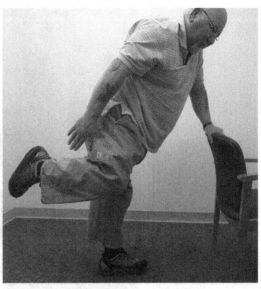

- Stand near a wall or a sturdy chair for balance.
- Steady yourself with the left hand against the wall or chair.
- Lift the right foot behind your back and grab it with the right hand.
- Stand straight with the thighs vertical and gently push the foot further toward the lower back toward the buttocks.
- Hold for 10 to 30 seconds before repeating on opposite leg.

FIGURE 12.2 *(continued)*

Groin Stretch

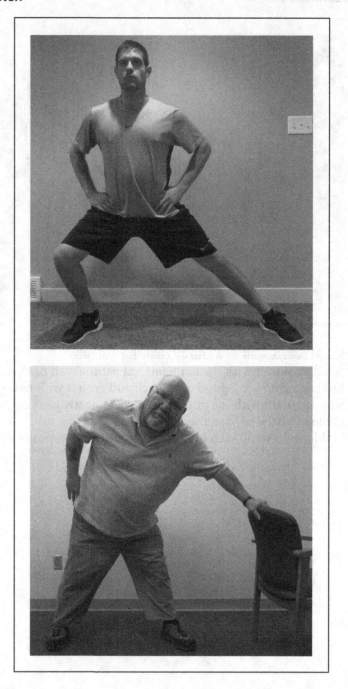

- Stand with feet slightly wider than shoulder-width apart.
- Lean to your right side and bend that right knee while keeping the left leg straight. You should feel a stretch on the inside of the thigh.
- Both feet should be pointing forward.
- Hands can be on your waist or resting on your thighs for balance.
- Hold for 10 to 30 seconds before switching to the left side.

FIGURE 12.2 (continued)

Calf Stretch

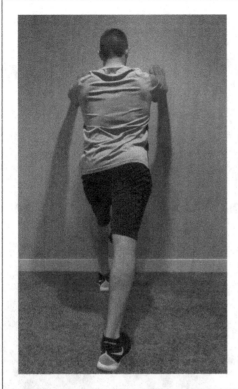 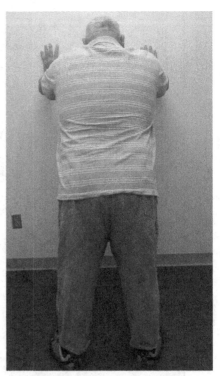

- Stand facing a wall with your hands on the wall at about eye level (like you are trying to push over a wall).
- Put the leg you want to stretch about a step behind your other leg.
- Keeping your back heel on the floor, bend your front knee until you feel a stretch in the back leg.
- Hold the stretch for 10 to 30 seconds.
- Repeat with opposite leg.

By moving your back leg farther away from the wall, you will feel the stretch in different parts of the lower leg.

FIGURE 12.2 (*continued*)

Chest Press

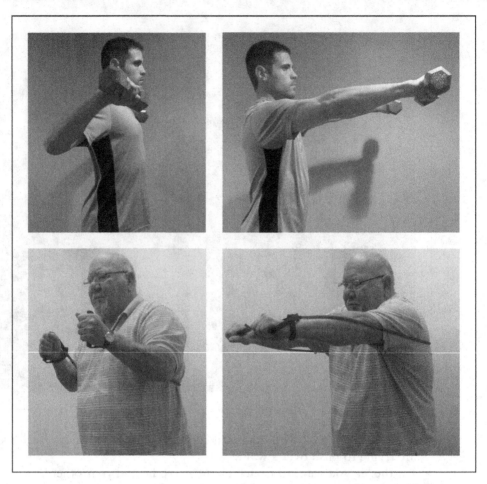

- If using a resistance band, place it around your back.
- Place band handles or weights in each hand with the hands at shoulder level.
- Engage your abdominal muscles and press arms out in front of you straight away from the chest.
- Keep wrists straight and keep arms at shoulder height.
- Hold for 2 seconds and return slowly to the starting position.
- Repeat.

FIGURE 12.3 Strengthening exercises.

Triceps Kickback

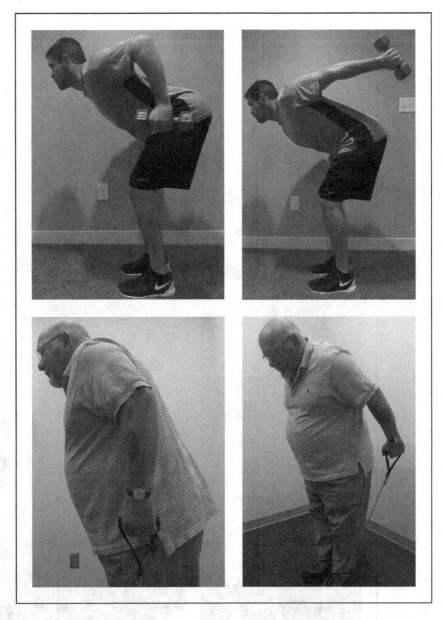

- Starting with the arms at the side, step on the band with both feet to create tension but make sure the tension is equal for both arms.
- Lean your body forward slightly, keeping your back straight. Pull abs in. Hold the band/weights in your hands with elbows bent at a 90° angle. Keep your elbow in the same spot throughout the exercise.
- Extend your forearm behind you, keeping your elbow still as you pass your hip in a fluid motion.
- Squeeze the back of your upper arm as you hold at the top for 2 seconds and then return slowly to the starting position.
- Repeat.

FIGURE 12.3 (*continued*)

Bent-Over Row

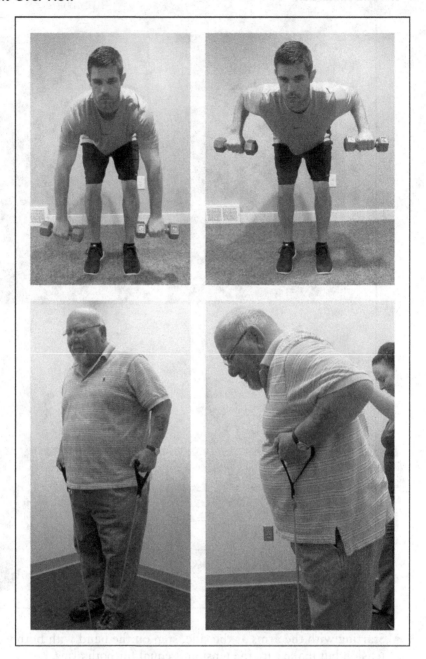

- Start with your arms at your side, with one foot or two feet on the band.
- Lean your body forward slightly, keeping your back straight and arms extended.
- Pull your elbows back until your hands are at your rib cage, squeezing your shoulder blades together. Hold for 2 seconds and return slowly to the starting position.
- Repeat.

FIGURE 12.3 (continued)

Biceps Curl

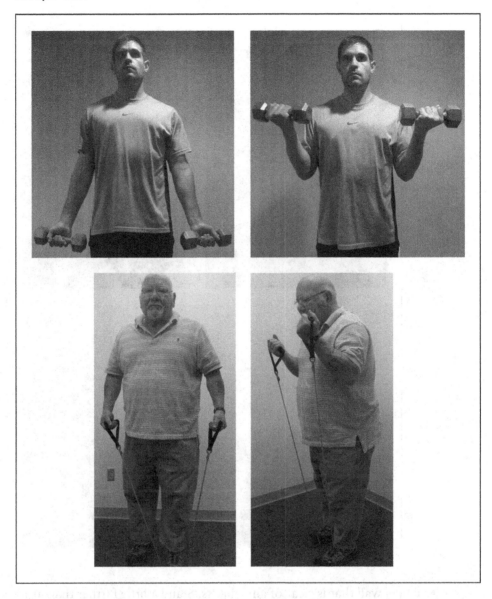

- Hold the band with both hands. To increase tension, stand on the band with both feet, shoulder-width apart.
- Start with your arms fully extended at your sides, palms facing forward.
- Pull up on the band/weights, with elbows glued to your side. Without bending your wrists, bring your hands up to your shoulder.
- Hold for 2 seconds, release, and slowly return to the starting position. Repeat.

FIGURE 12.3 *(continued)*

Wall Push-Ups

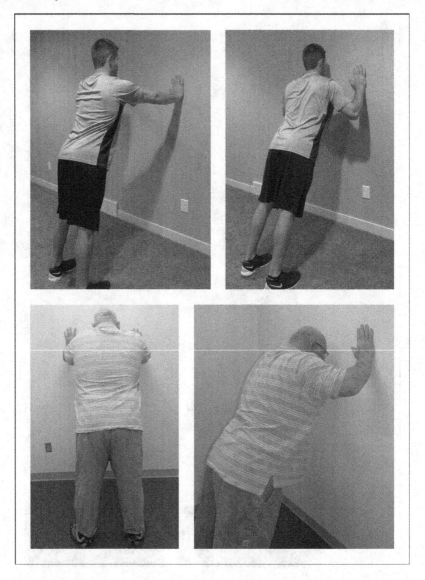

- Find a wall that is clear of any objects. Stand a little farther than arm's length from the wall.
- Facing the wall, lean your body forward and place your palms flat against the wall at about shoulder height and shoulder-width apart.
- Bend your elbows as you lower your upper body toward the wall in a slow, controlled motion, keeping your feet planted, until your elbows are bent to 90°.
- Slowly push yourself back until your arms are straight, but do not lock your elbows.

Make sure you do not round or arch your back.

FIGURE 12.3 (*continued*)

Seated Leg Extension

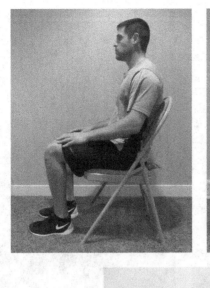
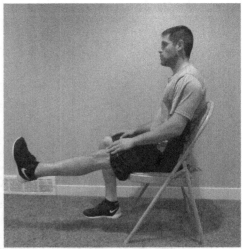
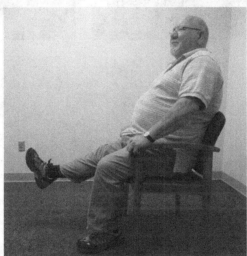

- Sitting up straight in a chair, plant both feet firmly on the ground.
- Tighten your abdominal muscles, then extend your leg until it is parallel to the floor (knee is straight), hold for 2 seconds, and slowly return to the starting position.
- Repeat and switch legs.
- To increase difficulty, use an ankle weight or resistance bands around ankles or perform the exercise while standing perpendicular to the chair, holding on for balance.

FIGURE 12.3 *(continued)*

Standing Hamstring Curl

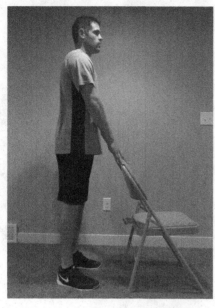
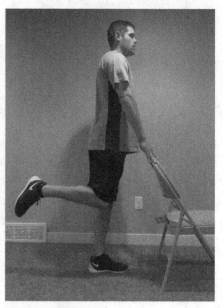
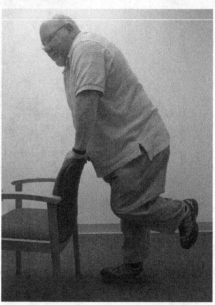

- Stand up, holding the back of a chair or wall for balance.
- Tighten the abdominal muscles. Keeping your upper body still and upright and your foot flexed, bend your knee to 90°, keeping your thigh stationary. Keep your knee pointing down. Hold for 2 seconds.
- Allow your leg to return slowly to the starting position.
- Repeat and switch legs.

FIGURE 12.3 *(continued)*

Hip Adduction

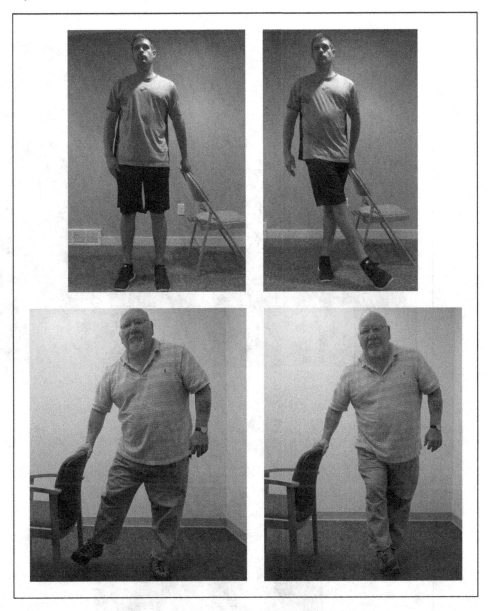

- Start by facing and holding the back of a chair or perpendicular to the back of a chair.
- Tighten your abdominal muscles and shift your weight to one foot (outside foot if perpendicular to chair). Keep your body still and upright, keep your toes pointing forward, then move your other leg (inside leg) across the front of your body.
- Repeat and switch legs.

FIGURE 12.3 *(continued)*

Hip Abduction

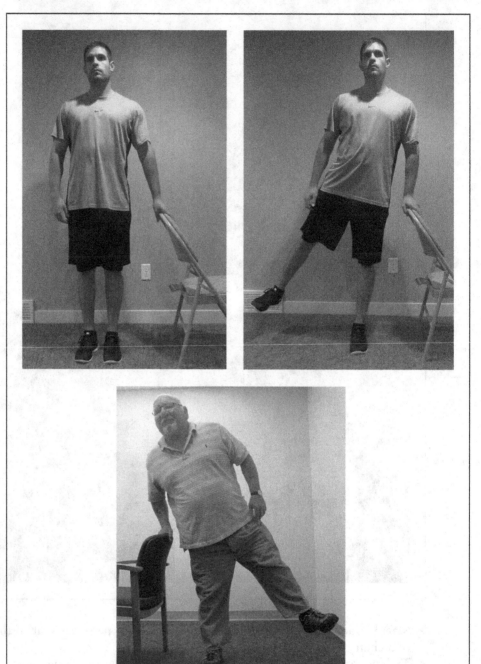

- Stand facing and holding onto a wall or door, or stand perpendicular to the back of a chair.
- Tighten your abdominal muscles, and keep your body still and upright. Keeping your toes pointed forward, slowly move your leg out to the side.
- Hold for 2 seconds, then return to the starting position.
- Repeat and switch legs.

FIGURE 12.3 (continued)

Hip Extension

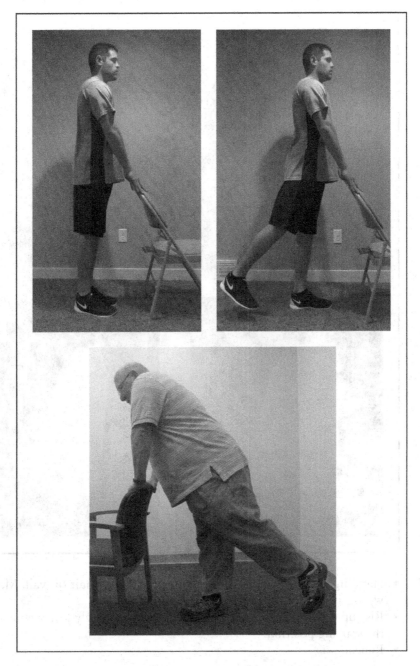

- Stand upright facing and holding the wall, door, or back of a sturdy chair.
- Tighten the abdominal, leg, and butt muscles; keep your body still and upright; lift one leg straight backward without bending the knee; and keep your foot flexed (do not point toes).
- Repeat and switch legs.

FIGURE 12.3 *(continued)*

Heel Raises (Calf Raises)

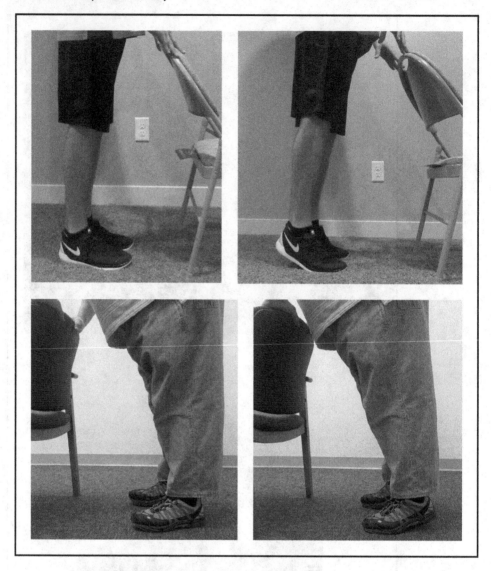

- Standing, balance yourself on both feet behind a chair or wall. Make sure the weight is evenly distributed between both feet.
- Rise up on your toes, hold for 5 seconds, then slowly lower yourself down to the starting position.
- Repeat.

FIGURE 12.3 *(continued)*

Squats

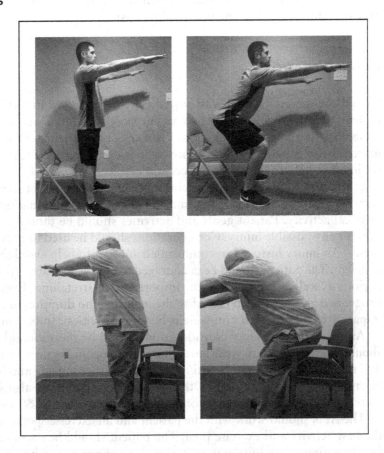

- In front of a sturdy chair, stand with feet slightly more than shoulder-width apart. Lean forward a little at the hips. You may put your arms straight out in front of you or on the arms of the chair for assistance.
- Making sure that your knees *never* come forward past your toes, lower yourself in a slow, controlled motion, to a count of four, until you reach a near-sitting position.
- Pause. Then, to a count of two, slowly rise back up to a standing position. Keep your knees over your ankles and your back straight.
- Repeat.
- If this exercise is too difficult, start off by using your hands for assistance. If you are unable to go all the way down, place a couple of pillows on the chair or only squat down 4 to 6 inches.
- Placing your weight more on your heels than on the balls or toes of your feet can help keep your knees from moving forward past your toes. It will also help to use the muscles of your hips more during the rise to a standing position.

Keep in mind the following:

Do not sit down too quickly.

Do not lean your weight too far forward or onto your toes when standing up.

FIGURE 12.3 *(continued)*

Again, this is a sample of what is given at one clinic. Changes or modifications may be made as needed on an individual basis.

SPECIAL CONSIDERATIONS

Special considerations exist with any patient and with any disease. With the obese patient, the end goal is weight loss and/or weight maintenance. The APN should remember that patient motivation is the key. The patient will not be successful in exercise or weight loss if the motivation is not there. Strategies, including goal setting, can help the patient be successful.

Injury prevention is also an important consideration with this patient population. Physical injury may be a primary reason for discontinuation of exercise or physical activity. Patient goals and activities should be thought out in order to prevent any possible injury. Considerations should be used to prevent an overuse injury. An injury history is recommended in order to help avoid the same type of problem. The patient should be encouraged to engage in warm-up and cool-down periods as well as be versed in the importance of stretching. Exercise should be progressed gradually with regard to the intensity and duration of activities. Low-impact activities or even non-weight-bearing activities can be considered.

Another patient safety consideration should be thermoregulation. Patients should be encouraged to wear loose-fitting clothing, maintain adequate hydration, and monitor the time of day and/or the temperature outside and humidity when engaging in physical activity. Other special considerations also depend on the associated comorbidity that accompanies obesity (Durstine & Moore, 2003).

The APN should work with the patient and an exercise specialist to determine the best activity and exercise plan. The patient should be encouraged to engage in any activity or additional activities throughout his or her daily life. Many patients with obesity feel that they cannot exercise because of the many hurdles that activity sometimes presents; however, with encouragement from the APN, they may be able to improve their overall health.

REFERENCES

Durstine, J. L., & Moore, G. E. (2003). *ACSM's exercise management for persons with chronic disease and disabilities* (2nd ed.). Champaign, IL: Human Kinetics.

Harvard School of Public Health. (2014). *Physical activity*. Retrieved from http://www.hsph.harvard.edu/obesity-prevention-source/obesity-causes/physical-activity-and-obesity/

Strath, S. J., Kaminsky, L. A., Ainsworth, B. E., Ekelund, U., Freedson, P. S., Gary, R. A., . . . Swartz, A. M. (2013). Guide to the assessment of physical activity: Clinic and research applications: A scientific statement from the American Heart Association. *Circulation*, *128*(20), 2259–2279. doi:10.1161/01.cir.0000435708.67487.da

Dietary Assessment and Patient Recommendations

Jennifer Roth

Healthy weight is about balancing food intake with physical activity. An individual's body weight is determined by a combination of genetic, metabolic, environmental, behavioral, and economic factors. These factors make treating obese individuals complex. The goals of weight management go beyond what the numbers on a scale say and should focus on developing healthful lifestyles with behavior modification. Goals of weight management may include prevention of weight gain, stopping weight regain, improvements in physical and emotional health, small maintainable weight losses, or more extensive weight losses. These should be achieved through modified eating and exercise behaviors along with improvements in eating, exercise, and other lifestyle behaviors.

The dietitian plays a crucial role in the delivery of the care to the patient for treatment of obesity. As an integral part of the health care team, the dietitian is responsible for helping to maintain good health and quality of life for the patients. The Academy of Nutrition and Dietetics Nutrition Care Process includes nutrition assessment, nutrition diagnosis, nutrition intervention, and nutrition monitoring and evaluation. Each of these steps is important in caring for a patient with obesity. Assessment is the first step in the Nutrition Care Process (American Dietetic Association, 2007; Lacey & Pritchet, 2003). This involves gathering all of the information needed to formulate a diagnosis and develop a care plan. Reviewing the patient's medical chart, including diagnosis, social history, medical history, medications, laboratory data, and evaluations by other medical professionals, is part of this step. The next step is to interview the patient to obtain diet history and other pertinent information to help provide the best nutrition intervention to address the problem. Once intervention is initiated, the next step is monitoring the patient to ensure that goals are met and the desired outcome is achieved. Interventions, outcomes, and any pertinent findings should be documented to help deliver the best care. Further guidance from the Nutrition Care Process can be found by visiting the Academy of Nutrition and Dietetics professional website at eatrightpro.org.

STARTING WITH A NEW PATIENT

It is important to schedule several sessions to begin working with patients toward losing weight. The sessions will involve monitoring goals, tracking progress, and offering accountability. The first session will help establish rapport and demonstrate to patients how small changes over time can make a big difference. Many patients typically try to make several habit changes at once and as a result often fail. Often, when big changes are made at one time, a patient may lose weight, but will regain it when going back to his or her previous ways of living. Once they realize that small changes can add up and produce significant results, they are more likely to be more perceptive and open to nutrition counseling. Before the first session, patients are sent a questionnaire to complete and bring along with them at the first visit. This will help with getting the most out of the appointment, offer insight into their mindset, and help them determine a starting point. A questionnaire may look like the example in Chapter 10 (Figure 10.2).

NUTRITION SCREENING

Body weight and changes in body weight nutrition screening should begin with measurement of height and weight along with calculation of body mass index (BMI). Please refer to Chapter 2 for further discussion of BMI. As part of the assessment, a patient-centered interview with supporting records from primary care providers and/or advanced practice nurses (APNs) is important. A medical examination should rule out any physiological causes of increased body weight, assess health risks, and evaluate for the presence of weight-related comorbidities. In addition to a medical assessment, a physiological evaluation will provide further information during this data-gathering stage. A physiological evaluation can screen for barriers to weight loss, such as depression, anxiety, bipolar disorder, binge-eating disorders, bulimia, and other personality disorders.

Nutrition screening should also include an assessment of dietary intake. The purpose of assessing the dietary intake is to evaluate the nutritional quality of the diet. Information on food intake can be obtained by a number of methods, including (a) 24-hour food recall; (b) food frequency questionnaire; (c) food record; and (d) diet history. Each method has its own advantages and limitations. Table 13.1 provides guidance for choosing the best dietary assessment method for the patient.

MONITORING PATIENTS' EATING PATTERNS AND HABITS

Two commonly used techniques to understand patients' eating patterns and habits are a 24-hour food recall and food journals. Twenty-four-hour recall involves interviewing a patient about his or her food and beverage consumption during the previous day or the preceding 24 hours. A single 24-hour recall is not considered to be representative of a habitual diet at an individual level (Raina, 2013). This is especially true for most patients, since diets are generally not consistent on a day-to-day basis. Some people find it easier to remember the most recent food or begin recalling from the previous day. Figure 13.1 gives an example of a 24-hour recall. If the 24-hour recall is used, questions about how dietary intake over the past

TABLE 13.1

STRENGTHS AND LIMITATIONS OF VARIOUS DIETARY ASSESSMENT METHODS USED IN CLINICAL SETTINGS		
	Strengths	Limitations
24-Hour food recall	Does not require literacy Relatively low burden on patient May be conducted in person or over the phone	Dependent on respondent's memory Relies on self-reported information Requires skilled staff Time consuming Single recall does not represent usual intake
Food record	Does not rely on memory Food portions may be measured at the time of consumption Multiple days of records provide valid measure of intake for most nutrients	Recording foods eaten may influence what is eaten Requires literacy Relies on self-reported information Time consuming

24 hours might differ from the usual dietary intake should be asked. The 24-hour food recall can be completed relatively quickly and with the combination of a food record/diary, a clearer picture of the patient's dietary routine can be obtained. The combination of the two can provide knowledge about consistency of diets with national dietary guidelines as well as sufficiency of energy and nutrient intakes.

DAILY FOOD RECORD OR JOURNAL

A daily food record or food journal involves documenting dietary intake as it occurs. It is often the most accurate and the most helpful to the individual if the food consumed is documented immediately after eating. According to a study published in the *American Journal of Preventative Medicine* involving 1,685 overweight or obese U.S. adults aged 25 and older, those who kept food records 6 days per week (documenting everything they ate and drank) for 6 months lost nearly twice as much weight as those who kept food records 1 day per week or less (American Dietetic Association, 2007). Food journals can bring to light patterns of overeating. They can also reveal food triggers. For some individuals, just recording every bite helps deter overeating. They may reconsider eating something because of not wanting to write it down. In the journal, the individual should be instructed to document time, food, amount/portions size, and degree of hunger. These details will provide insight into emotional triggers for eating habits, as well as times of day and places where healthy and unhealthy foods are the most likely to be consumed. Giving the patient a prepared journal with spaces to write these items is recommended; however, if another documenting system works better, it is encouraged as long as they are keeping track. Other ways of tracking may include online tools or personal notebooks. Food journals are the most helpful when they are reviewed by the individual and/or dietitian or APN who can help

Please be as specific as possible to review with the registered dietitian (RD).

Day 1

Food Item	Amount	Time	Where Was the Food Consumed?

FIGURE 13.1 24-Hour food recall.

point out patterns that may help in meeting weight-loss goals. Acknowledging and reflecting on the journal may be the most important piece in learning to make healthy choices for long-term lifestyle changes. Figure 13.2 is an example of a food and activity journal.

When discussing the concepts of the food journal, patients should be helped to understand that recording everything is important (if they do not want to write it down, they probably should not be eating it). They should be encouraged to be accurate, complete, and consistent by measuring portions, reading labels, including condiments and toppings, indicating how the food was prepared, and keeping the journal close at hand. By doing these things, a more complete picture will help the dietitian or care provider in assisting with reaching desired weight loss by the patient.

Date: _____

Nutritional Goal for the Day: _____

Time	Food Item	Amount	Why You Ate (hungry, bored, stressed, etc.)	Food Group

Please be as specific as possible with food items and portion sizes.

Activity Goal for the Day:

_____

Physical Activity	Minutes	How You Felt During/After

FIGURE 13.2 Food and activity journal.

ESTIMATING NEEDS FOR WEIGHT LOSS

Nutritional adequacy established from dietary history and food intake records coupled with anthropometric and biochemical measures provides baseline data. The Academy of Nutrition and Dietetics adult weight management guidelines advise measuring and including resting-energy expenditure as part of the dietary assessment. Estimated energy needs should be based on resting metabolic rate. If resting metabolic rate cannot be measured, then the Mifflin–St Jeor equations using actual weight are the most accurate for estimating resting metabolic rate for overweight and obese individuals (American Dietetic Association Evidence Analysis Library website, 2008). Figure 13.3 provides the Mifflin-St Jeor equations for both men and women.

Man: Basal metabolic rate (BMR) (10 × weight in kg) + (6.25 height in cm) –
   (5 × age in years) + 5.

Woman: BMR (10 × weight in kg) + (6.25 height in cm) – (5 × age in years) – 161.

FIGURE 13.3 Mifflin–St Jeor equations.

A negative energy balance is the most important factor affecting the weight-loss amount and rate. The first recommendation in obesity treatment is usually a reduction in energy intake: A reduction of 500 to 1,000 kcal/day is advised to achieve a weight loss of 1 to 2 pounds per week (American Dietetic Association Evidence Analysis Library website, 2008; U.S. Department of Health and Human Services [HHS], 1998). After calculating the energy needs of the patient for weight loss, it is important to talk to the patient about his or her needs, maintenance versus loss, and make the recommendation aloud. Reducing dietary fat and/or carbohydrates is a practical way to create a caloric deficit of 500 to 1,000 kcal below the estimated energy needs and should result in a weight loss of 1 to 2 pounds per week (American Dietetic Association Evidence Analysis Library website, 2008). A balanced energy-restricted diet is the most widely prescribed method of weight reduction. The diet should be nutritionally sound with decreased energy, so that fat stores are used to meet daily needs. Extreme energy-restricted diets provide fewer than 800 calories per day and are seldom prescribed as a treatment due to side effects, including urinary ketones, fatigue, lightheadedness, nervousness, constipation or diarrhea, dry skin, thinning hair, anemia, and menstrual irregularities.

DIET COMPOSITION

A low-fat, reduced-energy diet is the best studied weight-loss dietary strategy and is most frequently recommended by governing health authorities (American Dietetic Association Evidence Analysis Library website, 2008). Fat is the most energy-dense macronutrient, but is known to have a weak effect on both satiation and satiety (Blundell & Stubbs, 1999). These attributes make fat a useful target for reducing energy intake. Because diabetes and cardiovascular disease (CVD) are frequent comorbidities of obesity, reducing the dietary saturated and trans-fatty acid content is also recommended (Lichtenstein et al., 2006). The effectiveness of low-fat, low-energy diets in combination with lifestyle counseling and activity has been demonstrated in recent multicenter clinical trials where, in addition to 5% to 10% weight loss, the reduction or prevention of comorbidities such as diabetes and/or hypertension (HTN) has also occurred (Lindström et al., 2006).

PORTION CONTROL

Registered dietitians (RDs) typically recommend portion control to individuals trying to lose weight. They may do this in various ways, including providing information on the energy content of regularly consumed foods, use of premeasured foods, food models, or food labels. Other ways to teach about portion control include reviewing the difference in sizes of plates, bowls, and drinking glasses and encouraging individuals to choose the smaller options. The RD may recommend the individual consume more vegetables at a meal, therefore decreasing the size of the main entrée item at a meal. Reduced portions may be more or less satiating depending on the strategy used. These recommendations may affect their cognitive decisions to choose one food over another, possibly more palatable food. Effectively reducing portion sizes appears to be an important weight gain prevention strategy for everybody, as marketplace food and drink portions now exceed standard serving sizes by a factor of at least twofold (Young & Nestle, 2003). Discussing the proper portion sizes at both home and restaurants during the visit is vital to the educational piece of the appointment. *Portion distortion* is a term created to describe this perception of large portions as appropriate amounts to eat at a single eating occasion. This distortion is reinforced by packaging, dinnerware, and serving utensils that have also increased in size (Wansink & Van Ittersum, 2007).

RECOMMENDATIONS

Weight-loss programs should combine a nutritionally balanced dietary regimen with exercise and lifestyle changes. Selecting the best treatment strategy depends on the goals of the patient as well as on his or her health risks. Treatment options may include a low-calorie diet, increased physical activity and lifestyle modification, and the prevention of weight gain through energy balance. Recommendations for Americans have been made by many health organizations such as the United States Department of Agriculture (USDA), the American Heart Association (AHA), the American Cancer Society (ACS), and the Academy of Nutrition and Dietetics. The following are recommendations to help individuals achieve dietary goals and change lifestyle behaviors (Nutrition and Your Health: Dietary Guidelines for Americans, 2005):

- Make half your plate fruits and vegetables.
- Switch to skim or 1% milk.
- Make at least half your grains whole.
- Consume 25 to 30 g of fiber per day.
- Choose more low-fat protein choices such as skinless poultry, soy products, and lean cuts of beef and pork.
- Choose foods and drinks with little or no added sugars.
- Limit sodium intake to 2,400 mg per day.
- Eat fewer foods that are high in solid fats.

- Enjoy your food, but eat less.
- Cook more often at home, where you are in control of what is in your food.
- When eating out, choose lower-calorie menu options.
- Write down what you eat to keep track of how much you eat.
- If you drink alcoholic beverages, do so sensibly—limit to one drink a day for women or to two drinks a day for men.

Additional items to include in the conversation with the patient during an initial visit are as follows: Recommend the individual to think nutrient rich rather than "good" or "bad" foods, to eat a variety of foods from all of the food groups to get the nutrients a body needs, to increase the amount of dark green and orange vegetables, to vary protein choices with more fish, beans, and peas (as they are low in fat), and to eat at least three ounces of whole-grain cereals, breads, crackers, rice, or pasta every day.

COUNSELING TO IMPROVE BEHAVIOR CHANGE

The endpoint of obesity treatment is to help patients eat less and move more. Talking with patients about weight loss requires effective and compassionate treatment. Let us assume that obese individuals know that they are overweight. If they have not heard it from their health care professional, they have probably been told by family, friends, or even strangers. A phrase such as "what do you think about your weight?" will help you to assess the patient's interest in weight control in a nonjudgmental manner. This will also help with hearing the patient's perspective before making any recommendations for weight loss.

Be clear about weight-loss expectations in the initial appointment. Most times, patients desire rapid weight loss; however, healthy and ideal weight loss would be 10% in 6 months. Discussing a healthy weight-loss goal of 1 to 2 pounds per week with the patients may help identify any unrealistic expectations. One should focus on the non-weight changes such as improvements in laboratory values, blood pressure (BP), glucose levels as well as increased energy, and climbing stairs without being short of breath.

Some questions to ask include the following: What do you think about your weight? What strategies have worked for you in the past? How is your current weight affecting your life? Could you describe how your life might be different if you lost weight or adopted a healthier lifestyle? What would you like to do about your weight right now? How willing are you to make lifestyle changes at this time? These questions will help you gain more information and assess how willing they are to change.

When asking questions, one should take time and listen carefully to the patient. Listening creates a safe environment in which clients feel heard and the health professional discovers what clients want. It helps establish a comfortable relationship, build rapport, and alleviate stress and frustration. Reflective and active listening is the key to communication and, ultimately, helps the patient reach weight-loss goals. Reflective listening is a method of active listening where the listener illustrates comprehension by repeating, or parroting, what he or she has been told. It is designed to improve communication through empathy and paraphrasing. Active listening helps patients clarify what is working well and where they can make changes. It encourages them to set their own specific and realistic goals. Ask patients to state what they expect the visit. Part of active listening is reflecting back to the speaker, giving him or her plenty of time to talk without interjecting questions. Express empathy about dissatisfaction with weight and/or shape. Recognize and affirm past successes as well as current achieved goals at recurrent visits. Reframe negative thoughts and turn them into positive ones. "You have made some great goals. I'd like to see you back in one month to see how you are doing. Please don't worry if it doesn't go exactly as you planned. I'm here to help you problem-solve and come up with a new plan if this doesn't work."

Insightful questions prevent patients from giving short and pat answers and help raise awareness. Formatting the right questions can help make the patients take action and make their own decisions based on their own answers. One should avoid using the word *why*. Using this word implies that the patient should do something. Asking the same question using the word *how* or *what* changes the tone. One should ask questions that move clients forward instead of those that seek to justify what went wrong. For example, "What can you try next time you're hungry at night?" may prompt a solution, whereas "Tell me what you were thinking when you ate that bag of chips" focuses on what the client did wrong.

The nutrition assessment is an ongoing process that involves continual reassessment and evaluation. Assessment provides the foundation for the nutrition diagnosis. Treating individuals who are overweight and obese is complex, as body weight is determined by a combination of genetic, metabolic, behavioral, environmental, cultural, and socioeconomic influences. Health care providers should understand the importance of weight gain prevention and the challenge of weight-loss maintenance to effectively help them meet their goals.

REFERENCES

American Dietetic Association. (2007). *Nutrition diagnosis and intervention: Standardized language for the nutrition care process.* Chicago, IL: Author.

American Dietetic Association Evidence Analysis Library website. (2008). *Adult weight management evidence-based nutrition practice guideline.* Retrieved from http://www.adaevidencelibrary.com/topic.cfm?cat=2798

Blundell, J. E., & Stubbs, R. J. (1999). High and low carbohydrate and fat intakes: Limits imposed by appetite and palatability and their implications for energy balance. *European Journal of Clinical Nutrition, 53*(1), S148–S165.

Lacey, K., & Pritchet, E. (2003). Nutrition care process and model: ADA adopts road map to quality care and outcomes management. *Journal of the American Dietetic Association, 103,* 1061–1072.

Lichtenstein, A. H., Appel, L. J., Brands, M., Carnetho, M., Daniels, S., Franch, H. A., . . . Wylie-Rosett, J. (2006). Diet and lifestyle recommendations revision 2006: A scientific statement from the American Heart Association Nutrition Committee. *Circulation, 114,* 82–96.

Lindström, J., Ilanne-Parikka, P., Peltonen, M., Aunola, S., Eriksson, J. G., Hemiö, K., . . . Tuomilehto, J. (2006). Sustained reduction in the incidence of type 2 diabetes by lifestyle intervention: Follow-up of the Finnish Diabetes Prevention Study. *Lancet, 368,* 1673–1679.

Nutrition and Your Health: Dietary Guidelines for Americans. (2005). (6th ed., pp. 1–19). Washington, DC: U.S. Government Printing Office.

Raina, S. K. (2013). Limitations of 24-hour recall method: Micronutrient intake and the presence of the metabolic syndrome. *North American Journal of Medical Sciences, 5*(8), 498.

U.S. Department of Health and Human Services. (1998). *The clinical guidelines on the identification, evaluation, and treatment of overweight and obesity in adults: The evidence report* (NIH Publication no. 98-4083). Bethesda, MD: NHLBI Information Center.

Wansink, B., & Van Ittersum, K. (2007). Portion size me: Downsizing our consumption norms. *Journal of the American Dietetic Association, 107,* 1103–1106.

Young, L. R., & Nestle, M. (2003). Expanding portion sizes in the US marketplace: Implications for nutrition counseling. *Journal of the American Dietetic Association, 103,* 231–234.

Psychological Assessment

An initial psychological assessment should take place on the first appointment with the patient. This will allow open lines of communication with the patient. If any psychological history exists, a referral to a mental health nurse practitioner (MHNP), licensed counselor, or psychologist/psychiatrist is warranted. This chapter focuses on tools that are useful for the advanced practice nurse (APN) in an outpatient clinic setting.

By the year 2020, depression is projected to become the leading cause of disability, with the devastation caused by this disease surpassed only by heart disease. Screening tools are one way for the APN to identify depression. Several screening tools exist for use in an outpatient setting. These include the Beck Depression Inventory, the Center for Epidemiological Studies Depression scale, the General Health Questionnaire, and the Patient Health Questionnaire. The Beck Depression Inventory is used worldwide and is the most common self-reporting screening tool. Symptoms of sadness, guilt, failure, social withdrawal, and suicidal ideas are examined. The Center for Epidemiological Studies Depression scale and the General Health Questionnaire are less commonly used. The Patient Health Questionnaire is primarily used in primary care settings. Each screening tool should be reviewed by the APN for the best fit and individualized for each patient.

The following depressive disorders should be picked up by a screening tool for depression (Kerr & Kerr, 2001, p. 351):

- Major depressive disorder
- Chronic depressive disorder
- Dysthymic disorder
- Adjustment disorder with depressed mood
- Adjustment disorder with anxiety and depressed mood
- Melancholia
- Postpartum depressive disorder

The following somatic symptoms can also be seen with depression and could cause inadequate scoring in the screening tools (Kerr & Kerr, 2001, p. 352):

- Headache or migraines
- Sexual dysfunction
- Appetite changes
- Menstrual-related symptoms
- Chronic pain
- Chronic medical conditions (diabetes, Parkinson's disease, alcoholism)

- Digestive problems
- Sleep disturbances
- Fatigue

Many tools are available to use in order to screen patients for depression (Kerr & Kerr, 2001).

The Diagnostic and Statistical Manual of Mental Disorders, Fourth Edition (*DSM-IV*) is another resource that can be used to define the criteria for depression. Atypical depression can be seen with significant weight gain, increased appetite, and/or extreme sensitivity to perceived rejection.

The following questions could provide the basis for an evaluation of atypical depressive disorder: Are you eating more but not really enjoying your food? Are you sleeping longer than usual? Do your arms and legs feel leaden and heavy? Have you become more sensitive to criticism? Do you have more (than usual) displays of anger? (Kerr & Kerr, 2001, p. 352)

Along with depression, the APN should also screen for a possible eating disorder. Patients may be sensitive about weight, so one should approach this subject with care. During the initial patient examination, patients with any of the following conditions should be considered for a possible eating disorder:

- Amenorrhea
- Bradycardia
- Constipation
- Dehydration
- Elevated amylase
- Elevated creatinine
- Gastroesophageal reflux disease (GERD) or regurgitation
- Hypoglycemia
- Metabolic disturbance
- Syncope

While screening the patient, any or all of the following subjects may be approached (Maine & McCallum, 2015):

- Weight fluctuations (low weight, high weight, desired weight)
- Actions taken to maintain, control, or alter weight
- Diets or dieting
- Any use of medications to include supplements, appetite suppressants, laxatives, enemas, or diuretics
- Binge eating or purging
- Vomiting
- Report of food and liquid intake
- Exercise habits
- Excessive exercise
- Menstrual history
- Family history of:
  - Eating disorders
  - Obesity
  - Depression
  - Chemical dependence

The self-administered Questionnaire for Eating Disorder Diagnoses (Q-EDD) has been shown to have a 97% sensitivity and a 98% specificity. It has also been shown to be both valid and reliable by the *DSM-IV*. The Eating Disorder Screen for Primary Care (ESP) and the Sick, Control, One, Fat, and Food (SCOFF) clinical prediction guide questionnaires are also used in screening for eating disorders. Sample questions from ESP are as follows (Cotton, Ball, & Robinson, 2003, pp. 53–54):

- Are you satisfied with your eating patterns? (A "no" to this question was classified as an abnormal response.)
- Do you ever eat in secret? (A "yes" to this and all other questions was classified as an abnormal response.)
- Does your weight affect the way you feel about yourself?
- Have any members of your family suffered with an eating disorder?
- Do you currently suffer with or have you ever suffered in the past with an eating disorder?

The SCOFF clinical prediction guide uses five questions: They are as follows (Cotton et al., 2003, p. 54):

- Do you make yourself Sick because you feel uncomfortably full?
- Do you worry you have lost Control over how much you eat?
- Have you recently lost more than One stone (14 lb or 7.7 kg) in a 3-month period?
- Do you believe yourself to be Fat when others say you are thin?
- Would you say that Food dominates your life?

The Institute for Clinical Systems Improvement (ICSI; 2013) uses the following questions to screen for an eating disorder: "Do you eat a large amount of food in a short period of time—like eating more food than another person may eat in, say, a two-hour period of time? Do you ever feel like you can't stop eating even after you feel full? When you overeat, what do you do?" (p. 14). Several options for screening tools are available and again, the APN should tailor the tool or questions to each individual.

Motivational interviewing can be used to address weight, weight loss, and management. Motivational interviewing is a form of counseling that uses focused conversation in collaboration with the patient in order to strengthen his or her motivation toward a goal and commitment to change. "It is designed to strengthen an individual's motivation for and movement toward a specific goal by eliciting and exploring the person's own reasons for change within an atmosphere of acceptance and compassion" (Motivational Interviewing Website, 2013). The following suggestions could be used for motivational interviewing (Fitch et al., 2013, p. 83):

1. Why is now a good time for you to lose weight?
2. What have you tried in the past to lose weight?
3. How would you do things differently this time?
4. How would you feel if you were successful losing weight?
5. What is one thing we can do together to make a step toward your weight-loss goals?
6. Help me understand why you want to lose weight.
7. What could work? To what extent would this affect your life?

Sample scripts exist for conducting a 10-minute motivational interview. The following are points the APN can use to guide the patient interview:

1. Listen
2. Ask permission
3. Engage
4. Reflect
5. Ask-Tell-Ask
6. Elicit
7. Reflect
8. Provide
9. Elicit
10. Goal
11. Session close

Listening can be done using open-ended questions. Why Am I Talking? (W.A.I.T.) can be used to remind the APN to allow the patient to talk and refrain from any judgment. Asking permission allows the patient to open up and at times allows for the impossible to happen. Engaging the patient means looking at the situation from his or her perspective and forgetting the medical jargon. Reflection allows for clarification. One should be specific in questioning and ask what the patient wants to accomplish today. This helps devise the agenda. One should ask the patient about his or her weight concerns; then, one should elicit a response by using an active open statement that can allow for more than a one-word answer. One should use reflection again for clarification and provide the patient with nonjudgmental advice. "May I share with you what has worked for other patients to lose weight?" (p. 83). One should elicit a response from the patient by asking how he or she feels about the conversation. Setting a goal will allow the patient to focus on a change that the patient thinks he or she will be able to accomplish. The patient should be encouraged to rate the goal on a zero through ten scale to determine how confident the patient is that he or she will fulfill or meet this goal. One should write down the goals and send them home with the patient; one should also clarify the goals at the end of the session to make sure both parties agree. The session close should consist of highlighting the session and sending the patient forth with the encouragement to reach the goal. One should also remind the patient that the goals will be discussed again at the next session.

Shared decision making consists of *decisional conflict, decision support,* and *decision aids.* These terms are important to define so the APN and patient can move toward collaborative conversation. *Decisional conflict* is defined as options provided that do not satisfy all the patient's objectives or external influencers that exist, creating difficulty in making a choice. *Decision support* provides an assurance that a decision needs to be made. This is factual and provides clarity as to the patient's values, and it guides communication and progress. *Decision aids* are evidence-based tools that provide benefits, risks, harms, and scientific information to the patient. The essential steps of shared decision making that make up the SHARE approach is as follows (Agency for Healthcare Research and Quality [AHRQ], 2014, p. 2):

Step 1: Seek your patient's participation
Step 2: Help your patient explore and compare treatment options
Step 3: Assess your patient's values and preferences

Step 4: Reach a decision with your patient

Step 5: Evaluate your patient's decision

More information on shared decision making can be found in O'Connor, Stacey, and Jacobsen (2011).

Collaborative conversation encourages patients to take an active role in their health with nurture and guidance from the APN. This is a collaboration between the patient and APN in which both understand that each will play key roles in the decision making throughout the sessions. A certain skill set, including cognitive, affective, social, and spiritual, should be used in each decision-making process. Key communication skills used in collaborative conversation should include listening skills, questioning skills, and information-giving skills. Eye contact, appropriate body language, respect, empathy, and partnerships can aid in the effectiveness of collaborative conversation (Fitch et al., 2013).

"Weight loss requires frequent follow-up (initially weekly) with planned education/counseling by health care providers to be most effective (i.e., improve adherence)" (Chao et al., 2000; National Heart, Lung, and Blood Institute [NHLBI], 2000; Rejeski, Focht, & Messier, 2002; Tuomilehto et al., 2001). Again, it is important to assess for any depression and/or eating disorder on the initial visit and/or any time in which there is a change or cause for concern in patient symptoms that would warrant re-assessment. Referrals to a licensed mental health professional or a psychiatric mental health nurse practitioner (PMHNP) should be used as needed.

REFERENCES

Agency for Healthcare Research and Quality. (2014). *The SHARE approach. Essential steps of shared decision making: Expanded reference guide with sample conversation starters* (Workshop Curriculum: Tool 2). 1–14. Retrieved from http://www.ahrq.gov/sites/default/files/wysiwyg/professionals/education/curriculum-tools/shareddecisionmaking/tools/tool-2/share-tool2.pdf

Chao, D., Espeland, M. A., Farmer, D., Register, T. C., Lenchik, L., Applegate, W. B., & Ettinger, W. H. (2000). Effect of voluntary weight loss on bone mineral density in older overweight women. *Journal of the American Geriatric Society, 48*(7), 753–759.

Cotton, M., Ball, C., & Robinson, P. (2003). Four simple questions can help screen for eating disorders. *Journal of General Internal Medicine, 18*(1), 53–56. doi: 10.1046/j.1525-1497.2003.20374.x

Fitch, A., Everling, L., Fox, C., Goldberg, J., Heim, C., Johnson, K., . . . Webb, B. (2013). *Institute for clinical systems improvement: Prevention and management of obesity for adults*. Retrieved from https://www.icsi.org/_asset/s935hy/Obesity-Interactive0411.pdf

Institute for Clinical Systems Improvement. (2013). *Health care guideline: Prevention and management of obesity for adults*. Retrieved from https://www.icsi.org/_asset/s935hy/Obesity-Interactive0411.pdf

Kerr, L. K., & Kerr, L. D. (2001). Screening tools for depression in primary care: The effects of culture, gender, and somatic symptoms on the detection of depression. *Western Journal of Medicine, 175*(5), 349–352. Retrieved from http://www.ncbi.nlm.nih.gov/pmc/articles/PMC1071624

Maine, M., & McCallum, K. (2015). *Screening for eating disorders by primary care physicians*. National Eating Disorders Association (NEDA). Retrieved from https://www.nationaleatingdisorders.org/screening-eating-disorders-primary-care-physicians

Motivational Interviewing Website. (2013). Retrieved from http://www.motivational interviewing.org

National Heart, Lung, and Blood Institute. (2000). *The practical guide: Identification, evaluation, and treatment of overweight and obesity in adults* (NIH Publication No. 00-4084). Retrieved from http://www.nhlbi.nih.gov/files/docs/guidelines/prctgd_c.pdf

O'Connor, A., Stacey, D., & Jacobsen, M. (2011). Improving practitioners' decision support skills. Decision Support Tutorial. Ottawa Hospital Research Institute. Retrieved from https://decisionaid.ohri.ca/ODST/pdfs/ODST.pdf

Rejeski, W. J., Focht, B. C., & Messier, S. P. (2002). Obese, older adults with knee osteoarthritis: Weight loss, exercise, and quality of life. *Health Psychology, 21,* 419–426.

Tuomilehto, J., Lindstrom, J., Eriksson, J. G., Valle, T. T., Hämäläinen, H., Ilanne-Parikka, P., . . . Uusitupa, M. (2001). Prevention of type 2 diabetes by changes in lifestyle among subjects with impaired glucose tolerance. *New England Journal of Medicine, 344*(18), 1343–1350.

Case Study 3

This case study builds on information seen in Chapters 7 to 14 dealing with assessment.

- *Chapter 7: Overview of Genetics and Pathophysiology of Obesity*
- *Chapter 8: Behaviors, Addiction, and Eating Disorders*
- *Chapter 9: Which "Way" Is the Right "Weigh?"*
- *Chapter 10: Physical Assessment of the Adult Obese Patient*
- *Chapter 11: Physical Assessment of the Pediatric Obese Patient*
- *Chapter 12: Physical Activity, Exercise Assessment, and Patient Recommendations*
- *Chapter 13: Dietary Assessment and Patient Recommendations*—Jennifer Roth
- *Chapter 14: Psychological Assessment*

Mrs. Smith, a 68-year-old Caucasian woman, presents to the clinic with a goal of wanting to lose weight. She also wants to feel better, be less short of breath, play with her grandchildren, and be able to wear "normal" and not "baggy" clothes. She reports she has been either overweight or obese ever since she graduated high school and started having children. She is married with four grown children and 10 grandchildren.

She reports that her weight fluctuates, but over the past 10 years it has just gone up. She reports that she has tried to "eat healthy" and exercise. She reports that sometimes if she feels that she eats too much she gets "sick" and vomits.

She reports that she would walk more, but her knee and/or hip bothers her when she tries to walk "too much." She enjoys riding a bike, but only enjoys doing this outside. She lives in the Midwest and cannot ride her bike outdoors year round. She reports that she has an indoor stationary bike, but says that she "gets bored staring at the wall for too long." She has a history of depression and says that the only medication she takes is Prozac.

She says that this clinic is her "last hope." She reports that she would like to lose at least 100 pounds in 6 months. She reports that she is willing to do "anything" to lose weight. She reports trying to lose weight in the past, but states that it has either not worked or she gave up and just tried making herself get sick.

She has a family history of obesity in her mother, father, and two brothers. She reports that she has a sister who is of normal weight. She also has a family history of depression in her father and one of her brothers. Her father also has type 2 diabetes mellitus (T2DM), hypertension (HTN), and high cholesterol. Her mother has a history of breast cancer.

Today, her vitals are as follows:

Blood pressure: 150/88
Pulse: 70 bpm
Respirations: 12
Height: 5 feet, 6 inches
Weight: 376 pounds
Body mass index (BMI): 60.7 kg/m^2
Pulse oximetry: 90% on room air
Neck circumference: 16 inches

Her physical examination shows the following:

General: Looks stated age, appropriate conversation, in no acute distress
Head, Eyes, Ears, Nose, Throat (HEENT): PERRLA, extraocular muscles intact.
    Conjunctiva normal, anicteric
Neck: Supple, no jugular vein distension (JVD)
Skin: Warm. Pink. Dry
Mucosa: No cyanosis, moist
Cardiovascular: Normal S1 and S2. No murmur
Lungs: Good bilateral air entry
Abdomen: Obese, soft, and nontender. Normal bowel sounds. No rebound pain
    or rigidity
Extremities: No edema, no cyanosis or clubbing
Neurological: Alert and oriented ×3. No motor or sensory deficit

She had fasting laboratory work drawn before her appointment today and brought in copies. The results are as follows:

Basic Metabolic Panel (BMP)

Sodium: 138
Potassium: 4.2
Chloride: 101
CO_2: 25
Blood urea nitrogen (BUN): 24
Creatinine: 0.9
Glucose: 122

Complete Blood Count (CBC)

White blood cells: 7.0
Hemoglobin: 14.7
Hematocrit: 44.5
Platelets: 211

Thyroid-stimulating hormone (TSH): 3.2

Fasting Lipid Panel

Total cholesterol: 223
Triglycerides: 155
High-density lipoprotein (HDL): 30
Low-density lipoprotein (LDL): 155

Is she overweight or obese? What category does her BMI fall into?

How would you address her weight?

What has led to her obesity?

Is she a candidate for weight loss?

Is her weight loss of 100 pounds in 6 months feasible? Why or why not? What would you recommend?

How would you present her with a plan for weight loss? What would this include?

How would you address her "getting sick" or vomiting?

Would you make any additional referrals?

Would you order any testing? If yes, what testing and why?

What dietary advice would you provide?

What lifestyle changes would you suggest?

What physical activity would you encourage? Please include mode/type, frequency, duration, and time.

Would you recommend stretching and strengthening activities? Please include mode/type, frequency, duration, and time.

Would you recommend any family lifestyle counseling?

Would you continue her current medication—Prozac? Would there be a better choice?

Would you consider any additional medications? If yes, what?

Would you order any other laboratory work? If yes, what?

When would you repeat laboratory work?

When would you schedule her next follow-up appointment?

Would you involve any other advanced practice nurses (APNs) in her care?

What additional education, if any, would you provide?

Disease Management

Disease Management and the Role of the Advanced Practice Nurse

Disease management focuses on the concept of reducing health care costs while improving the quality of treatment for chronic diseases. This concept utilizes integrated or collaborative care to prevent or minimize the effects of these diseases. Health improvement and cost containment are the focus of disease management. This concept also empowers self-care with the help of a coordinated health care team and interventions. Many times, people suffering with chronic health care conditions see multiple providers and often receive poor care coordination. With disease management, the advance practice nurse (APN) works with other providers as well as with a health care team to provide the best overall care for the treatment of the overweight and/or obese individual and his or her comorbid conditions.

A proactive approach with multidisciplinary providers is developed from evidence-based practice guidelines. Multiple components are used in the makeup of disease management programs. These can include, but are not limited to, the following (Academy of Managed Care Pharmacy, 2015):

- Population identification
- Chronic diseases
- Costly medical conditions
- Collaboration with a multidisciplinary team:
  - APNs, physicians, psychologists, pharmacists, dietitians, exercise specialists, physical therapists, and nurses
- Risk stratification and management
- Implementation of self-management:
  - Education, behavior modification, and support groups
- Outcome measurement
- Outcome evaluation
- Reporting feedback loops
- Use of electronic charting and information technology

Chronic disease management commonly includes diseases such as diabetes mellitus (DM), hypertension (HTN), coronary artery disease (CAD), congestive heart failure (CHF), chronic obstructive pulmonary disease (COPD), and asthma. Although obesity is not commonly listed as a chronic disease, this condition can play a major role in the diseases listed earlier. It is thought of as an additional complication in the treatment of other chronic diseases.

Indicators such as clinical, humanistic, and economic outcomes can determine the quality and success of the program. Health care utilization also plays a role in outcome measurement. Success can be measured by the change in incidence of the problem, the patient's quality of life, or the determination of any cost savings (Academy of Managed Care Pharmacy, 2015).

Multiple practice specialties may be involved in effective team care of chronic illness and disease management. Primary and specialty care as well as a community organization or agency can work together to provide adequate patient care. Team collaboration has been shown to be more effective with patients who have received both clinical and self-management support services. The following strategies are used for effective patient treatment: population-based care, treatment planning, evidence-based clinical management, self-management support, more effective consultations, and sustained follow-up.

Effective disease management starts with population-based care. High-quality patient care and effective interventions given to a defined patient population constitute population-based care. An established protocol providing guidelines for assessment and treatment as well as specific duties are provided to team members for a comprehensive approach. Treatment planning is effective in formal treatment of chronic illness; it also provides navigation for a multidisciplinary approach. Plans should be designed according to patient preferences for overall better satisfaction.

The use of evidence-based clinical management allows for data-driven, effective treatment regimens and practices. A team or multidisciplinary approach has been shown to improve outcomes in regards to chronic conditions. This approach has also been proved successful when it comes to self-management support. A behavioral counselor is one such team member who can encourage self-support and inspire more patient confidence. Team members help in encouraging and reinforcing patient skills in managing a chronic illness rather than just focusing on a protocol or treatment plan.

The use of group consultations or specialty clinics is also valuable when it comes to treatment of chronic disease (Wagner, 2000). Beck et al. (1997) found that group consultations, comprising more than one patient at a time, led to more patient satisfaction as well as lowered the number of overall health services used in comparison to those who did not receive group consultation. These consultations were held on a monthly basis with a physician and a nurse. Sessions provided patient education, as well as discussion on prevention, socialization, and support. They also provided the opportunity for one-on-one consultation, as needed (Beck et al., 1997). Lastly, sustained follow-up ensures continued patient care in a timely, appropriate manner. This allows for better flow and can ensure patient compliance and/or the possibility of treatment failure. Follow-up care for chronic illness is best with routine, scheduled appointments; however, telephone follow-up by team members has also been shown to be effective in treatment of chronic diseases (Wagner, 2000).

The Chronic Care Model (CCM), developed by the Group Health Cooperative of Puget Sound, Washington, provides six elements that are used to address chronic illness care. Delivery system design, self-management support, decision support, clinical information system, community resources and policies, and health care organizations are used to provide guidance and optimal care for chronic illness management. As is similar to Wagner (2000), this six-element model also uses a team approach as defined in the delivery system design. This allows for altering of the "normal" structure of practice while allowing each subspecialty provider to have a distinct role in the treatment of chronic illness.

Self-management support, as described by Wagner (2000), encourages the patient to take an active role in his or her own treatment. Decision support is the use of evidence-based practice guidelines in the daily and long-term treatment plans. The clinical information system utilizes technology to ensure guidelines are met and to promote performance quality. Community resources and policies serve as the connection between the provider, patient, and specialty services. These services could include coordinating home care, food services, physical therapy or rehabilitation, and/or clinical appointments. The six-element, health care organization identifies chronic care as a priority. This element strives to provide continuous quality health care improvement (Boville, Saran, Salem, Clough, & Jones, 2007).

> **QUICK TIPS—WAGNER (2000) STRATEGIES FOR CHRONIC ILLNESS MANAGEMENT**
>
> - Population-based care
> - Treatment planning
> - Evidence-based clinical management
> - Self-management support
> - More effective consultations
> - Sustained follow-up

> **QUICK TIPS—CHRONIC CARE MODEL (CCM)**
>
> - Delivery system design
> - Self-management support
> - Decision support
> - Clinical information system
> - Community resources and policies
> - Health care organization

There are many models that exist in regards to treatment of chronic illness. Many models have slight differences; however, all of them are intended to provide guidelines for treatment and management of chronic illness. The Strategies for Chronic Illness Management Model and the CCM have similarities and have been in use for years. There is no one set of standards or guidelines that exist to treat chronic disease. The APN must use a combination of models and find what works best for him or her. There is commonality among a majority of the models that identifies that a team approach for treatment is the best. "It is becoming increasingly clear that care of chronic geriatric conditions is better when it's done in teams" (Rivero, 2013, n.p.).

Many studies have examined the team approach in regards to doctors versus nurse practitioners (NPs). A recent study examines the team approach of geriatricians and NPs to comanage care of the chronic illness in the primary care setting. Researchers screened a total of 1,084 patients in two primary care facilities in Southern California. Of these patients, 658 had at least one chronic condition (falls, urinary incontinence, dementia/Alzheimer's disease, or depression). Of the 658 patients, 485 were randomly selected for the medical review. According to the study, NPs have spent more time on treatment of chronic disease in comparison to physicians. This study found that a higher percentage of patient quality measures were met by those who received care comanaged by an NP and a physician, compared with those seen by a physician alone. NPs were thought to be more detailed in regards to patient history taking and assessment. Limitations existed with any study and further research was recommended, including a longer time, more facilities taking part, and a larger geographic area (Rivero, 2013).

APNs play an integral role in management of chronic disease. Although obesity is not identified as a chronic disease, it coexists with these diseases. A team approach and routine follow-up are essential for long-term success.

REFERENCES

Academy of Managed Care Pharmacy. (2015). *Concept series paper on disease management*. Retrieved from http://www.amcp.org/WorkArea/DownloadAsset.aspx?id=9295

Beck, A., Scott, J., Williams, P., Robertson, B., Jackson, D., Gade, G., & Cowan, P. (1997). A randomized trial of group outpatient visits for chronically ill older HMO members: The Cooperative Health Care Clinic. *Journal of the American Geriatrics Society*, 45, 543–549.

Boville, D., Saran, M., Salem, J. K., Clough, L., & Jones, R. R. (2007). An innovative role for nurse practitioners in managing chronic disease. *Nursing Economics*, 25(6), 359–364.

Rivero, E. (2013). *Nurse practitioners can help boost quality of care for older patients with chronic conditions*. UCLA Newsroom. Retrieved from http://newsroom.ucla.edu/releases/nurse-practitioners-can-significantly-246956

Wagner, E. H. (2000). The role of patient care teams in chronic disease management. *British Medical Journal*, 320(7234), 569–572.

Obesity-Related Diseases

This chapter addresses common diseases associated with obesity and focuses on how to treat these conditions in the overweight or obese patient. These diseases include hypertension (HTN), dyslipidemia, cardiovascular disease (CVD), diabetes mellitus (DM), obstructive sleep apnea (OSA), osteoarthritis (OA), polycystic ovary syndrome (PCOS), and metabolic syndrome. Many of these conditions are treated as per standard medical guidelines; however, the treatment plan must be individualized and tailored for each patient. With each new diagnosis or chronic disease treatment, primary approaches to weight loss should be considered as initial treatment. Again, these diseases are common in the overweight or obese patient; thus, first-line treatment must be aimed at weight loss and/or weight management. Many obese patients will have more than one of these diseases and require multiple medications. Dual-purpose medications, especially those that are "weight-neutral," are preferred to ensure better medication and treatment compliance without the worry of additional weight gain.

Obtaining a thorough, accurate, and current medical history, as well as a past patient medical history, is essential when treating the patient and examining his or her comorbid conditions. First, one should inquire about how long the condition has been present. This will aid in determining the treatment approach. Second, one should ask about associated symptoms that may exist with the medical condition. One should inquire about weight history in relation to the disease as well as ask about sedentary lifestyle, physical activity, and tobacco abuse. Asking about dietary intake is also essential in order to assess for needed dietary changes. One should inquire about sodium, saturated fat, and cholesterol consumption as well as about alcohol and caffeine. One should examine the use of any previous medications, including any use of illegal drugs. It is also essential to obtain a complete and accurate medication list from the patient and/or pharmacy for further evaluation and accurate treatment. Stress or psychological conditions must also be examined, as these too can aid in weight gain. Lastly, inquiring about the patient's family history of any current conditions or past medical history is essential.

HYPERTENSION

The more the patient weighs, the more likely he or she is to have HTN. This is due to the fact that overweight or obese patients require more blood volume to supply the extra tissue. Sleep apnea, physical inactivity, alcohol intake, smoking, polycythemia vera, and hyperuricemia are also risk factors associated with HTN (Nixon, 2011). According to the Centers for Disease Control and Prevention

(CDC), nearly 67 million or one in three adults are diagnosed with HTN. Fifty-three million of those adults are aware of their HTN, whereas only 47 million are being treated. Out of those 67 million adults with HTN, only 31 million are considered to have controlled blood pressure. (Centers for Disease Control and Prevention [CDC], 2012).

Basics

HTN is defined as "a common disorder characterized by elevated blood pressure (BP) persistently exceeding 149/90 mmHg" (Mosby's Medical, Nursing, & Allied Health Dictionary, 2002, p. 849). According to the Joint National Committee on Prevention, Detection, Evaluation, and Treatment of High BP (Seventh Report of Joint National Committee [JNC-7]; National Institutes of Health National Heart, Lung, and Blood Institute [NIHNHLBI], 2004), *normal BP* is defined as systolic BP (SBP) less than 120 mmHg and diastolic BP (DBP) is less than 80 mmHg. *Prehypertension* is defined as an SBP ranging from 120 to 139 mmHg and a DBP ranging from 80 to 89 mmHg. *Stage I HTN* is defined as an SBP ranging from 140 to 159 mmHg and a DBP ranging from 90 to 99 mmHg. *Stage II HTN* is defined as an SBP greater than 160 mmHg and a DBP greater than 100 mmHg (National Institutes of Health National Heart, Lung, and Blood Institute [NIH-NHLBI], 2004).

New guidelines from the 2014 Evidence-Based Guidelines for the Management of High BP in Adults' Report From the Panel Members Appointed to the Eighth Joint National Committee (JNC8) were released in December 2013 and published in *The Journal of the American Medical Association (JAMA)* in February 2014. Various medical groups speculated about what changes might appear in the updated guidelines, although they felt the cutoff definition of *HTN* would remain 140/90, based on the European Society of Hypertension/European Society of Cardiology (ESH/ESC) 2013 guidelines. The National Institute for Health and Clinical Excellence (NICE) 2011 guidelines maintained the same cutoff as previously listed; however, they also recommended confirming the clinic BP with an ambulatory reading or home BP measurement. Speculations arose as to not only the BP cutoffs but also the recommendations for those in special populations, including DM, chronic kidney disease (CKD), coronary artery disease (CAD), heart failure (HF), peripheral arterial disease (PAD), and those older than age 80 (Davis, 2013). Table 16.1 addresses BP recommendations from JNC7 and ESH/ESC.

JNC8 consists of nine guidelines for the treatment of HTN. Recommendation 1 focuses on treatment of the patient older than or equal to 60 years. Pharmacological treatment should be initiated for those with an SBP less than 150 mmHg or a DBP less than 90 mmHg. Recommendation 2 concentrates on the patient younger than 60 years. Pharmacological treatment should be initiated for those with a DBP greater than or equal to 90 mmHg. Treatment goals should work to reduce a DBP less than 90 mmHg. Recommendation 3 focuses again on the patient less than 60 years. An SBP greater than or equal to 140 mmHg should be given pharmacological therapy with a goal of less than 140 mmHg. Recommendation 4 discusses the patient with CKD who is older than or equal to 18 years. Pharmacological treatment should be aimed at reducing the patient's SBP to less than 140 mmHg and DBP to less than 90 mmHg. Recommendation 5 addresses the patient older than or equal to 18 years with DM. Treatment recommendations are identical to those in recommendation 4—those patients with CKD (treatment to reduce SBP to less than 140 mmHg and DBP to less than 90 mmHg). Recommen-

TABLE 16.1

CLASSIFICATION OF HTN			
Classification of BP	SBP (mmHg)[a]	DBP (mmHg)[a]	Treatment Recommendations
Normal[b]	Less than 120	Less than 80	Continue healthy eating habits and exercise therapy. Monitor BP on a routine basis.
Prehypertension[b]	120 to 139	80 to 89	Monitor sodium intake; consider dietary approaches to stop HTN-DASH diet. Moderate physical activity and stop smoking. Limit alcohol consumption. Conduct routine medical follow-up.
Stage I hypertension[b]	140 to 159	90 to 99	Continue earlier suggested recommendations and medication therapy.
Grade 1[c]	140 to 159	90 to 99	Continue earlier suggested recommendations and medication therapy.
Stage II hypertension[b]	Greater than or equal to 160	Greater than or equal to 100	Continue earlier suggested recommendations and medication therapy.
Grade 2[c]	160 to 179	100 to 109	Continue earlier suggested recommendations and medication therapy.
Grade 3[c]	Greater than or equal to 180	Greater than or equal to 110	Continue earlier suggested recommendations and medication therapy.

BP, blood pressure; DASH, Dietary Approaches to Stop Hypertension; DBP, diastolic blood pressure; HTN, hypertension; SBP, systolic blood pressure.
[a]Millimeters of mercury.
[b]JNC-7 Recommendations for hypertension.
[c]ESH/ESC 2013 Recommendations for hypertension.

dation 6 discusses initial pharmacological treatment. "In the general nonblack population, including those with diabetes, initial antihypertensive treatment should include a thiazide-type diuretic, calcium channel blocker (CCB), angiotensin-converting enzyme inhibitor (ACEI), or angiotensin receptor blocker (ARB)" (James et al., 2014). Recommendation 6 addresses the non-Black population, whereas recommendation 7 addresses the general Black population. Treatment of HTN, including those with DM, should be given with either a thiazide-type diuretic or CCB serving as first-line treatment. Recommendation 8 is as follows: "In the population aged ≥18 years with CKD, initial (or add-on) antihypertensive treatment should include an ACEI or ARB to improve kidney outcomes. This applies to all CKD patients with HTN regardless of race or diabetes status" (James et al., 2014). Recommendation 9, the last recommendation, discusses the main objective of HTN treatment—to attain and maintain adequate BP. The patient should be seen, and BP should be checked within 1 month of treatment. If the goal of BP is unattained, a second drug should be added from the list given earlier. If the goal cannot be reached with two drugs, a third should be added (again from the earlier list). An ACEI and ARB should not be used together. If more than three drugs are needed to reach the goal of BP, other classes of antihypertensive medications as well as referral to an HTN specialist could be considered (James et al., 2014).

Left untreated, HTN is commonly associated with CAD, myocardial infarction (MI), congestive heart failure (CHF), arrhythmias, cerebral vascular accident (CVA) or transient ischemic attacks (TIAs), carotid artery disease, PAD, renal failure, retinopathy, and aneurysms.

Pathophysiology

HTN is thought to be caused by an increased total peripheral resistance due to arteriolar constriction. This is because of the inappropriate retention of salt and water by the renal system or an increase in cardiac output. Other causes could be the regulation of body fluid volume or the renin–angiotensin system. Primary or essential HTN, considered the most common type of HTN, is not defined by one identifiable cause; however, it is commonly linked to obesity and sedentary lifestyle. Some estimate that greater than 90% to 95% of HTN falls into this category. Family history of HTN and dyslipidemia are also possible associated causes (Mosby's Medical, Nursing, & Allied Health Dictionary, 2002; Widmaier, Raff, & Strang, 2006).

Less than 5% to 8% of the adult population has an identifiable cause of their HTN. This is referred to as secondary HTN. Three causes of secondary HTN are vasoconstriction due to the increase in catecholamines, the renin–angiotensin cascade, or expansion of blood volume secondary to retention of sodium and water (Uphold & Graham, 2003). Secondary HTN could be caused by any of the following: acute stress, vascular disorders, dissecting aortic aneurysm, endocrine disorders, neurological disorders, problems with pregnancy, renal disorders, medications, severe anemia, and/or tyramine-containing foods (beer or wine, chicken, liver, yeast extract, and/or an aged cheese; Uphold & Graham, 2003).

After primary or secondary HTN is diagnosed, identification of cardiovascular risk factors and assessment of presence or absence of target organ damage should take place. Cardiovascular risk factors include HTN, DM, age (men older than or equal to 55 years and women older than or equal to 65 years), elevated total cholesterol or low-density lipoprotein (LDL) or low high-density lipoprotein (HDL), estimated glomerular filtration rate (GFR) less than 60 mL/min, microalbuminuria, obesity, physical inactivity, family history of premature CVD (men less than 55 years and women less than 65 years), and tobacco abuse. Target organ damage to the heart could include the following: angina, prior MI, HF, prior coronary revascularization, and/or left ventricular hypertrophy (LVH). Damage to the brain such as dementia, TIA, or stroke could also be a result of HTN. CKD, retinopathy, and peripheral vascular disease (PVD) are other complications of longstanding HTN (NIHNHLBI, 2004).

Signs and Symptoms

Many patients with HTN are asymptomatic; however, some symptoms can include headache, dyspnea, edema, angina, lightheadedness or syncope, tinnitus, and palpitations.

Diagnostic Tests

A new diagnosis of HTN must be obtained by two or more BP measurements in a seated position. The measurements should occur after at least 5 minutes of rest. The patient should be seated in a chair with both feet on the floor and the arm supported at the level of the heart. For an accurate reading, no smoking or intake of caffeine should occur within 30 minutes of the BP being taken. Appropriate cuff fit should also be evaluated with at least 80% of the bladder of the BP cuff encircling the patient's arm.

When there is difficulty obtaining an accurate BP reading, an ambulatory BP monitoring should be considered. This is frequently used to aid in an accurate diagnosis of HTN, especially with those considered to have "white-coat" HTN, nocturnal pressure changes, hypotensive symptoms, and/or drug resistance. Another form of measuring BP is by self-monitoring. The patient should be instructed to keep track of the measurements throughout different times during the day. A BP more than 135/88 mmHg recorded at home is considered HTN.

Other diagnostic tests before medication therapy should include the following laboratory data: basic metabolic panel (BMP), complete blood count (CBC), and lipid panel. An electrocardiogram (EKG) and urinalysis should also be considered. If secondary causes of HTN are being considered, ordering additional labs such as thyroid-stimulating hormone (TSH), erythrocyte sedimentation rate (ESR), glycosylated hemoglobin (HgA1c), C-reactive protein (CRP), uric acid, creatinine clearance, and brain natriuretic peptide (BNP) can prove helpful in proper diagnosis. A 24-hour urine and microalbumin can also determine proper diagnosis. Radiology tests, including a vascular angiogram, CT scan, and/or ultrasound, could identify suspected organ involvement. Lastly, a graded treadmill stress test and ECG could identify any cardiac involvement (Uphold & Graham, 2003).

Treatment

First-line treatment of HTN includes lifestyle modification. One such modification is weight loss or aiming for a normal body mass index (BMI). Second, it is important to talk to one's patient about reducing sodium intake. One should consider the DASH diet (Table 16.2) for teaching one's patient about low sodium foods, whole grains, a high intake of fruits and vegetables, low-fat dairy, and reduced consumption of saturated fat. Recommendations for sodium intake are approximately 2,400 mg of sodium or 6,000 mg of sodium chloride per day. Also, initiating exercise is essential. One should remember to start slow in exercise therapy. Lifestyle modification also includes encouraging smoking cessation. This may provide extra stress, as many times food can be a substitute for cigarettes. Having a plan for smoking cessation will aid in further stress reduction. Lastly, patients should be educated to limit alcohol consumption.

Medication treatment is also essential in the treatment of HTN. When deciding what medication is best, there are many considerations. Comorbid conditions DM, HF, CKD, post-MI, stable angina, acute coronary syndrome (ACS), and recurrent stroke prevention should be considered with selection of an antihypertensive agent. The elderly population as well as the African American population should also be considered when selecting treatment.

TABLE 16.2

DASH DIET	
Food	**Recommended Servings**
Grains	Six to eight servings daily
Fruits	Four to five servings daily
Vegetables	Four to five servings daily
Dairy	Two to three servings daily
Meats, poultry, and fish	Two or fewer or six ounces or less daily
Nuts, seeds, and legumes	Four to five times per week
Fats and oils	Two to three servings daily
Sweets	Five or less per week

DASH, Dietary Approaches to Stop Hypertension.

Thiazide diuretics are the first line of treatment in HTN. ACEIs, ARBs, and CCB therapies are recommended for use in the JNC8 guidelines given earlier. Renin inhibitors, beta blockers (BBs), alpha blockers, alpha-beta blockers, central acting agents, and vasodilators can be used if the previous medications are unable to control BP (Uphold & Graham, 2003).

Patient Education

It is important to educate the patient on the significance of routine BP monitoring and follow-up. This includes education on low sodium foods and appropriate exercise therapy. The patient should also be instructed on what signs and symptoms to monitor for. Medication compliance, including the importance of dosing and timing of medications, is essential. Lastly, the patient should be educated on the comorbid conditions of untreated HTN. This helps them understand why appropriate treatment is crucial.

QUICK TIPS FOR HTN

Symptoms: Headache, dyspnea, edema, angina, tinnitus, lightheadedness, syncope, and palpitations

- **Prehypertension: 120-139/80-89**

Consider medical treatment **aimed at weight loss** and DASH dietary changes

- **HTN: 140-159/90-99**

Medication therapy: Thiazide diuretics, ACE, ARB, BB, CCB, alpha blockers, alpha-beta blockers, central acting agents, and vasodilators

DYSLIPIDEMIA

Almost as common as HTN is dyslipidemia. The overweight and obese patient is at an increased risk for development of dyslipidemia. As many as 12.9% of adults in the United States have been diagnosed as having elevated total cholesterol (Carroll, Kit, Lacher, & Yoon, 2012). Smith (2007) states that more than 100 million Americans have total cholesterol levels higher than 200 mg/dL.

Morbidity and mortality in those with dyslipidemia is also very high secondary to the high relation to coronary heart disease (CHD). More than 4 million deaths per year are associated with dyslipidemia as well as with more than half the cases of ischemic heart disease (Smith, 2007). Those with a past medical history of any type of renal, liver, or vascular disease or those with DM, hypothyroidism, Cushing's syndrome, or immunological disease are at a higher risk of development of dyslipidemia (Uphold & Graham, 2003).

Basics

Dyslipidemia is defined as an "abnormality in, or abnormal amount of, lipids and lipoproteins, in the blood" (Mosby's Medical, Nursing, & Allied Health Dictionary, 2002, p. 561). Uphold and Graham (2003) also define this condition as an elevation of cholesterol and/or triglycerides. The Adult Treatment Panel (ATP) III classifies cholesterol levels into total cholesterol, LDL, and HDL. Desirable total cholesterol is less than 200 mg/dL, whereas borderline high is 200 to 239 mg/dL and greater than or equal to 240 is considered high. LDL cholesterol is separated into five categories: optimal, near or above optimal, borderline high, high, and very high. Optimal LDL is less than 100 mg/dL, whereas near or above optimal is 100 to 129 mg/dL. Borderline high is 130 to 159 mg/dL. High LDL is 160 to 189 mg/dL, and very high is greater than or equal to 190 mg/dL. HDL cholesterol has two categories: low and high. Low is considered less than 40 mg/dL, and high is defined as greater than or equal to 60 mg/dL.

Many diseases can contribute to the increased incidence of dyslipidemia. Obesity, DM, Cushing's syndrome, PCOS, hypothyroidism, lipodystrophies, anorexia nervosa, acute intermittent porphyria, uremia and nephrotic syndrome, obstructive liver disease, primary biliary cirrhosis, acute hepatitis, hepatoma, and systemic lupus erythematosus are such diseases. Other secondary factors that can contribute to this disease include stress; low activity levels; increased caloric intake; diets high in saturated fat, cholesterol, and increased carbohydrates; and increased alcohol consumption. Certain medications are also said to increase the incidence of dyslipidemia. These can include diuretics (thiazide and loop), BB, progestins, corticosteroids, anabolic steroids, and HIV protease inhibitors (Uphold & Graham, 2003).

Pathophysiology

Dietary cholesterol and cholesterol in the body are the two sources of cholesterol. Dietary cholesterol comes from the food we ingest, especially animal sources (see Table 16.3). Not all of the ingested animal sources are absorbed into the bloodstream. Some of this ingested cholesterol passes through the gastrointestinal system and is excreted through feces out of the body. Most cells in the body can produce their own cholesterol for their plasma membranes; however, not all of these cells can produce enough and thus rely on getting some from the blood cholesterol. The liver is the center for cholesterol synthesis. It is responsible for adding cholesterol to the bloodstream as well as for the removal of cholesterol that distributes it into the bile or creates bile salts. Hepatic synthesis is inhibited as increased amounts of cholesterol are ingested, whereas hepatic synthesis is stimulated when lower amounts of dietary cholesterol are consumed. Low levels of dietary cholesterol lead to a reduction of overall plasma cholesterol. As systemic cholesterol levels fall below a certain threshold, increased cholesterol production is initiated through intracellular processes. This action produces a negative feedback and is considered a primary reason as to why cholesterol is difficult to reduce by only dietary means. As part of the plasma cholesterol, LDL and HDL are also part of the lipoprotein complexes. Although LDL is considered a "bad" type of cholesterol, it is needed to bind to specific plasma membrane receptors for synthesis. The HDL is responsible for removing excess cholesterol, especially atherosclerotic plaque. It is essential to assess the total plasma cholesterol levels, but more important to look at the ratio of LDL to HDL. The risk of atherosclerotic heart disease is lower with an overall reduced ratio (Widmaier, Raff, & Strang, 2006).

Signs and Symptoms

As with HTN, most patients with dyslipidemia are asymptomatic. If severe dyslipidemia is present, the patient could present with early CHD, dermatological conditions, certain gastrointestinal conditions, aortic stenosis (AS), hyperinsulinemia, hyperuricemia, arthritis, Achilles tendinitis, and arcus cornea. Xanthomas may arise over areas of skin folds, the buttocks, or knees. Pancreatitis or severe abdominal pain, hepatomegaly, splenomegaly, or cholelithiasis may also be a result of severe hypertriglyceridemia. The patient should also be monitored for metobolic syndrome, which includes atherogenic dyslipidemia (Uphold & Graham, 2003).

Diagnostic Tests

A fasting lipid panel is used to diagnose dyslipidemia. This lab panel includes total cholesterol, LDL cholesterol, HDL cholesterol, and triglycerides. This test is recommended for all adults older than or equal to age 20. If normal, the recommendation is to be repeated every 5 years. Again, fasting is recommended; however, if this test is not done while the patient is fasting, only total cholesterol and HDL are considered valid. With the diagnosis of obesity, it is recommended that all patients be screened for dyslipidemia, no matter their age. If the patient has DM, HTN, is a current smoker, has an unknown family history, and is younger than age 20, screening with a fasting lipid panel is also recommended (Uphold & Graham, 2003).

Treatment

Risk reduction therapy is always recommended. It is aimed at reducing lifestyle risk factors and encourages therapeutic lifestyle changes (TLC). This includes reducing weight, increasing physical activity, and aiming at proper nutrition. These recommendations should be encouraged routinely even if the patient requires further medication treatment. Nutrition recommendations are shown in Table 16.3.

New dyslipidemia treatment guidelines were released by the American College of Cardiology (ACC) and the American Heart Association (AHA) in November

TABLE 16.3

CHOLESTEROL NUTRITION RECOMMENDATIONS			
Choose This	Recommended Servings	Examples	Choose This Only Occasionally
Fruits	Two to four servings	Fresh or frozen is best. Buy canned fruits in their own juice or lite syrup.	Avoid heavy syrup, creams, or fried food.
Vegetables	Three to five servings	Fresh or frozen is best. Buy canned vegetables low in sodium or sauce and rinse off with water.	Avoid creams, fried, or buttered food.
Grains	Greater than six servings	Whole wheat, oat, or corn. Whole grain or unsweetened cereal.	Cookies, cakes, pies, Danish croissants, muffins, biscuits, doughnuts, chips, crackers, buttered popcorn.
Dairy	Two to three servings	Skim or 1% mild. Low-fat yogurt, low-fat cottage cheese, low-fat cheese.	Whole milk, ice cream, heavy cream, cheese.
Meat	Less than six ounces per day	Fish, chicken, or pork. Lean cuts or loin cuts. Choose less beef. Lean meats.	Higher fat cuts of meat, sausage, hot dogs, salami, bologna, T-bone steak, fried meats, poultry with the skin, organ meats.
Fats	Sparingly	Choose unsaturated fats: olive oil, canola oil, vegetable oil, peanut oil. Nuts.	Butter, stick margarine, coconut oil.

2013. The guidelines allow for estimation of a patient's 10-year and lifetime risk for atherosclerotic cardiovascular disease (ASCVD). The downloadable spreadsheet can be found at: http://my.americanheart.org/cvriskcalculator and www.cardiosource.org/science-and-quality/practice-guidelines-and-quality-standards/2013-prevention-guideline-tools.aspx. Four major groups were identified in which the ASCVD risk reduction outweighs adverse effects. These groups are patients (a) with ASCVD, (b) with an elevation of LDL greater than 190 mg/dL, (c) aged 40 to 75 with diabetes, without ASCVD, and an LDL from 70 to 189 mg/dL, and (d) without ASCVD or diabetes but having an estimated 10-year ASCVD risk of greater than 7.5% and an LDL from 70 to 189 mg/dL.

The Expert Panel did not make recommendations for or against the use of target-specific LDL-C goals. The panel focused on four groups. Recommendations are made for secondary prevention as well as for primary prevention in those with an elevated LDL-C greater than or equal to 190 mg/dL, with and without DM, and LDL-C from 70 to 189 mg/dL. These guidelines differ from previous theories of thought that focused on specific LDL-C targets.

In secondary prevention, high-intensity statin therapy should be continued or initiated in people who have ASCVD and are older than 75 years. If high-dose statin therapy is contraindicated in these people, then moderate-intensity statin therapy should be considered. The risks versus benefits for this age group should also be reviewed, and the best treatment option should be discussed individually with the patient.

Patients older than or equal to 21 years with an LDL greater than or equal to 190 mg/dL should be screened for other causes of hyperlipidemia, that is, familial hypercholesterolemia. Those with triglyceride levels greater than or equal to 500 mg/dL should be screened as well. Both of these recommendations fall under primary prevention. High-intensity statin therapy should be used in these patients unless contraindicated. If the patient is unable to tolerate high-dose therapy, the maximum tolerated statin should be used. The goal of statin therapy should be at least a 50% reduction in LDL-C. Once the patient is maximized on statin therapy, addition of non-statin medication should be considered for risk reduction.

Primary prevention for those with DM and an LDL-C from 70 to 189 includes three recommendations. The first recommendation is for the use of moderate-intensity statin therapy. Adults aged 40 to 75 years are included. High-intensity statin therapy is recommended for those with DM and an ASCVD risk greater than or equal to 7.5%. For those outside the age range, the ASCVD score should be evaluated and the risks versus benefits to statin therapy should be weighed.

There are five recommendations under primary prevention for those without DM and an LDL-C from 70 to 189. Statin therapy initiation should be based on the ASCVD risk score for those without ASCVD to further determine therapy. Moderate- to high-intensity statin therapy should be used for adults aged 40 to 75 with an ASCVD risk score greater than or equal to 7.5%, without ASCVD and without DM. Moderate-intensity statin therapy should be used for those with an ASCVD risk score of 5% to less than 7.5%, without ASCVD or DM. Discussion should take place prior to initiation of statin therapy for those without ASCVD or DM to determine the best option for patient treatment. Lastly, a discussion should also take place as to possible treatment options for those patients who have an LDL-C less than 190 mg/dL and who are not otherwise in one of the categories mentioned earlier (Stone et al., 2013).

Statin dose references, including "high-intensity," "moderate-intensity," and "lower-intensity," are used throughout the guidelines. It is important to understand and differentiate, as these were derived from Critical Question 1 (CQ1) and Critical Question 2 (CQ2). The following medications fall under the treatment categories:

- High-Intensity Statins
  - Atorvastatin 40 (80) mg
  - Rosuvastatin 20 *(40)* mg
- Moderate-Intensity Statins
  - Atorvastatin 10 *(20)* mg
  - Rosuvastatin *(5)* 10 mg
  - Simvastatin 20 to 40 mg
  - Pravastatin 40 *(80)* mg
  - Lovastatin 40 mg
  - Fluvastatin XL 80 mg
  - Fluvastatin 40 mg BID
  - Pitavastatin 2 to 4 mg

- Low-Intensity Statins
  - Simvastatin 10 mg
  - *Pravastatin 10 to 20 mg*
  - Lovastatin 20 mg
  - Fluvastatin 20 to 40 mg
  - *Pitavastatin 1 mg*

Statins and doses listed in *italics* are approved by the Food and Drug Administration (FDA); however, they were not in the reviewed randomized controlled trials (RCTs) by the Expert Panel (Stone et al., 2013).

Statin therapy or HMG-CoA reductase inhibitors are recommended for patients as previously described. This class of medications is known for its LDL reduction. Chronic or active liver disease is a contraindication for this group of medications. Myalgias or myopathies are also a common patient complaint. Medication should be monitored with routine lipid and liver testing. Patients should be advised to report any side effects. Bile acid sequestrants, nicotinic acids, fibric acid derivatives, and ezetimibe are also used in treatment of dyslipidemia (Uphold & Graham, 2003).

Patient Education

It is important to educate patients on the significance of routine cholesterol monitoring and follow-up. This includes education on low cholesterol foods, exercise, and medication therapy. The patient should also be educated on the possible signs of muscle pain or myalgias. Again, medication compliance, including the importance of dosing and timing of medications, is essential. Lastly, the patient should be educated on the comorbid conditions associated with dyslipidemia.

QUICK TIPS FOR DYSLIPIDEMIA

Symptoms: Usually asymptomatic in presentation

- Desirable total cholesterol is less than 200 mg/dL
- Desirable LDL is less than 100 mg/dL
- Desirable HDL is greater than or equal to 60 mg/dL

Consider TLC: Reducing weight, increasing physical activity, and maintaining proper nutrition

Medication therapy: Statin therapy or HMG-CoA reductase inhibitors, bile acid sequestrants, nicotinic acids, fibric acid derivatives, and ezetimibe

---

CARDIOVASCULAR DISEASE

The overweight and obese patient is at a higher risk for CVD. CVD can include the following: atherosclerosis, rheumatic heart disease, cardiomyopathy, syphilitic endocarditis, and systemic venous HTN. This section focuses on atherosclerosis related to CAD and cardiomyopathy or HF.

Approximately one in every four deaths per year is related to heart disease—that is approximately 600,000 U.S. deaths each year. The leading type of CVD is CAD—which is responsible for 385,000 deaths per year. Present in both men and women, CAD is the leading cause of death in both sexes. Cost containment is another factor to consider when focusing on obesity prevention and treatment. The cost of CAD in the United States alone is more than $108 billion (CDC, 2013b).

In the United States, approximately 5.7 million people have been diagnosed with HF. In 2008, approximately 280,000 persons had HF listed as a contributing cause of death. The cost of HF is not as high annually as CAD; however, it still accounts for a total of more than $34 billion (CDC, 2013a).

Basics

CVD is defined as "any abnormal condition characterized by dysfunction of the heart and blood vessels" (Mosby's Medical, Nursing, & Allied Health Dictionary, 2002, p. 297). CAD refers to the narrowing of epicardial arteries related to atherosclerosis. Common risk factors of CAD include age, HTN, DM, hyperlipidemia, family history of CAD, and tobacco abuse. Other, less common risk factors include use of oral contraceptives, sedentary lifestyle, obesity, stress, and personality type (Uphold & Graham, 2003).

Cardiomyopathy is a condition that can weaken the heart muscle, characterized by left ventricular (LV) enlargement and/or right ventricular (RV) enlargement. In other words, the heart cannot pump enough blood and oxygen to supply the other body organs. Over time, it can cause a reduction of systolic LV dysfunction, progression of HF, and increased risk of sudden death. Dilated cardiomyopathy is the most common type; however, many potential etiologies exist with most being idiopathic in nature (Nixon, 2011). Heart failure with reduced ejection fraction (HFrEF) is also commonly known as HF with a poor systolic function and an ejection fraction (EF) of less than 40% to 50%, depending on the study.

Previously, HF with a normal LV function was referred to as diastolic HF; however, now it is called heart failure with preserved ejection fraction (HFpEF). HFpEF is diagnosed with a preserved LV systolic function and the presence of clinical HF symptoms. Diastolic dysfunction as evidenced by an ECG, change in cardiac biomarkers, or documentation by cardiac catheterization must also be present without any noted evidence of valvular disease. HTN, DM, ischemia aging, amyloidosis, sarcoidosis, idiopathic cardiomyopathy, hypertrophic cardiomyopathy, pericardial effusion, and constrictive pericarditis are common causes of diastolic dysfunction with HFpEF (Castro, n.d.).

It is important to recognize and report HF signs and symptoms through staging. The ACC/AHA developed the staging system to help reliably evaluate with objectivity. Stages A through D are used, but only stages C and D are used in supporting the clinical diagnosis of HF. These stages were first developed in 2001, but they were last revised in 2005. Stage A describes those at high risk for the development of HF. This includes not only those with a family history of cardiomyopathy but also those with risk factors. Risk factors include HTN, DM, CAD, metabolic syndrome, history of drug or alcohol abuse, and/or rheumatic fever. Stage B describes those with known systolic LV dysfunction, but no apparent HF symptoms. Stage C includes those with documented systolic LV dysfunction with HF symptoms, including shortness of breath, reduced exercise ability, or fatigue. Stage D encompasses those with the diagnosis of systolic HF with reduced LV function with the reoccurrence of symptoms even after optimal medical treatment.

The New York Heart Association Functional Classification (NYHA) is used as subjective information for providers. Because patients' symptoms with HF change frequently, so do their functional class. Stages I to IV describe the extent of HF symptoms. Stage I demonstrates no limitation in normal day-to-day activities. In stage II, patients demonstrate mild symptoms with activities. Stage III describes marked limitations with minimal activity whereas stage IV describes severe limitations, with symptoms present at rest (Uphold & Graham, 2003).

Pathophysiology

CAD is caused primarily by atherosclerosis of the coronary vessels. Atherosclerosis is caused by a thickening of the arterial wall due to an excess of macrophages and/or lymphocytes, cholesterol, or connective tissue. This plaque reduces the blood flow through the coronary arteries by causing increased resistance of flow. Also, the release of excess vasoconstrictors and deficient vasodilators at the atherosclerotic area hinders blood flow. Over time, progression occurs and at times leads to total occlusion. This is usually thought to be secondary to a coronary thrombosis and can lead to an MI. Because of the complexity of atherosclerosis, this progression is not totally understood. Damage to the endothelial tissue and proliferative and inflammatory response are thought to initiate a protective mechanism, but excess is thought to cause further injury. Overall, assessing and reducing risk factors is essential to eliminate any further incidence.

An inadequate cardiac output is noted in both HFrEF and HFpEF. HFrEF is a reduction in systolic function. This type of HF is caused by myocardial damage and results in a decrease in cardiac contractility and a reduction in stroke volume. Arterial baroreceptor reflexes also play a large part in reduced cardiac output. With HF, these baroreceptors are less sensitive and result in a fall in pressure, causing an increased heart rate and an increased total peripheral resistance. This is due to increased amounts of angiotensin II and vasopressin. If continued during a prolonged period, extracellular volume is present in the form of fluid retention. The kidneys then reduce their excretion of sodium and water, causing even more extracellular fluid and increased plasma volume. Decreased cardiac output causes an increase in venous pressure and end-diastolic ventricular pressure. Stroke volume is restored by the Frank–Starling mechanism.

As fluid retention continues, the LV becomes distended with blood, reducing the force of contraction. The elevation of venous pressure causes the capillaries to drain fluid to the veins. As venous pressure increases, so does the capillary pressure, causing increased interstitial fluid and an increase in peripheral edema. As with increased overall capillary pressure, the pulmonary capillary pressure, too, is increased, causing a filtration out into the pulmonary system. Thus, this increases the incidence of pulmonary edema (Widmaier, Raff, & Strang, 2006).

The pathophysiology of HFpEF is under continued investigation, as the etiology is still in question. The Ibersartan in HFpEF trial (I-PRESERVE) evaluated diagnostic ECG studies in an attempt to better understand this condition. This study demonstrated an increase in left atrium (LA) area, concentric LV remodeling, LVH, and diastolic dysfunction, which indicated structural remodeling. This study concluded similar results as those previously conducted (Castro, n.d.).

Reduced stroke volume due to abnormal relaxation and decreased passivity of the LV due to stiffness are two causes of diastolic dysfunction. During diastole, when the cardiac cycle is lengthened or incomplete, diastolic dysfunction occurs. Isovolumetric relaxation and early ventricular filling occur at the end of the systole. This is part of the active relaxation process. Calcium is removed from the cytosol, resulting in the initiation of the sarcoplasmic reticulum calcium ATP-ase (SERCA) pump. If part of the SERCA pump fails, so does the action of the LV. The SERCA pump is affected by several conditions: LVH, AS, ischemia, and hypothyroidism. Passive stiffness of the ventricle can occur with the aging process due to fibrosis or focal scarring after an MI. Because of this process, the diastolic pressure–volume relationship is affected, decreasing the stroke volume (Castro, n.d.).

Signs and Symptoms

To assess signs of CAD, one must look at the symptoms, complete a full assessment, and use diagnostic testing. One common symptom of CAD is chest pain. Chest pain or angina is usually midsternal and described as a pain, pressure, heaviness, fullness, tightness, burning, aching, or squeezing sensation. Patients may also complain of radiation of pain to the arm, neck, jaw, or back. Angina is usually related to exertion and relieved with rest. It can have accompanying symptoms such as shortness of breath or dyspnea on exertion (DOE), nausea, vomiting, diaphoresis, dizziness, and/or syncope or palpitations.

Signs of HF include peripheral edema, jugular vein distension (JVD), pallor, and/or cyanosis. Symptoms of HF include shortness of breath, DOE, paroxysmal nocturnal dyspnea (PND), or orthopnea. Other symptoms patients may complain of are fatigue, weakness, weight gain, and edema. A cough, dizziness, chest pain, or cold hands or feet may also be symptoms of HF (see Table 16.4 for a more thorough review of the signs and symptoms of HF).

Diagnostic Tests

When determining any new or underlying evidence of any CAD, it is important to get a baseline 12-lead EKG. This can determine if further testing is needed or if referral to cardiology is necessary. If the patient is having active chest pain, cardiac enzymes or biomarkers should be drawn. This would include a troponin, creatine kinase muscle brain (CKMB), and creatine kinase (CK) levels. A chest x-ray (CXR) is also used to further define the heart size. Prior to recommending the patient to exercise, a treadmill stress test may be beneficial to look for any underlying ischemia. Further stress testing, which can include a nuclear stress test, cardiac CT, or an angiogram, may be needed. An ECG may also be helpful to determine the patient's LV function (Uphold & Graham, 2003).

When examining a patient with HF, one should evaluate for any tachycardia, tachypnea, and/or JVD. A third or fourth heart sound—S3 or S4—can be present.

TABLE 16.4

HF—SIGNS AND SYMPTOMS	
HF Signs	**HF Symptoms**
Peripheral edema, JVD, pallor, cyanosis, tachycardia, hepatomegaly, hepatojugular reflux, abdominal ascities, respiratory problems, crackles, rales, S3 or S4	Shortness of breath, DOE, PND, orthopnea, fatigue, weakness, weight gain, weight loss, cough, frothy sputum, dizziness, syncope, chest pain, cold hands or feet, nausea, bloating, constipation, anorexia, nocturia

DOE, dyspnea on exertion; HF, heart failure; JVD, jugular vein distension; PND, paroxysmal nocturnal dyspnea.

The presence of lower-extremity edema, ascites, or diminished lung sounds should be documented. Laboratory testing should include CBC with differential, comprehensive metabolic panel (CMP), BNP, TSH, hepatic function, troponin, and lipid panel. Imaging should consist of a CXR and a 2-D ECG. The CXR can evaluate for any fluid overload or pulmonary vascular congestion. An ECG will help evaluate the LV and/or RV dilatation, identify the presence of any thrombus, and assess for any valvular regurgitation (Nixon, 2011).

Treatment

Treatment of CAD includes modifying risk factors and treatment of the comorbid conditions. As always, weight loss, nutritional recommendations, and exercise therapy should be encouraged. Aspirin should be used for primary prevention in all men older than the age of 55, women older than the age of 65, and anyone diagnosed with CAD unless contraindicated. One should consider BB, ACE, or ARB long-acting nitrates, and/or CCB therapy as per individual patient. The patient should also carry sublingual nitroglycerin for emergent angina as needed.

Treatment of both HFrEF and HFPER is aimed at symptom management with a goal to improve activities of daily living (ADLs). Pharmacological treatment of HFrEF is essential. One should work with the patient's cardiology provider to maximize medication. Treatment with BB, ACE, or ARB, diuretics, and digitalis is considered a first-line treatment. Additional medications, including spironolactone, potassium, hydralazine, and long-acting nitrates, may also prove beneficial. In patients with HFrEF, use of CCB should be avoided. The goal of treatment for those with HFpEF includes reducing the elevated filling pressures. This includes controlling heart rate, BP, blood volume, and ischemia to the myocardium (Uphold & Graham, 2003).

Patient Education

Patients with CAD should be educated on the importance to watch for any new change in symptoms. Anginal pain during exercise should be monitored, and nitroglycerin, as needed, should be used. One should refer back to cardiology for routine follow-up on an as-needed basis. Low-fat and low-cholesterol medications as well as routine activity should be encouraged. Also, referral to cardiac rehabilitation if the patient qualifies should be considered. The routine use of aspirin therapy and all prescribed medications should be encouraged. As patients lose weight, they should be monitored for hypotension and medications should be adjusted as needed. Also, smoking cessation should be encouraged.

Patients with HFrEF and HFpEF should be educated on the disease itself, symptoms to watch for, and the importance of medication therapy. The importance of daily weighing and weight loss in the obese patient should be stressed. Routine exercise and low-sodium foods should be encouraged. Fluid intake should be monitored. If weight increases by 2 to 3 pounds in less than 4 days, the patient should be advised to contact appropriate providers. If the patient feels more shortness of breath, he or she should be instructed to call the office. He or she should be encouraged to avoid tobacco and reduce alcohol consumption. Stress management should be taught. Patients should be taught to avoid medications that can cause exacerbation of HF. These include nonsteroidal anti-inflammatories, anti-arrhythmics, glucocorticoids, androgens, and estrogens (Uphold & Graham, 2003).

> ## QUICK TIPS FOR CVD—CAD
>
> **Symptoms:** Angina, shortness of breath, DOE, nausea, vomiting, diaphoresis, dizziness, syncope, and palpitations
>
> - **Diagnostic tests:** EKG, labs (troponin, CKMB, & CK), CXR, treadmill stress test, nuclear stress test, CT, ECG, and an angiogram
> - **Encourage weight loss**, foods low in fat and cardiovascular exercise
>
> **Medication therapy:** ASA; BB; ACE or ARB; long-acting nitrates; CCB; and sublingual nitroglycerin

> ## QUICK TIPS FOR CVD—HF
>
> **Signs and symptoms:** Shortness of breath, DOE, PND, orthopnea, fatigue, weakness, weight gain, edema, cough, dizziness, chest pain and cold hands or feet, peripheral edema, JVD, pallor, and cyanosis
>
> **Diagnostic tests:** CBC, CMP, BNP, TSH, hepatic function, troponin, lipid panel, CXR, and ECG
>
> - **Encourage weight loss** and low sodium diet
>
> **Medication therapy:** BB, ACE, ARB, diuretics, digitalis spironolactone, potassium, hydralazine, and long-acting nitrates

DIABETES MELLITUS

DM is on the rise, especially in overweight and obese individuals. The classification of DM includes type 1 diabetes mellitus (T1DM), type 2 diabetes mellitus (T2DM), gestational diabetes mellitus (GDM), impaired glucose tolerance (IGT), impaired fasting glucose (IFG), or other specific types of diabetes: genetic defects, diseases of the exocrine pancreas, endocrinopathies, drug- or chemical-induced diabetes, infections, immune-mediated diabetes, and certain genetic disorders (Uphold & Graham, 2003). This section addresses T2DM only in relation to the overweight or obese patient. Obesity, especially increased abdominal fat, increases a patient's chance for DM. According to the CDC (2011b), diabetes affects more than 11% of adults aged 20 and older. More than 7 million Americans do not even know that they have the disease. Alarming statistics indicate that by 2050, one in three Americans could have a diagnosis of diabetes, especially if unhealthy lifestyle trends continue. Recent studies show that the progression of T2DM could be slowed and even prevented with weight loss as well as with an exercise program. As little as a 5% to 7% weight loss could reduce the risk of DM by as much as 60% (CDC, 2011b).

Basics

DM is defined as "a complex disorder of carbohydrate, fat, and protein metabolism that is primarily a result of a deficiency or complete lack of insulin secretion by the beta cells of the pancreas or resistance to insulin" (Mosby's Medical,

Nursing, & Allied Health Dictionary, 2002, p. 511). Widmaier, Raff, and Strang (2006) also state that there is not a problem with the amount of insulin produced, but rather a lack of sensitivity in response to insulin. Micro- and macrovascular complications, such as retinopathy, nephropathy, neuropathy, and CVD, are seen in long-standing DM. Cognitive impairment, increased risk of infection, and digit contractures are also seen in DM (Uphold & Graham, 2003).

Pathophysiology

Obesity is a cause of T2DM. Excess weight places the patient at increased risk for insulin resistance due to the excess adipose tissue and muscle cells present. It is thought that the insulin is blocked because of the excess adipose tissue. This tissue causes downregulation of glucose transporters; thus, the insulin action is denied. Along with the insulin resistance, those with T2DM have defective beta cells that do not allow secretion of insulin in response to hyperglycemia (Widmaier, Raff, & Strang, 2006).

Signs and Symptoms

To assess the signs of T2DM, further testing should be considered. Many times, people with T2DM do not have noticeable symptoms. Polydipsia, polyuria, and polyphagia are the most common symptoms seen. Weight loss, fatigue, nausea, slow healing sores, yeast infections, or itching skin are other common symptoms of DM. Women with vaginal infections should also be checked for DM (American Diabetes Association [ADA], 2013).

Diagnostic Tests

Diagnostic criteria for DM include monitoring the patient for symptoms and identifying fasting plasma glucose (FPG) or assessing 2-hour plasma glucose. *FPG* is defined as a lab value greater than or equal to 126 mg/dL. An oral glucose tolerance test (OGTT) is performed using a 75-g anhydrous glucose load. A positive OGTT is a 2-hour plasma glucose greater than or equal to 200 mg/dL (Uphold & Graham, 2003). Glycosylated hemoglobin (HgA1c) is also used to determine 2- to 3-month glucose levels. The American Diabetes Association (ADA) recommends a level of 7% or less (ADA, 2013).

Patient examination should include height, weight, and orthostatic BP. A thorough skin examination, including assessing for the presence of acanthosis nigricans, eye examination, mouth and dental examination, thyroid palpation, complete neurological examination, and abdominal examination with assessment for liver enlargement, should also be completed. A complete cardiac examination as well as joint mobility testing should also be included. Lastly, a foot exam, including the use of Semmes–Weinstein monofilament, is essential (Uphold & Graham, 2003).

Treatment

First-line treatment for T2DM is initially aimed at weight loss and weight reduction through exercise and dietary modification. Exercise is thought responsible for an increased number of glucose transporters, thus reducing glucose levels. Patients should be recommended to have a dietary consult with a registered dietitian (RD). Patients could achieve weight loss of 1 pound per week by reducing total caloric intake by 500 calories daily. Dietary recommendations for weight reduction and weight loss of 1 to 2 pounds per week are provided in Chapter 13.

Another important tool for patients with DM is the glycemic index (GI). This determines how fast blood sugars rise. Foods with a high GI level (based on a score of 0 to 100) digest quickly and can cause blood sugars to rise. Low GI foods absorb at a slower rate, thus causing a slower rise in blood sugars. Combining portion size and GI provides an equation called glycemic load (GL). A number higher than 20 is a high GL, 11 to 19 is moderate, and less than or equal to 10 is considered low. The GL is calculated by taking the carbohydrate content of the serving multiplied by the food's GI, then divided by 100. GI is not the perfect system, but it provides a reference for nutrient-dense foods versus those higher in carbohydrates, allowing for better blood pressure control (Kimball, 2013).

There is no one specific diet for those with DM. It is important to monitor eating healthy to keep blood sugar levels as stable as possible. Eating routinely and regularly is important. Patients should be encouraged to eat three meals per day with appropriate snacks in between as needed. They should be encouraged to eat about the same portion size at each meal or snack. It is important to recommend dietary and nutrition advice from an RD, as they can help determine the appropriate amount of caloric intake, carbohydrate needs, and adequate servings from each food group. Educating patients on the exchange list and carbohydrate counting is also a vital part of patient education on DM. The exchange list utilizes six food groups: vegetables, fruits, meats, starchy foods, dairy, and fat. Foods can be "exchanged" for another food that has a similar content of carbohydrate, protein, and fats. Carbohydrate counting is essential to control blood sugar levels. Meeting with an RD will determine the number of carbohydrates appropriate for each patient and his or her specific dietary needs (Academy of Nutrition and Dietetics, 2012).

If these changes are unsuccessful, then medication therapy along with the recommended dietary and activity changes are encouraged. Oral therapy is usually initiated as a first-line medication therapy. Metformin, a biguanide, is considered a good medication for DM control, as it is a weight-neutral medication. Sulfonylureas, non-sulfonylurea secretagogues, alpha-glucosidase inhibitors, thiazolidinediones, combination sulfonylurea and biguanide, and combination thiazolidinedione and biguanide are other oral hypoglycemic agents. If single-agent therapy is not enough to sustain good blood sugar control, one should consider adding another

---

QUICK TIPS FOR T2DM

Symptoms: Polydipsia, polyuria, polyphagia, weight loss, fatigue, nausea, and slow-healing sores

- **Diagnostic tests:** FPG greater than or equal to 126 mg/dL, OGTT greater than or equal to 200 mg/dL, and HgA1c lesser than or equal to 7%
- **Encourage weight loss** and carbohydrate counting

Medication therapy: Biguanide, non-sulfonylurea secretagogues, alpha-glucosidase inhibitors, thiazolidinediones, sulfonylurea and biguanide, thiazolidinedione and biguanide, insulin, exenatide, and liraglutide

medication or consider a combination oral antidiabetic agent. If the combination oral antidiabetic agents fail, one should consider substituting insulin for one of the medications or add insulin in addition to the treatment plan (Uphold & Graham, 2003).

Incretin mimetics, including exenatide (Byetta and Bydureon) and liraglutide (Victoza), are given in the form of an injection, similar to insulin. This class of medication mimics glucagon-like peptide 1 (GLP-1). These medications are also known for their ability to suppress appetite and lead to weight loss. Appetite suppression is seen as food movement is delayed in the stomach before moving to the small intestine, thus producing a feeling of satiety (Collazo-Clavell, 2015).

Patient Education

Patients should be educated to look for signs and symptoms of hypoglycemia. One should consider referral to an RD for further dietary education. It is important for baseline information to include carbohydrate counting, the exchange list, GI, and GL. Patients should be encouraged to check blood sugars frequently, keep track of the levels, and bring in a record of this for review at each visit. Medication compliance should also be encouraged. Patients should also monitor for the presence of nonhealing wounds or foot ulcers and be instructed to report this as soon as noted.

OBESITY AND THE PULMONARY SYSTEM

This section focuses on the relationship between obesity and OSA. Obesity is one of the leading conditions associated with OSA. The word *apnea* is a Greek word that means "without breath." Obstructive, central, and mixed or complex sleep apnea are three types of sleep apnea (American Sleep Apnea Association, 2015). Those with a secondary pulmonary issue are more often affected. Untreated sleep apnea can lead to central sleep apnea (CSA), pulmonary failure, HTN—systemic or pulmonary, cardiac dysfunction—CAD, CHF, arrhythmias, decreased HDL, increased CRP, increased blood glucose, and increased homocysteine, CVA, and/or death. Differential diagnoses should include obesity-hypoventilation syndrome (Pickwickian syndrome) and tracheal stenosis. Neuromuscular disorders or parenchymal lung disorders should also be considered (Nixon, 2011).

Basics

OSA is defined as "a form of sleep apnea involving a physical obstruction in the upper airways" (Mosby's Medical, Nursing, & Allied Health Dictionary, 2002, p. 1208). This obstruction usually is caused by a prolapse of the tongue or soft palate (Nixon, 2011). This condition is usually marked by extreme fatigue and drowsiness, snoring, gasping or choking, and/or frequent interruptions in sleep with frequent awakenings. *CSA* is defined as "a form of sleep apnea resulting from decreased respiratory center output" (Mosby's Medical, Nursing, & Allied Health Dictionary, 2002, p. 318). The primary brainstem medullary depression is thought to be involved due to a loss of ventilator motor output (Mosby's Medical, Nursing, & Allied Health Dictionary, 2002; Nixon, 2011). These patients have a lower arterial carbon dioxide ($PaCO_2$) and oscillation of ventilation between apnea and hyperapnea (Nixon, 2011). Possible causes of the central apnea include idiopathic central hypoventilation, poliomyelitis, or a possible tumor of the posterior fossa (Mosby's Medical, Nursing, & Allied Health Dictionary, 2002).

The third type of sleep apnea, *mixed sleep apnea*, is defined as "a condition marked by signs and symptoms of both CSA and OSA" (p. 1111). This type of sleep apnea is thought to begin as a central form and develops into an obstruction; however, it may also be vice versa, starting as an obstructive form and developing into a central apnea. The latter is thought to occur as a result of hypoxia and hypercapnia (Mosby's Medical, Nursing, & Allied Health Dictionary, 2002).

Pathophysiology

Hypoxia occurs in OSA and is considered the main causative factor. Several mechanisms of action are seen as a result of the hypoxia, thus increasing one's risk for the development of CHF, which is both systolic and diastolic in nature. The hypoxia and hypercapnia can increase heart rate caused by the interaction of chemoreceptors and baroreceptor reflexes. Hypoxemia is also seen as a cause of nocturnal sympathetic activation. Ventricular transmural wall afterload is present due to increased intrapleural pressure. Stimulation of the parasympathetic nervous system is seen as bradycardia and asystole as a result of respiratory acidosis, hypoventilation, and hypoxemia. Lastly, proinflammatory and prothrombic factors are seen causing an increased risk for development of CVD (Nixon, 2011).

Signs and Symptoms

A large variety of signs and symptoms exist in sleep apnea. These can include snoring with periodic cessation of breath, frequent awakenings, excessive daytime sleepiness and fatigue, daytime somnolence, insomnia, morning headache, PND, Cheyne–Stokes respirations, nocturnal angina, and nocturnal desaturation. Obesity, lack of concentration, systemic or pulmonary HTN, right HF (cor pulmonale), and polycythemia may also be seen. Several types of cardiac arrhythmias also exist in sleep apnea. Sinus bradycardia, premature atrial contractions (PACs), atrial fibrillation, premature ventricular contractions (PVCs), and ventricular tachycardia (VT) can also be seen. CHF, ischemic stroke or TIA, and MI can also be detected with sleep apnea (Nixon, 2011).

Diagnostic Tests

Diagnostic tests can include an ambulatory overnight oximeter, which monitors the oxygen saturation while sleeping. An in-home portable monitoring system is available; however, the gold-standard treatment is still considered a formal laboratory polysomnography (PSG) or sleep study. Suggested laboratory testing can include arterial blood gases (ABGs), serum bicarbonate, hemoglobin and hematocrit, and BNP. An ECG may be done to assess for any evidence of severe pulmonary HTN, reduced RV systolic function, elevated pulmonary artery systolic pressure, tricuspid regurgitation, and/or right atrial enlargement (Nixon, 2011).

Treatment

No pharmacological therapy is available for treatment of sleep apnea. Again, a primary approach is aimed at weight loss, as this is a risk factor of OSA. "Consequently, maintenance of ideal weight and weight loss might be important strategies for the management of OSA, either together with other therapies or as stand-alone treatments" (Morgenthaler et al, 2006, p. 1031). Weight reduction, including successful dietary weight loss and/or consideration of bariatric surgery, is stressed as primary treatment. The Task Force and the Standards of Practice Committee recommend bariatric surgery, as it shows improvement in AHI and offers an alternative to positive airway pressure (PAP). Positional therapy is also recommended, as most obstructions occur in the supine position (Morgenthaler et al., 2006). Continuous positive airway pressure (CPAP) or nasal bilevel positive airway pressure (BiPAP) is also recommended for treatment. CPAP and BiPAP are recommended for routine nightly use, as they improve nocturnal oxygenation. They can improve EF and reduce pulmonary artery pressure. Improvement is noticed in BP, cardiac function, and quality of life (QOL). It is important for frequent follow-up with these patients to ensure compliance. Issues with claustrophobia, pressure intolerance, and fit should be addressed (Nixon, 2011). New PAP devices are equipped with humidifiers, usage monitors, apnea and hypopnea monitors, leak detection, and gradual pressure onset, also known as the "ramp" feature (Kushida et al., 2006). If not tolerated, low-flow oxygen administration via nasal cannula can be used. This is not considered effective for OSA, but is for hypoxia or CSA. Dental devices or oral appliances are also being utilized as a form of treatment for OSA. Most oral appliances are designed to advance the mandible and hold it forward with sleeping. Some oral appliances hold the tongue forward. All oral appliances have the goal of clearing the airway so it is not obstructed. Many of these devices are ordered and fitted through a dentist; however, some are "boil and bite," which can be done by the patient themselves at home (Ferguson, Cartwright, Rogers, & Schmidt-Nowara, 2006). Surgical options for OSA that are noncompliant with CPAP therapy can be considered. These options include tracheostomy, uvulopalatopharyngoplasty (UPPP), geniohyoid (jaw) adjustment, or laser palatoplasty (Nixon, 2011).

Patient Education

Patients should be educated about the importance of sleep hygiene. They should be encouraged to have a bedtime routine that includes going to bed at the same time and arising at the same time. Patients should be taught to avoid caffeine, alcohol, and nicotine before bed and to avoid eating prior to bed (CDC, 2013c). Nightly use of the CPAP or BiPAP therapy or dental device should be encouraged. Patients should be educated on the importance of treatment and routine follow-up in relation to the numerous comorbid conditions.

QUICK TIPS FOR SLEEP APNEA

Symptoms: Snoring, frequent awakenings, excessive daytime sleepiness, fatigue, daytime somnolence, insomnia, morning headache, PND, Cheyne–Stokes respirations, nocturnal angina, and nocturnal desaturation

- Types: OSA, central and mixed or complex sleep apnea
- Diagnostic tests: overnight oximeter, in-home monitoring system, and PSG
- **Primary treatment is aimed at weight loss**

Treatment: CPAP, BiPap, or dental devices

OSTEOARTHRITIS

OA is the most common form of chronic arthritis. This too is a disease associated with the increased incidence of obesity, as two in every three people who are obese are expected to have symptomatic knee OA. People identified as overweight and obese have more doctor-diagnosed OA at 66% (CDC, 2011a). Age is also a common factor associated with OA, as most people do not see symptoms until age 60 or older. The joints most affected include the distal interphalangeal (DIP), hip, and knees. The cervical and lumbar spine and first metacarpophalangeal can also be affected. Knee pain is the most common with hip pain reported as the most painful (Uphold & Graham, 2003). Currently in the United States, an estimated 50 million adults have been diagnosed with arthritis, with an estimated 27 million diagnosed with OA. This is expected to increase up to 67 million by the year 2030 (CDC, 2011a).

Basics

OA is defined as "a form of arthritis in which one of many joints undergo degenerative changes, including subchondral bony sclerosis, loss of articular cartilage, and proliferation of bone spurs (osteophytes) and cartilage in the joints" (Mosby's Medical, Nursing, & Allied Health Dictionary, 2002, p. 1242). There are several factors associated with the development of OA. These include chemical, mechanical, genetic, and metabolic. Age and occupational overuse are two conditions frequently associated with OA. Certain endocrine disorders, muscle weakness, and congenital musculoskeletal disorders also go along with OA. No general OA diagnostic criteria exist; however, certain criteria exist for the hip and knee. Patients should have a head-to-toe examination, including range of motion, palpation, and muscle strength testing. The patient's gait as well as site of pain should be examined. They should be assessed for any tenderness, edema, redness, and warmth (Uphold & Graham, 2003).

Pathophysiology

Articular cartilage that lines the joints is the beginning of a progressive breakdown. Marginal osteophytes are made as the bone is formed as the cartilage base, thus resulting in synovial inflammation (Uphold & Graham, 2003).

Signs and Symptoms

The pain associated with OA often presents gradually. Pain is usually worsened with physical activity and improved with rest. Swelling and redness may also be present over the joint site. Stiffness or crepitus as well as joint tenderness can be present. Heberden's nodes are present in some individuals. Bony cysts or subluxation may also occur (Uphold & Graham, 2003).

Diagnostic Tests

Basic lab work, including ESR, CBC, BMP, calcium, phosphorus, alkaline phosphatase, iron saturation, ferritin, and uric acid, should be drawn. A urinalysis should also be collected. X-rays of the affected joint should also be ordered (Uphold & Graham, 2003).

QUICK TIPS FOR OA

Signs and symptoms: Pain, swelling, redness, stiffness, crepitus, joint tenderness, Heberden's nodes, bony cysts, or subluxation

- **Encourage weight loss** with a combination of exercise and nutrition therapy

Medication therapy: Acetaminophen, Cox-2 selective NSAIDs, nonselective NSAIDs, Tramadol, and opioids

- **Other therapies:** Hot and cold, TENS, ultrasound therapy, total joint replacement, arthrodesis, osteotomy, bone removal procedures, and soft tissue procedures

Treatment

First-line treatment should be aimed at weight loss with a combination of exercise and nutrition therapy. A 50% reduction of OA in women can occur with 11 pounds lost (CDC, 2011a). Exercise recommendations include at least 30 minutes of activity most days of the week. Referral to physical or occupational therapy should be considered, especially if the patient is reducing activity levels. Low-impact activities that take pressure off the affected joint should be recommended. One should consider swimming or water activities to reduce joint impact. Supplements such as glucosamine and chondroitin can be considered. Pharmacological pain management is also important. Oral medications acetaminophen, COX-2 selective nonsteroidal anti-inflammatory drugs (NSAIDs), nonselective NSAIDs, Tramadol, and opioids are important for pain management as well as for reducing inflammation. Capsaicin 0.025% cream applied to the affected area may also provide pain relief. Hyaluronic acid (HA) viscosupplementation or intra-articular injection with corticosteroids are also used for pain treatment. Hot and cold therapy, transcutaneous electrical nerve stimulation (TENS), and ultrasound therapy may also prove beneficial for some patients. Surgery, including total joint replacement, arthrodesis, osteotomy, bone removal procedures, and soft tissue procedures, are also good options for patients. Referral to a surgeon should be considered if the patient is deemed a good surgical candidate; however, the patient must be educated that he or she may have a higher-than-usual risk for surgery due to obesity (Uphold & Graham, 2003).

Patient Education

Patient education should include a plan for weight loss. The importance of consistent and routine physical activity should be stressed. The patient should be educated to avoid strenuous activities that aggravate the affected site. Focus should be on low-impact activities. Appropriate pain management is necessary for better mobility. Lastly, referrals to physical and/or occupational therapies and surgery should be discussed with the patient to determine the best overall treatment plan.

POLYCYSTIC OVARY SYNDROME

This section focuses on PCOS in relation to obesity. Between 5% and 10% of women are affected with PCOS, whereas up to 80% of women with PCOS are obese (American College of Obstetricians and Gynecologists [ACOG], 2011; Pannill, 2002). This disease is seen in obese women and can cause infrequent (less than eight cycles per year) or persistent, long (less than 35 days) menstruation (Pannill, 2002). Acne and additional hair growth can also be seen. Although PCOS is primarily observed in obese women, this condition can also cause or further weight gain. Difficulty becoming pregnant may also be a first telltale sign of this disease. If pregnancy does occur, the patient is at higher risk for gestational DM or pregnancy-induced HTN. Those with untreated PCOS are at higher risk of other diseases. T2DM, HTN, dyslipidemia, and metabolic syndrome are common conditions reported. Elevated CRP, nonalcoholic steatohepatitis (NASH), and OSA are also seen. Endometrial cancer and abnormal uterine bleeding are seen as a result of elevated estrogen levels (Mayo Foundation for Medical Education and Research, 2011).

Basics

PCOS is defined as "the presence of hyperandrogenism (clinically and/or biochemically) and/or chronic anovulation in the absence of specific adrenal and/or pituitary disease" (Sheehan, 2004, p. 15). PCOS affects women during reproductive age due to a hormone disorder. This disease refers to the enlargement of the ovaries and the significant number of cysts on the outer edge, hence its "polycystic appearance" (Mayo Foundation for Medical Education and Research, 2011). Between 67% and 87% of the women diagnosed with PCOS have polycystic ovaries; however, polycystic ovaries are not necessary to complete the PCOS diagnosis. Differential diagnoses for an abnormal menstrual cycle could include rapid weight loss, low BMI, anorexia nervosa, extreme physical exertion, pregnancy, premature ovarian failure, post-pill amenorrhea, hypo- or hyperthyroidism, or a pituitary adenoma. Other causes could include Cushing's syndrome, a tumor of the adrenal gland or ovaries, or adrenal hyperplasia (Pannill, 2002).

Pathophysiology

The exact cause of PCOS is not known; however, insulin resistance, low-grade inflammation, heredity, and abnormal fetal development are seen in this condition. This condition is thought to start initially after menarche. Elevated luteinizing hormone (LH) is seen with PCOS; however, the cause of this elevation is not known. Neither the LH nor the insulin resistance can explain the PCOS; however, it is known that the elevation in LH and the increased insulin work together and cause ovarian growth and cyst formation as well as increased androgen creation. High levels of insulin are found in obese women compared with nonobese individuals; however, hyperandrogenism and oligo-ovulation or anovulation are seen in both groups (Pannill, 2002).

Signs and Symptoms

Initial signs and symptoms vary in severity and are usually seen at menarche; however, they are also seen in later years in response to weight gain. At least two of the following are needed for a diagnosis: menstrual abnormality, excess androgen, and/or polycystic ovaries. Menstrual abnormalities can include either the presence or absence of menstruation (Mayo Foundation for Medical Education and

Research, 2011). Infertility is also common. Hirsutism, acne, oily skin, and acanthosis nigricans can also be seen in those with PCOS (ACOG, 2011).

Diagnostic Tests

No one test can diagnose PCOS. A pelvic examination should be done as well as laboratory data drawn. Laboratory data include those tests performed for the underlying condition. TSH, prolactin, 17-hydroxyprogesterone (17OH-progesterone), total testosterone, luteinizing hormone/follicle-stimulating hormone (LH/FSH) ratio, and dehydroepiandrosterone-sulfate (DHEA-S) should be drawn to look for an underlying disorder or endocrinological condition. These tests as well as a pregnancy test should be done in every patient. A 24-hour urine-free cortisol should also be done if one suspects underlying Cushing's syndrome (Sheehan, 2004). Endometrial aspiration should be done to rule out endometrial carcinoma in any patient with persistent, sustained amenorrhea or oligomenorrhea (Pannill, 2002).

Treatment

Treatment is recommended to control the PCOS-associated conditions. Further treatment is recommended to control irregular menstruation, treatment of hirsutism, management of infertility, and management of insulin and/or T2DM. Weight loss is the first-line treatment recommended for those with PCOS. This is because even a small weight loss can help regulate menstruation.

Oral contraceptives and Metformin therapy are also used in treatment of irregular menstruation. Periodic progesterone withdrawal is also used in treatment of PCOS. Medroxyprogesterone in a 7- to 10-day course every 3 months is often given to ensure menstruation four times per year. Treatment of hirsutism is divided into two categories—biochemical and mechanical. Biochemical consists of two goals: decreasing testosterone production and action. Testosterone production is decreased by the use of oral contraceptives, progesterone withdrawal, metformin, and weight loss. Anti-androgens and weight loss are used to decrease testosterone action. Plucking, shaving, laser treatment, or electrolysis removal of excess hair is one of the mechanical treatments of hirsutism. Vaniqa cream can also be used. Medications used for management of infertility include clomiphene citrate (Clomid), metformin, and thiazolidinedione. Again, lifestyle modification and weight loss are recommended for treatment (Sheehan, 2004). An ovarian wedge resection was previously done for PCOS; however, it is not used any more. Now, ovarian

QUICK TIPS FOR PCOS

Signs and symptoms: Menstrual abnormality, excess androgen, and/or polycystic ovaries, hirsutism, acne, oily skin, and acanthosis nigricans

- **Diagnostic tests:** No one test can diagnose PCOS. A pelvic examination should be done. Laboratory data include those used to diagnose the underlying condition
- **Weight loss is first-line treatment**

Medication therapy: Oral contraceptives, metformin, medroxyprogesterone

drilling is a surgical procedure that involves cauterizing ovarian follicles, thus decreasing androgen production (Pannill, 2002).

Patient Education

Patient education includes proper identification and treatment of PCOS and its associated conditions. After a treatment plan is determined, the patient should be educated on the importance of medication and/or treatment compliance. Initial education should again focus on lifestyle modification, including good dietary and exercise choices aimed at weight loss.

METABOLIC SYNDROME

Metobolic syndrome is a cluster of risk factors associated with an increase of CVD and T2DM. Although these conditions increase the risk for CVD, it cannot assess overall risk. This condition is more common in certain ethnic groups, such as Native Americans, Hispanics, and Asians (Nixon, 2011). Metabolic syndrome increases with BMI and age (Ervin, 2009). Risk factors include childhood obesity, sedentary lifestyle, and poor dietary choices, including a diet high in fat and carbohydrates. Tobacco abuse, especially cigarette smoking, increases the risk of metabolic syndrome as does a family history of T2DM. NASH and OSA are two commonly associated conditions. Other conditions that often appear in combination with metabolic syndrome are PCOS, hyperuricemia, and primary hyperlipidemias (Nixon, 2011).

Basics

Metabolic syndrome is defined by a set of criteria, including abdominal obesity, dyslipidemia, elevated BP, insulin resistance, T2DM, a fasting blood glucose greater than or equal to 110 mg/dL, and a prothrombotic and proinflammatory state (Ervin, 2009; Uphold & Graham, 2003). Nixon (2011) provides a stricter number for fasting blood glucose at greater than or equal to 100 mg/dL. At least three or more of the criteria must be met for a diagnosis. *Abdominal obesity* is defined as a waist circumference greater than 102 cm and greater than 88 cm for men and women, respectively. Dyslipidemia includes the diagnosis of hypertriglyceridemia greater than or equal to 150 mg/dL and low HDL. A *low HDL* is defined as less than 40 mg/dL for a man and less than 50 mg/dL for a woman. *HTN* is defined as treatment with medication to control BP or a BP greater than or equal to 130/85 mmHg. Forty percent of people older than the age of 60 are affected with metabolic syndrome. The highest prevalence of metabolic syndrome—54.4%—is found in women older than the age of 60. Individual component contribution is also broken down into percentages. The highest component is abdominal obesity at 53%. HTN is the next highest at 40%, followed by hyperglycemia at 39%, then hypertriglyceridemia at 31%, and low HDL at 25% (Nixon, 2011).

Pathophysiology

The pathophysiology is not specific for metabolic syndrome itself, but rather for the multiple conditions that combine to make up this disease. HTN, dyslipidemia,

QUICK TIPS FOR METABOLIC SYNDROME

Symptoms: Specific for each individual component of the disease

- **Criteria:** Abdominal obesity, dyslipidemia, elevated
- BP, insulin resistance, T2DM, or a fasting blood glucose greater than or equal to 110 mg/dL, and prothrombotic and proinflammatory state
- Consider medical treatment **aimed at weight loss**

Medication therapy: Treatment focuses on the underlying causes

and insulin resistance with DM are explained in the previous sections under these specific conditions. Abdominal obesity is caused by an increased production of hormones involved in the inflammation process. Glucose and lipid metabolism are altered as a result of this. Also, the increase of free fatty acids due to heightened hepatic concentration upsurges hepatic glucose and lipoprotein production. Prothrombic changes, including amplified fibroinogen, plasminogen, activator inhibitor-1, asymmetric dimethylarginine, and endothelial dysfunction, are affected. Also seen are microabluminuria, low-grade chronic inflammation, and diminished fibrinolysis (Nixon, 2011).

Signs and Symptoms

Signs and symptoms are specific for each individual component of the disease. Please refer to each individual disease in the previous sections.

Diagnostic Tests

Diagnostic testing should be aimed at risk stratification for CVD. Lab work should include a fasting lipid profile, AST, ALT, ALP, uric acid, CRP, and microalbuminuria. OGTT should also be considered (Nixon, 2011). For further diagnostic testing for each specific condition, please review the diagnostic tests under the previous sections.

Treatment

Treatment focuses on the underlying causes. Treatment of lipids—including elevated triglycerides and low HDL—and HTN is essential. Aspirin is recommended to reduce the prothrombotic state (Uphold & Graham, 2003). General treatment measures should also focus on risk reduction of CVD. Lifestyle management goals include physical activity, dietary modification, and smoking cessation. Consider referrals to an endocrinologist, lipid specialist, or gastroenterologist, as needed (Nixon, 2011).

Patient Education

Patient education should be focused on lifestyle modification. Primary prevention is focused on early lifestyle changes, whereas secondary prevention is focused on the treatment and management of each of the risk factors and associated conditions.

It is important for the APN to have a thorough understanding of the disease associated with obesity. Treatment of these diseases is essential. The primary focus should be aimed at lifestyle modification, but some of these diseases will need further pharmacological management. The APN should monitor, address, and treat these diseases on an individualized patient basis.

REFERENCES

Academy of Nutrition and Dietetics. (2012). *Diabetes and diet.* Retrieved from http://www.eatright.org/Public/content.aspx?id=6813

American College of Obstetricians and Gynecologists (ACOG). (2011). *Frequently asked questions faq121 gynecologic problems polycystic ovary syndrome.* Retrieved from http://www.acog.org/~/media/For%20Patients/faq121.pdf?dmc=1&ts=20131130T1343398557

American Diabetes Association (ADA). (2013). *Living with diabetes: A1C and eAG.* Retrieved from http://www.diabetes.org/living-with-diabetes/treatment-and-care/blood-glucose-control/a1c

American Sleep Apnea Association. (2015). *Sleep apnea.* Retrieved from http://www.sleepapnea.org/learn/sleep-apnea.html

Carroll, M. D., Kit, B. K., Lacher, D. A., & Yoon, S. S. (2012). Total and high-density lipoprotein cholesterol in adults: National health and nutrition examination survey, 2011–2012. Centers for Disease Control and Prevention. Retrieved from http://www.cdc.gov/nchs/data/databriefs/db132.pdf

Castro, R. (n.d.). *Heart failure with preserved ejection fraction (HFpEF).* American Association of Heart Failure Nurses, 1–16.

Centers for Disease Control and Prevention (CDC). (2011a). *Arthritis-related statistics.* Retrieved from http://www.cdc.gov/arthritis/data_statistics/arthritis_related_stats.htm

Centers for Disease Control and Prevention (CDC). (2011b). *Get the facts on diabetes.* Retrieved from http://www.cdc.gov/features/diabetesfactsheet

Centers for Disease Control and Prevention (CDC). (2012). *Getting blood pressure under control.* Retrieved from http://www.cdc.gov/vitalsigns/Hypertension/index.html

Centers for Disease Control and Prevention (CDC). (2013a). Division for heart disease and stroke prevention: Heart failure fact sheet. Centers for Disease Control and Prevention. Retrieved from http://www.cdc.gov/dhdsp/data_statistics/fact_sheets/fs_heart_failure.htm

Centers for Disease Control and Prevention (CDC). (2013b). *Heart disease: Heart disease facts.* Retrieved from http://www.cdc.gov/heartdisease/facts.htm

Centers for Disease Control and Prevention (CDC). (2013c). *Insufficient sleep is a public health epidemic.* Retrieved from http://www.cdc.gov/features/dssleep

Collazo-Clavell, M. (2015). *Diseases and conditions: Tell me about the diabetes drugs Byetta, Victoza and Bydureon. Can they really help people who have diabetes lose weight? Are there side effects?* Retrieved from http://www.mayoclinic.org/diseases-conditions/type-2-diabetes/expert-answers/byetta/FAQ-20057955

Davis, L. L. (2013). Using the latest evidence to manage hypertension. *Journal for Nurse Practitioners, 9*(10), 621–628.

Ervin, R. B. (2009). Prevalence of metabolic syndrome among adults 20 years of age and over, by sex, age, race and ethnicity, and body mass index: United States, 2003–2006. *National Health Statistics Report, 13,* 1–8. Retrieved from http://www.cdc.gov/nchs/data/nhsr/nhsr013.pdf

Ferguson, K. A., Cartwright, R., Rogers, R., & Schmidt-Norwara, W. (2006). Oral appliances for snoring and obstructive sleep apnea: A review. *Sleep, 29*(2), 244–262.

James, P. A., Oparil, S., Carter, B. L., Cushman, W. C., Dennison-Himmelfarb, C., Handler, J., . . . Ortiz, E. (2014). 2014 Evidence-based guideline for the management of high blood pressure in adults report from the panel members appointed to the Eighth Joint National Committee (JNC8). *Journal of the American Medical Association, 311*(5), 507–520. doi:10.1001/jama.2013.284427

Kimball, M. (2013). *What is glycemic index? Academy of Nutrition and Dietetics.* Retrieved from http://www.eatright.org/Public/content.aspx?id=6442478158

Kushida, C. A., Littner, M. R., Hirshkowitz, M., Morgenthaler, I., Alessi, C. A., Bailey, D., . . . Wise, M. S. (2006). Practice parameters for the use of continuous and bilevel positive airway pressure devices to treat adult patients with sleep-related breathing disorders. *Sleep, 29*(3), 375–380.

Mayo Foundation for Medical Education and Research. (2011). *Polycystic ovary syndrome.* Retrieved from http://www.mayoclinic.com/health/polycystic-ovary-syndrome/DS00423

Morgenthaler, T. I., Kapen, S., Lee-Chiong, T., Alessi, C., Boehlecke, B., Brown, T., . . . Swick, T. (2006). Practice parameters for the medical therapy of obstructive sleep apnea. *Sleep, 29*(8), 1031–1035.

Mosby's Medical, Nursing, & Allied Health Dictionary. (2002). (6th. ed). St. Louis, MO: Mosby.

National Institutes of Health National Heart, Lung, and Blood Institute (NIHNHLBI). (2004). JNC 7 The seventh report of the Joint National Committee on Prevention, Detection, Evaluation, and Treatment of High Blood Pressure. NIH Publication Number 04-5230. Retrieved from http://www.nhlbi.nih.gov/guidelines/hypertension/jnc7full.htm

Nixon, J. V. (2011). *The AHA clinical cardiac consult* (3rd ed.). Philadelphia, PA: Lippincott Williams & Wilkins.

Pannill, M. (2002). Polycystic ovary syndrome: An overview. Topics in advanced practice. *Nursing eJournal, 2*(3). Retrieved from http://www.medscape.com/viewarticle/438597_1

Sheehan, M. T. (2004). Polycystic ovarian syndrome: Diagnosis and management. *Clinical Medicine and Research, 2*(1), 13–27.

Smith, D. (2007). Epidemiology of dyslipidemia and economic burden on the healthcare system. *American Journal of Managed Care, 6*(13). Retrieved from http://www.ajmc.com/publications/supplement/2007/2007-06-vol13-n3Suppl/Jun07-2502pS69-S71/#sthash.adVJN9VA.dpuf

Stone, N. J., Robinson, J., Lichtenstein, A. H., Merz, C. N. B., Blum, C. B., Eckel, R. H., . . . Wilson, P. W. F. (2013). 2013 ACC/AHA guideline on the treatment of blood cholesterol to reduce atherosclerotic cardiovascular risk in adults: A report of the American College of Cardiology/American Heart Association task force on practice guidelines. *Circulation.* Retrieved from http://circ.ahajournals.org/content/early/2013/11/11/01.cir.0000437738.63853.7a.citation

Uphold, C. R., & Graham, M. V. (2003). *Clinical guidelines in family practice* (4th ed.). Gainesville, FL: Barmarrae Books.

Widmaier, E. P., Raff, H., & Strang, K. T. (2006). *Vander's human physiology: The mechanisms of body function* (10th ed.). New York, NY: The McGraw-Hill Companies.

Obesity-Related Diseases: A Pediatric Focus

This chapter addresses obesity-related diseases found in pediatric patients. These diseases can be found in childhood or place the individual at high risk in adulthood. Immediate health effects of obesity can include hypertension (HTN), hypercholesterolemia, prediabetes or diabetes, bone or joint problems, obstructive sleep apnea (OSA), pseudotumor cerebri, and social or psychological problems. Such social or psychological problems could include poor self-esteem or stigmatization. Long-term diseases can include cardiovascular disease (CVD), type 2 diabetes mellitus (T2DM), cerebral vascular accident (CVA), osteoarthritis (OA), and/or several forms of cancer: for example, breast cancer, as well as cancer of the esophagus, thyroid, kidney, pancreas, gallbladder, colon, endometrium, ovary, cervix, or prostate. Overweight or obesity can also place a child at higher risk for multiple myeloma or Hodgkin's lymphoma (Centers for Disease Control and Prevention [CDC], 2014).

The incidence of metabolic syndrome is as high as 50% in adolescents with a body mass index (BMI) greater than 40.6 kg/m^2 and is 4.2% among 12- to 19-year-olds in the United States. Obese pre- or mid-pubertal girls have a higher increase in hyperandrogenemia, hyperinsulinism, and polycystic ovary syndrome (PCOS). Focal segmental glomerulosclerosis (FSGS) is also more common in obese adolescents and may lead to end-stage renal disease (ESRD).

Nonalcoholic fatty liver disease (NAFLD) affects primarily alanine aminotransferase (ALT) with an estimated 10% to 25% of obese pediatrics at risk for elevated ALT. NAFLD affects up to 52% of all obese children. NAFLD increases the child's risk for progression of cirrhosis. An increased incidence of gallstones is also seen in obese children. This increased incidence of gallstones also correlates with metabolic syndrome and hyperinsulinemia. Rapid weight loss can also increase one's risk for gallstones.

Growth, musculoskeletal health, and bone health are also affected by pediatric obesity. The pediatric patient is also at risk for spondylolisthesis, scoliosis, OA, slipped capital femoral epiphysis, genu valga, tibia vara (Blount disease), flat kneecap pressure or pain, and flat foot (August et al., 2013).

There are many comorbid conditions that can coexist with obesity; however, this chapter only addresses the following top five diseases found in pediatric obesity: HTN, dyslipidemia, T2DM, OSA, and asthma.

HYPERTENSION

HTN is a serious disease in overweight and obese children. If left untreated, it can lead to complications later in childhood or progress into adolescence and adulthood. Evidence has shown that elevated blood pressure (BP) and HTN in childhood are precursors to the disease in adulthood. Both prehypertension and HTN have been on the rise since 1990. Estimated at 14% in boys and 6% in girls from 2003 to 2006, prehypertension was seen in those aged 8 to 17 years. The prevalence of HTN is also present and estimated at 3% to 4% in children. One in three individuals with a childhood diagnosis of HTN is found to have accompanying target organ damage—most common left ventricular hypertrophy (LVH). "An analysis of the National Childhood Blood Pressure database found that 14% of adolescents with prehypertension developed elevated BP within 2 years" (George, Tong, Wigington, Gillespie, & Hong, 2014, p. 47).

Basics

When measuring a child's BP, there are several considerations used to determine a normal range. These include the child's age, height, and gender. Rather than expressing this range in systolic over diastolic numbers, the range is expressed as a percentile. Table 17.1 defines the different BP stages and ranges. Three categories are used to express percentages: normal BP, prehypertension, and HTN. The category of HTN is further divided into stage 1 HTN and stage 2 HTN. *Normal BP* is defined as systolic and diastolic readings less than the 90th percentile. *Prehypertension* is defined as systolic and/or diastolic pressures greater than or equal to the 90th percentile but less than the 95th percentile. In adolescents, *prehypertension* can also be defined as BP greater than 120/80 mmHg. *HTN* is defined as greater than or equal to the 95th percentile and must also be measured on at least three separate visits or occasions. Adolescent BP can also be considered if numbers are greater than 140/90 mmHg. *Stage 1 HTN* is defined as a BP of the 95th to 99th percentile plus 5 mmHg, whereas stage 2 HTN is greater than or equal to the 99th percentile plus 5 mmHg.

BP is commonly classified as primary, secondary, or white-coat HTN. Primary HTN refers to that without an identifiable cause. Primary HTN is more likely seen

TABLE 17.1

ADOLESCENT BP RECOMMENDATIONS	
BP Stage	**BP Range**
Normal BP	<90th percentile
Prehypertension	>90th to 94th percentiles >120/80 mmHg
HTN	>95th percentile >140/90 mmHg
Stage 1 HTN	95th to 99th percentile + 5 mmHg
Stage 2 HTN	>99th percentile + 5 mmHg

in those children who are overweight or obese. Secondary HTN is that with a known or identifiable cause. "White coat" HTN is that which is thought to be caused by anxiety secondary to entering the office, clinic, or hospital.

Pathophysiology

The pathophysiology of HTN can be found in Chapter 16.

Signs and Symptoms

Signs and symptoms of HTN in children and adolescents are similar to those in adults. Further signs and symptoms are discussed in Chapter 16.

Diagnostic Testing

All children older than the age of 3 should have their BP measured during routine office visits at least once per year. Children should have a couple of minutes of quiet time before their BP is taken. Infants are measured while lying flat, whereas children who are able to sit should have their back and feet supported. If a child is upset or crying, his or her BP will be inaccurate. It is also important to have the correct size of cuff. According to Mattoo (2013), BP should also be measured in the right arm. For an official diagnosis of HTN to be made, the readings greater than the 95th percentile should have occurred on at least three isolated occasions. These visits should be separated by a period of days or even weeks.

Treatment

One of the first steps in treating HTN is to determine and treat any possible underlying cause. Once this is done, then it is essential to focus on lifestyle changes, which are particularly helpful with the diagnosis of prehypertension and HTN. Along with exercise and dietary changes, weight loss is considered a first-line treatment for HTN related to obesity.

If lifestyle changes are not enough to control BP, medications may be needed. Medication treatment is recommended for any of the following situations (Mattoo, 2013):

- Symptoms of headaches and/or seizures are present or signs of ventricular hypertrophy are noted.
- Prehypertension and more than one risk factor for CVD (obesity) are noted.
- Stage 1 HTN with diabetes mellitus (DM) or other risk factors for CVD (obesity) are noted.
- Stage 1 or stage 2 HTN that persists after 4 to 6 months of lifestyle or nonpharmacological therapy is noted.
- Stage 2 HTN is noted.

Five classes of antihypertensives are commonly used in the treatment of child or adolescent HTN. These can include, but are not limited to, thiazide diuretics, angiotensin-converting enzyme (ACE) inhibitors, angiotensin receptor blockers (ARBs), beta blockers (BBs), and calcium channel blockers (CCBs), These medications are commonly prescribed in this order; however, each provider may vary somewhat.

These medications, dosages, and common side effects can be found in Chapter 16. Additional pediatric medication information is as follows (Mattoo, 2013):

- Hydrochlorothiazide (HCTZ) and chlorothiazide are the most commonly used thiazide diuretics.
- Enalapril and lisinopril are the most commonly used ACE inhibitors.
- Losartan is an approved ARB for children.
- ACE inhibitors and ARBs are not recommended for girls who are sexually active secondary to potential harm to the fetus.
- Metoprolol, atenolol, and bisoprolol are the most common recommended BBs.
- BBs should not be prescribed with asthma or heart block.

Medications should be used as long as needed to control and treat HTN. Continued nonpharmacological treatments should also be encouraged throughout the treatment process.

Patient Education

BP should be monitored in the obese patient on a routine basis. For those with a diagnosis of prehypertension, BP should be monitored every 4 to 6 months. Those with a diagnosis of HTN should have this monitored more often. The long-term BP goal for HTN is greater than the 95th percentile. If another comorbid condition such as obesity exists, the BP goal should be redefined to greater than the 90th percentile (Mattoo, 2013).

DYSLIPIDEMIA

Similar to HTN, dyslipidemia is a common disease found in obese children. It is important for the advanced practice nurse (APN) to work toward better understanding of the screening process, treatment, and patient education. Ten percent of children had cholesterol levels greater than 200 mg/dL from 1994 through 1998 according to the National Health and Nutrition Examination Survey. This number has now risen to more than 13% (13.3) in children aged 9 to 10 according to the Child and Adolescent Trial for Cardiovascular Health (Gauer, 2010).

Basics

An ongoing discussion on what age to begin screening for dyslipidemia remains for debate. According to the U.S. Preventive Services Task Force (USPSTF), an extensive literature review found insufficient evidence in regards to screening recommendations. Although this task force found insufficient evidence, many providers continue to use the following algorithm for the management of dyslipidemia in children and teenagers. In reviewing the patient's risk assessment, if a positive family history exists, recommendation is made to draw a fasting lipid panel and then repeat and average. If the risk assessment is reviewed and a parent's total cholesterol is greater than 240 mg/dL, the recommendation is to measure the total blood cholesterol (Spiotta & Luma, 2008). Both the screening recommendations and the lipid clinic at Cincinnati Children's Hospital Medical Center categorize cholesterol levels as normal, borderline, and high. The lipid clinic at Cincinnati Children's recommends further evaluation for all children and/or adolescents with triglycerides greater than or equal to 200 mg/dL or a low-density lipoprotein (LDL) greater than or equal to 130 mg/dL.

A normal total cholesterol level is less than 170 mg/dL, and an LDL level is greater than 100 mg/dL. A diagnosis of borderline total cholesterol is defined between 170 and 200 mg/dL, and an LDL is defined between 100 and 130 mg/dL. High total cholesterol is measured as greater than 200 mg/dL. Men with a high-density lipoprotein (HDL) less than 45 mg/dL and women with HDL less than 50 mg/dL are at increased risk for future cardiac events and should be considered for treatment (Cincinnati Children's, 2013). If the cholesterol is considered borderline, the recommendation is made to repeat and average. A repeat level less than 170 mg/dL indicates the need for further lab repeat in 5 years and the need to provide diet and education. If the repeat average is greater than or equal to 170 mg/dL, a fasting lipoprotein analysis is recommended along with a repeat and average.

From the total lipid panel, LDL levels are further examined. If the LDL level is found acceptable (less than 110 mg/dL), a repeat lipoprotein analysis is recommended within 5 years. Education is recommended on the importance of good dietary choices. If the LDL is found to be borderline (110–130 mg/dL), risk factor advice is given along with the Step-1 diet. Recommendation is given to repeat the lipoprotein analysis in 1 year. If the LDL level is greater than or equal to 130 mg/dL, a clinical evaluation is recommended to include a history and physical examination as well as further laboratory analysis. Evaluation should be done to rule out any secondary causes as well as any familial disorders. Intensive clinical intervention and screening of all family members is recommended as well. Setting an LDL goal less than 130 mg/dL with an ideal less than 110 mg/dL is also suggested.

The Step-1 and Step-2 diets are encouraged (Spiotta & Luma, 2008). The Step-1 diet is used as a first-line treatment for children older than the age of 2 to treat high cholesterol. The Step-2 diet is a more restrictive diet used to treat high cholesterol. It is used if one has completed the Step-1 diet and continues to have high cholesterol or if one has evidence of atherosclerosis (Gateway Health Alliance, Inc., 2011).

Despite the difference in recommendation for cholesterol screening, a 2008 clinical report by the American Academy of Pediatrics (AAP) Expert Committee has recommended that a cholesterol screening be done for those considered overweight. This includes children aged 2 through 10 years regardless of family history. Weight management was recommended as the treatment of choice (Spiotta & Luma, 2008).

Pathophysiology

The pathophysiology of dyslipidemia can be found in Chapter 16.

Signs and Symptoms

Signs and symptoms of dyslipidemia in children and adolescents are similar to those in adults. Further signs and symptoms are discussed in Chapter 16.

Diagnostic Testing

The diagnostic testing for cholesterol in children is similar to that in adults—a lipid panel. Further information about diagnostic testing can be found in Chapter 16.

Treatment

Treatment should be set with reasonable, attainable goals in mind. First-line treatment should focus on the child's and family's diet. According to the National Cholesterol Education Program (NCEP), total dietary fat should not exceed 30% of the total caloric intake. This should be on average 50 to 80 g of total fat per day. Daily dietary cholesterol intake should also be monitored and be kept to no more than 200 to 300 mg per day (Spiotta & Luma, 2008).

There have been no trials to date that have examined the use of statin therapy in nonfamilial hypercholesterolemia patients. Concerns regarding the safety and efficacy of long-term statin use have not been established (Eiland & Luttrell, 2010). Current treatment is therefore focused on dietary and exercise management without the use of medications.

Patient Education

Family counseling should take place when educating on reducing cholesterol intake. Individuals should eat 25 to 30 g of fiber daily. Simple sugars should be limited. This includes reducing or eliminating sugary beverages. Education on saturated fats should also take place. The fats primarily found in animal fats should be limited to less than 10% of daily calories (Spiotta & Luma, 2008).

DIABETES MELLITUS

DM is a complex disease that is commonly seen in obese or overweight children. Type I DM (T1DM) is a disease found in childhood; however, this section focuses on T2DM, as this is more common in obese children. T2DM was previously thought of as a disease only found in adults. It was previously called adult-onset diabetes. Children diagnosed with DM are also more at risk for several complications from the disease. These can include hypoglycemia, HTN, dyslipidemia, CVD death rates, heart attack, stroke, blindness or eye problems, kidney disease, and/or amputations (American Diabetes Association [ADA], 2014).

Basics

As childhood obesity continues to rise, so does the incidence of T2DM. Approximately 0.25% or 208,000 Americans younger than the age of 20 are estimated to have DM (this includes both type I and type 2) (ADA, 2014). An estimated 13,000 cases of DM are diagnosed each year (Peterson, Silverstein, Kaufman, & Warren-Boulton, 2007). From 2008 through 2009, the annual incidence of T1DM was still seen in more youth (estimated at 18,436) whereas T2DM was estimated at 5,089 (ADA, 2014). The prevalence of T2DM continues to increase among Black, Hispanic, and White youth. These numbers were statistically significant as seen in 2009 at 1.20 per 1,000 (American Indian), 1.06 per 1,000 (Black), 0.79 per 1,000 (Hispanic), and 0.17 per 1,000 (White). Between 2001 and 2009, significant increases in this condition occurred no matter the age or sex. An overall 30.5% increase in T2DM was noted during this time frame (Dabelea et al., 2014). Acanthosis nigricans and skin tags are more common in obese adolescents. African Americans have a greater incidence of acanthosis nigricans (51%) in comparison to Caucasians (8%) (August et al., 2013).

Childhood T2DM is typically found in children with certain characteristics. These commonalities can include, but are not limited to, the following:

- An elevated BMI (overweight or obese)
- A strong family history of T2DM

A considerable residual insulin capacity found at the time of initial diagnosis is seen with normal or elevated insulin and C-peptide levels (Copeland et al., 2013). A diagnosis of T2DM consists of the following (Copeland et al., 2013):

- An "insidious onset of disease" (Copeland et al., 2013, p. 365)
- Demonstration of insulin resistance
- Clinical evidence of acanthosis nigricans or PCOS
- Deficient evidence for T1DM autoantibodies

Pathophysiology

The pathophysiology of DM can be found in Chapter 16.

Signs and Symptoms

Signs and symptoms of DM in children and adolescents are similar to those in adults. Further signs and symptoms are discussed in Chapter 16.

Diagnostic Testing

Copeland et al. (2013) define *diabetes* according to the ADA criteria and four laboratory tests. They are HgA1c, fasting plasma glucose, 2-hour plasma glucose, and a random plasma glucose. H1A1c is positive if greater than or equal to 6.5%. Fasting (no caloric intake in 8 hours prior to testing) plasma glucose greater than or equal to 126 mg/dL is also an abnormal or positive finding. A 2-hour plasma glucose test during an oral glucose test is positive when the lab value is greater than or equal to 200 mg/dL. The patient must also ingest 75 g of anhydrous glucose 2 hours prior to the test. Those with symptoms of hyperglycemia and a random plasma glucose level greater than or equal to 200 mg/dL are also positive for the diagnosis (Copeland et al., 2013).

Treatment

The USPSTF states insufficient evidence to recommend for or against adverse health outcomes in overweight youth to include DM (Peterson et al., 2007). Most medications used for T2DM have not been tested on children or adolescents, and most current research exists for those patients older than the age of 18. Scant scientific evidence exists, and new guidelines exist after a review of medical data from January 1, 1990, through July 1, 2008 (Copeland et al., 2013). However, the latest clinical practice guidelines by Copeland et al. (2013) recommend six key action statements that APNs are to follow for treatment of T2DM.

The first key statement discusses the use of insulin therapy. Insulin therapy is recommended for those with T2DM and who have a random plasma blood glucose greater than or equal to 250 mg/dL or whose HgA1c is greater than 9%. It is also recommended for children or adolescents with diagnosed T2DM who are ketotic or in diabetic ketoacidosis. Insulin is also recommended in cases where the distinction between T1DM and T2DM is unclear. One oral medication, metformin, is also addressed. The guidelines state that metformin is considered first-line therapy for children and/or adolescents upon diagnosis. Because of the association of gastrointestinal side effects with metformin, the guidelines recommend low and slow titration of the medication to its maximum dose of 2,000 mg (in divided doses) daily. Initiating the dose of 600 mg daily with an increase of 500 mg every 1 to 2 weeks is recommended. A dose higher than the recommended 2,000 mg daily has not been shown to provide any additional benefit. The addition of rosiglitazone to metformin is currently under investigation in the use in the pediatric population. The National Institute of Diabetes and Digestive and Kidney Diseases-supported Treatment Options for Type 2 Diabetes in Adolescents and Youth (TODAY) trial is still ongoing at the time of this book's publication.

The second key statement recommends that APNs encourage lifestyle modifications, including proper dietary choices and physical activity, whereas the sixth key statement discusses exercise therapy. Appropriate exercise recommendations include moderate to vigorous exercise for at least 60 minutes on a daily basis. "Nonacademic screen time" should also be limited to no more than 2 hours per day. Copeland et al. (2013) also recommend incorporation of the Academy of Nutrition and Dietetics' *Pediatric Weight Management Evidence-Based Nutrition Practice Guidelines* in continued nutrition counseling as stated in the fifth key statement. The third key statement also recommends close monitoring of HgA1c (every 3 months). Patients should monitor finger-stick blood glucose if they are on insulin, have hypoglycemic symptoms, have recently changed or initiated treatment, have not met goals, or have other concurrent illnesses as stated in the fourth key statement (Copeland et al., 2013).

Patient Education

A joint plan should be discussed with patients and their families. The plan should include reducing sedentary behavior and increasing physical activity. Exercise plans should be specific and include the activity, timing, and duration. The activity does not need to be a continuous 60 minutes, but can be divided into shorter interval periods totaling 60 minutes daily. Parents can encourage structured activity through games or sports. Activity can also include everyday activities such as walking or general play. Nonacademic screen time should be reduced to less than 2 hours per day. Television sets or video games should be avoided in the children's bedrooms (Copeland et al., 2013).

OBSTRUCTIVE SLEEP APNEA

This section focuses on pediatric and childhood OSA, also known as obstructive sleep apnea syndrome (OSAS). It is a common condition and can result in severe complications if not recognized and left untreated.

Basics

The 2012 APA Clinical Practice Guideline for the Diagnosis and Management of Childhood OSA Syndrome defines *OSA* in children as "a disorder of breathing

during sleep characterized by prolonged partial upper airway obstruction and/
or intermittent complete obstructions (obstructive apnea) that disrupts normal
ventilation during sleep and normal sleep patterns" (Marcus et al., 2012, p.577).
According to Lipton and Gozal (2003), OSA is estimated at 2% of the pediatric
population whereas snoring is seen in 8% to 27%.

Pathophysiology

The pathophysiology of OSA can be found in Chapter 16.

Signs and Symptoms

Signs and symptoms of OSA in children and adolescents are similar to those in
adults; however, daytime sleepiness is uncommon. All children should be screened
for snoring on initial and subsequent appointments. Neurobehavioral problems
such as neurocognitive impairment, behavioral problems, and failure to thrive may
also be seen (Marcus et al., 2012). Further signs and symptoms are discussed in
Chapter 16.

Diagnostic Testing

Diagnostic testing is discussed in Chapter 16. The gold standard for pediatric
testing for OSA is a formal, attended, laboratory polysomnography (PSG). If PSG
is not available, alternative diagnostic tests can be considered. These include nocturnal oximetry, daytime nap or ambulatory PSG, or nocturnal video recording.

Treatment

Treatment of OSA may be referred to a sleep specialist. First-line treatment consists of weight loss for those who are overweight or obese. Weight loss should be
done in addition to further treatment, as this is sometimes a slow process. Adenotonsillectomy is recommended as first-line treatment for children with adenoton-
sillar hypertrophy. Postoperative care should include continued monitoring for
ongoing symptoms that are suggestive of continued OSA. Continuous positive
airway pressure (CPAP) is recommended for those who are not eligible for adenotonsillectomy or in whom symptoms persist postoperatively. Those with mild OSA
may benefit from intranasal corticosteroids. This is recommended for children
with mild OSA (apnea-hypopnea index [AHI] less than five). This treatment can
be considered when adenotonsillectomy is contraindicated or when mild OSA
remains postoperatively.

Patient Education

Extensive patient and family discussion needs to take place regarding treatment
of OSA. It is important for the family to be aware of all the treatment options
available to make an informed decision. Discussion regarding long-term compliance
in order to reduce risk for further comorbid conditions also needs to take place.
No quick treatment for this condition exists; therefore, it is important for continued education at each subsequent appointment.

ASTHMA

Asthma is discussed in this section in relation to pediatric obesity. Rates of both asthma and obesity are on the rise. The Centers for Disease Control and Prevention (CDC) document the prevalence of asthma from 3.6% in 1980 to 5.8% in 2003. The relationship between asthma and obesity has been studied more in recent years. Many researchers feel that obesity precedes the diagnosis of asthma. Obesity is also thought to increase not only the prevalence but also the harshness of the disease. It is also thought to lessen the effectiveness of medications used in asthma treatment (Delgado, Barranco, & Quirce, 2008).

Basics

Asthma is defined as a chronic inflammatory disease of the airways. Obesity, too, is considered an inflammatory disease. In the United States, an estimated 6.8 million children carry an active diagnosis of asthma, whereas 9 million children younger than the age of 18 have been diagnosed with asthma at some point in life. Children aged 5 through 17 have a greater prevalence of this disease in comparison to all other age groups. Ranked in the top 10 of conditions limiting activity, asthma is also the third highest cause of hospitalizations for those younger than the age of 15. Asthma is a widespread and costly disease affecting many low-income families, inner-city communities, and ethnic minorities (Rance & O'Laughlen, 2011).

Pathophysiology

Central and excessive body fat affects the lungs and disrupts breathing. Breathing is affected as the fat restricts air movement and compresses the lungs. Airway narrowing is also thought to be caused by long-term restriction of deep breathing secondary to obesity. This narrowing is caused by reduction of bronchial smooth muscle expansion, leading to the lack of deep breathing and thus the restrictive lung pattern and obesity. This predisposes a child to asthma. Researchers have found that obesity may lead to the development of asthma and vice versa—asthma may increase the incidence of obesity.

The lung of an obese child may be impacted in multiple ways, both intrinsically and extrinsically—through the inflammatory process and excessive body fat that restrict breathing, respectively (Rance & O'Laughlen, 2011). Reduction in pulmonary compliance, lung volumes, and the diameter of the peripheral airways can be affected. The volume of the blood in the lungs and the ventilation–perfusion relationship can also be affected as a result of obesity. With a limitation in airflow, reduction in both forced expiratory volume (FEV_1) and forced vital capacity (FVC) is seen; many times, this is symmetrical with the FEV_1/FVC ratio remaining unchanged. The changes in lung physiology can cause superficial respiration and reduction in lung volumes. Expiratory reserve volume leads to a reduced diameter of peripheral airways, thus reducing the function of bronchial smooth muscle. An increase in obstruction and bronchial hyperreactivity can be observed with a change in the actin–myosin cross-bridge cycle.

A systemic proinflammatory state can be observed in an obese individual with an increase in normal functioning of adipose tissue. Increased concentrations of cytokines, as well as soluble fractions of receptors and chemokines, are seen. Adipokines are derived from a group of cells synthesized and secreted from adipose tissue to include IL-6, IL-10, eotaxin, tumor necrosis factor (TNF)-α, TGF-β1, C-reactive protein, leptin, and adiponection. Linked to the production of T_H2 cytokines (IL-4, IL-6) in the bronchial epithelium, TNF-α is a known marker elevated in asthma; it also provides a direct link to body fat. IL-6 is also seen in both obesity and asthma, and elevation of these levels is thought to have a direct correlation with the severity of asthma.

Leptin, a hormone produced by adipocytes, is found in obese patients and also plays a role in inflammation, thus affecting asthma. Leptin possesses a considerable structural homology and can regulate the proliferation and activation of T cells. Thus, angiogenesis and recruitment of both macrophages and monocytes occur as a result of this process. Leptin is critical in the development of the lungs. It is considered a mediator among fibroblasts and lipofibroblasts and can play a role in the production of surfactant. Higher levels of leptin have been found in women with asthma, and further studies suggest that leptin may be used to predict childhood asthma.

Genetic and hormonal factors are also under investigation regarding the correlation between obesity and asthma. Specific genetic regions are under investigation to include chromosomes 5q, 6, 11q13, and 12q of the human genome. The role of hormones has also shown evidence that links obesity and asthma, more so in women than men. The complexity between obesity and asthma suggests more than one biological mechanism is involved (Delgado et al., 2008).

Signs and Symptoms

Signs and symptoms of asthma can include, but are not limited to, wheezing, shortness of breath, coughing, and at times chest tightness. There can also be signs of chest congestion, which are especially noticeable after a cold or viral illness. Fatigue and poor sleep can also be seen. Trouble tolerating activities or play time can also be seen. Symptoms can be worse at night or in the early morning (Mayo Clinic Staff, 2013; Rance & O'Laughlen, 2011). In children younger than age 5, the most common symptom is a viral respiratory infection (Potter, 2010).

Diagnostic Testing

The diagnosis of asthma is difficult, as there is no one, true diagnostic test in children. Confirmation of the presence of airway inflammation is not usually possible with the current clinical tools. Large broncho-alveolar specimens with elevations in inflammatory mediators and cells have been obtained. Some experts recommend a trail of medications in children aged 0 through 4 to aid in diagnosis, whereas a simple lung function test can be performed in children aged 5 through 11 (Potter, 2010).

Treatment

Weight loss has resulted in improvement in patients' asthma outcomes. The Nurse Health Study looked at weight gain from age 18 and older. This study found that the risk of asthma increased by 4.7% due to weight gain in comparison to those who maintained weight. As much as a 15% loss of body weight led to better pulmonary function test (PFT) results in FEV_1 and FVC (Delgado et al., 2008). Physical activity as well as dietary changes can help focus on weight loss and thus reduce asthma complications. Clinical intervention and treatment recommendations of overweight and obese children are offered by several organizations, including the National Association of Pediatric Nurse Practitioners (NAPNAP), AAP, and the American Heart Association (AHA). NAPNAP encourages a program initiative called Healthy Eating and Activity Together (HEAT). Designed by and for use by APNs, the HEAT Clinical Practice Guideline, "Identifying and Preventing Overweight in Childhood," provides recommendations for those who work with children in an outpatient setting (Rance & O'Laughlen, 2011).

Four major guidelines are currently available that address the management of asthma is children: the (1) the EPR3 of the National Asthma Education Programme (NAEPP) published in 2007, (2) the PRACTALL consensus report published by the European Academy of Asthma and Allergy, (3) an evidence-based approach compiled by the European Respiratory Society task force, published in 2008, and (4) the Global Initiative (GINA) published in 2009. These guidelines primarily focus on the treatment of asthma in people aged 0 to 4 and/or 0 to 5. Because patient symptoms vary, the APN can choose and tailor each guideline to the patient specifics.

Each guideline has specific recommendations for treatments as well as classifications of asthma severity and asthma control. As needed, treatment focuses on use of an inhaled short-acting β_2-agonist (SABA), whereas preferred treatment for long-term management uses low-dose inhaled corticosteroid (ICS), Cromolyn or Montelukast, medium-dose ICS, an inhaled long-acting β_2-agonist (LABA), a high-dose ICS, and/or an oral systemic corticosteroid.

Anytime a step-up is needed, the APN should first check adherence to medication and compliance, inhaler technique, and environmental control. A step-down may be initiated if the asthma is well controlled for at least 3 months. Patient education and environmental control are also recommended at each step before a medication change. If an alternative treatment is used and the response appears inadequate, it should be discontinued and a preferred treatment should be used prior to stepping up. Apart from this, if a clear benefit is not observed in a 4- to 6-week period, one should consider adjusting treatment (Potter, 2010). Additional research is needed on the relationship that exists between obesity and childhood asthma. Further guidelines for evaluation methods, suggested dietary choices and healthy eating lifestyles, and the role of physical activity levels are needed (Delgado et al., 2008; Rance & O'Laughlen, 2011).

Patient Education

Patients and families require ongoing education in regards to the diagnosis and treatment of asthma. Many times, further education is needed in regards to physical activity and dietary choices. Children should be seen at least every 3 months by the APN and sooner if exacerbations occur. Treatment is aimed at reducing the number of exacerbations as well as at reducing hospital admissions and readmissions. Proper use of inhalers as well as an explanation of when and how to take the medications is essential. Patients and families should be encouraged to call or make an appointment if they have any questions or concerns.

Metabolic syndrome, NAFLD, early puberty or menstruation, depression, and even some cancers can also be linked to childhood obesity. These conditions should also be addressed and treated; however, due to the numerous diseases associated with obesity, this chapter is devoted to only the top five conditions. Metabolic syndrome, however, is addressed in detail in Chapter 16.

REFERENCES

American Diabetes Association (ADA). (2014). *Statistics about diabetes: National diabetes statistics report, 2014*. Retrieved from http://www.diabetes.org/diabetes-basics/statistics

August, G. P., Caprio, S., Fennoy, I., Freemark, M., Kaugman, F. R., Lustig, R. H., . . . Montori, V. M. (2013). Prevention and treatment of pediatric obesity: An endocrine society clinical practice guideline based on expert opinion. *Journal of Clinical Endocrinology and Metabolism*, 93(12). Retrieved from http://press.endocrine.org/doi/full/10.1210/jc.2007-2458

Centers for Disease Control and Prevention. (2014). *Childhood obesity facts*. Retrieved from http://www.cdc.gov/healthyyouth/obesity/facts.htm

Cincinnati Children's. (2013). *Hyperlipidemia/cholesterol problems in children*. Retrieved from http://www.cincinnatichildrens.org/health/h/hyperlipidemia

Copeland, K. C., Silverstein, J., Moore, K. R., Prazar, G. E., Raymer, T., Shiffman, R. N., . . . Flinn, S. K. (2013). Management of newly diagnosed type 2 diabetes mellitus (T2DM) in children and adolescents. *Pediatrics*, 131(2), 364–382. Retrieved from http://pediatrics.aappublications.org/content/131/2/364.full.pdf+html

Dabelea, D., Mayer-Davis, E. J., Saydah, S., Imperatore, G., Linder, B., Divers, J., . . . Hamman, R. F. (2014). Prevalence of type 1 and type 2 diabetes among children and adolescents from 2001 to 2009. *Journal of the American Medical Association*, 311(17), 1778–1786. Retrieved from http://jama.jamanetwork.com/article.aspx?articleid=1866098

Delgado, J., Barranco, P., & Quirce, S. (2008). Obesity and asthma. *Journal of Investigative Allergology and Clinical Immunology*, 18(6), 420–425.

Eiland, L. S., & Luttrell, P. K. (2010). Use of statins for dyslipidemia in the pediatric population. *Journal of Pediatric Pharmacology and Therapeutics*, 15(3), 160–172. Retrieved from http://www.ncbi.nlm.nih.gov/pmc/articles/PMC3018249

Gateway Health Alliance, Inc. (2011). *Healthy solutions*. Retrieved from http://www.gatewayhealth.com/images/uploads/general/36_-_Low_Cholesterol_Diet.pdf

Gauer, R. (2010). Hyperlipidemia treatment in children: The younger, the better. *American Family Physician*, 1(82), 460–467.

George, M. G., Tong, X., Wigington, C., Gillespie, C., & Hong, Y. (2014). Hypertension screening in children and adolescents—National ambulatory medical care surgery, national hospital ambulatory medical care survey, and medical expenditure panel survey, United States, 2007–2010. *Supplements*, 63(02), 47–53. Retrieve from http://www.cdc.gov/mmwr/preview/mmwrhtml/su6302a8.htm

Lipton, A. J., & Gozal, D. (2003). Treatment of obstructive sleep apnea in children: Do we really know how? *Sleep Medicine Reviews*, 7(1), 61–80. doi:10.1053/smrv.2001.0256

Marcus, C. L., Brooks, L. J., Draper, K. A., Gozal, D., Halbower, A. C., Jones, J., . . . Shiffman, R. N. (2012). Diagnosis and management of childhood obstructive sleep apnea syndrome. *Pediatrics*, 130, 576–584. doi: 10.1542/peds.2012-1671

Mattoo, T. K. (2013). *Patient information: High blood pressure in children (Beyond the Basics)*. UpToDate. Retrieved from http://www.uptodate.com/contents/high-blood-pressure-in-children-beyond-the-basics

Mayo Clinic Staff. (2013). *Diseases and condition: Childhood asthma*. Retrieved from http://www.mayoclinic.org/diseases-conditions/childhood-asthma/basics/symptoms/con-20028628

Peterson, K., Silverstein, J., Kaufman, F., & Warren-Boulton, E. (2007). Management of type 2 diabetes in youth: An update. *American Family Physician*, 1(76), 658–664.

Potter, P. C. (2010). Current guidelines for the management of asthma in young children. *Allergy, Asthma and Immunology Research*, 2(1), 1–13. doi:10.4168/aair.2010.2.1.1

Rance, K., & O'Laughlen, M. (2011). Obesity and asthma: A dangerous link in children—An integrative review of the literature. *Journal for Nurse Practitioners*, 7(4), 287–292.

Spiotta, R. T., & Luma, G. B. (2008). Evaluating obesity and cardiovascular risk factors in children and adolescents. *American Family Physician*, 78(9), 1052–1058.

Prevention

Obesity prevention is a difficult task. If it were easy, it would not even need to exist; people would just automatically do it and be thin. Causes of obesity (social, environmental, and governmental) have become so intertwined that they are difficult to combat. Prevention strategies are gaining popularity; however, they still have a difficult climb. Changes need to focus on all levels and parts of society. This includes government and school involvement, communities, businesses, nonprofits, families, and individuals. Policies need to be changed to encourage and encompass a healthier environment. The following key behaviors focus on prevention and are needed to turn the epidemic around (Harvard School of Public Health, 2014g):

- Choosing healthier foods
- Limiting unhealthy foods
- Increasing physical activity
- Limiting sitting or sedentary time
  - Television, screen, computer, and video games
- Improving sleeping patterns
- Limiting stress

PREVENTION GUIDELINES

The Endocrine Society made prevention of obesity recommendations in the updated *Prevention and Treatment of Pediatric Obesity: An Endocrine Society Clinical Practice Guideline Based on Expert Opinion*. The three prevention recommendations are as follows:

- A minimum of 6 months of breastfeeding
- Advanced practice nurse (APN) promotion and participation in education, patient and family guidance, and promotion of dietary needs and physical activity
- APN community education on healthy dietary and activity choices

Breastfeeding and Infant Influences

Breastfeeding has been proven to reduce the risk for overweight and obese children. Studies have shown that school-age children are up to 35% less likely to be obese if they were breastfed for at least 3 to 5 months. Odds ratios are reduced at 3, 6, and 9 months of breastfeeding. After the 9-month period, this risk plateaus.

Caloric intake, although different in infants, should be based on appetite. Most infants are instinctive in the fact that they understand how much they need. Because of this, they will not over- or undereat. Infants should not be pressured to finish their food and should only be fed when hungry.

School and community-based interventions demonstrated a positive effect on weight control; these interventions were focused on preventing childhood obesity and were aimed at healthy eating patterns and increased physical activity. Pediatric patients as well as family members should be educated on healthy lifestyle guidelines. Culturally sensitive materials as well as avoidance of any language barriers should be presented so that materials reach a greater amount of people (August et al., 2008).

Family Influence on Prevention

Families, early child care, schools, health care, worksites, healthy food environments, and healthy activity environments play a role in obesity prevention. This section addresses these areas and provides ideas of how to incorporate changes into current practices and communities. APNs are at the forefront for preventive health education.

Families, one of the most important influences on life choices, have a lasting effect on children. Parents have the potential to make a lifelong impact in regards to healthy choices. They can provide both the tools and experience to foster healthy eating and to promote physical activity. They can also give guidance to disregard unhealthy signals (Harvard School of Public Health, 2014b).

Child Care and School Involvement

Obesity prevention can begin in early childhood; this is a time of critical growth and learning. Learning to crawl, walk, and play, as well as developing taste preferences, is also seen during this period. It is known that families and parental support are important during this time, but many times other caregivers may be involved, such as a babysitter or a children care development center. As many as 75% of children spend an average of at least 35 hours per week in child care.

Child care providers play an essential role in parental education of healthy eating and activity. Limiting junk food and serving age-appropriate foods are things that can enhance a child's life. Offering a variety of activities throughout the day is another way to entice a child's interest. Keeping that interest is also important. Therefore, activity times should not be too long as the child loses attention or becomes bored. Turning the television off and having a separate sleeping room without a television are imperative. Encouragement of adopting these or similar practices at home also inspires healthy lifestyles (Harvard School of Public Health, 2014a).

Children spend a majority of their time outside of their home life at school. Schools have a unique opportunity to focus on and improve children's health. They can provide a foundation for healthy lifestyles that can last lifelong.

SCHOOL OPPORTUNITIES FOR PREVENTION FOCUS

Education is one of the main objectives of any school. This principle provides a unique opportunity to educate on both nutrition and physical education/activity.

The core curriculum should focus on evidence-based nutrition and regular activity. Healthier food options in the cafeteria as well as snack options and concession options are ways in which schools can promote healthier lifestyles. Activity during recess time as well as encouraging walking or biking to school promotes an energetic lifestyle.

School meal planning is also an essential part of obesity prevention. The following recommendations are given in regards to school meal programs:

- Students should be encouraged to participate in meal programs. This includes breakfast, lunch, and after-school programs.
- The U.S. Dietary Guidelines should determine national nutritional standards.
- Caloric levels should be set for each meal and determined by each age group.
- Cafeteria facilities should include display cases as well as room to store and prepare food.
- Food staff should be trained in regards to food safety.
- Adequate time should be given for eating.
- Children who participate in free and/or reduced-price meals should have a judgment-free zone.
- Nutrition education should be provided along with each meal.
- Local, state, and federal governments should be involved and help fund school meal programs.

Competitive foods and beverages sold within the schools should also be addressed. Schools in Boston went as far as banning sugary drinks in 2004. Studies done since have shown that this led to a reduction in overall sugary drinks. Sugary beverages should be limited within schools. Classroom parties and school functions are occasions when healthy food and drink options can be served. Food should never be used as either a reward or punishment; it should be used to provide a fuel source for the body.

The school food environment should also be addressed. Students should feel comfortable in this environment, and cafeterias should be clean. Drinking water should also be accessible and offered throughout the day. Healthy foods should be marketed, whereas unhealthy foods should be limited. Support should also be given for school gardens. Lastly, staff should be encouraged to be role models for healthy eating (Harvard School of Public Health, 2014i).

Incorporating wellness programs within the school for faculty and staff can also bolster further enthusiasm for healthy changes (Harvard School of Public Health, 2014h). Along with providing a wellness program for staff, wellness program policies that encompass and focus on students, school nutrition, and physical education should be implemented. Health education should also be a priority within schools. The health education curriculum should do the following (Harvard School of Public Health, 2014d):

- Address nutrition and physical activity
- Align with national standards
- Focus on healthy standards and incorporate them into other subject areas
- Train teachers on health education
- Measure student learning in health education classes

In a world with information overload, it is easy to see where it is hard to decipher the truth. APNs are at the forefront to provide accurate information about obesity—both its prevention and treatment. It is important to get all medical providers on board in regards to prevention. It is also important to encourage health care facilities and insurance plans to work toward obesity prevention. Along with encouragement for prevention, it is important to encourage and paint a picture for inspiration of healthy choices and behavior.

Promoting healthy environments should be at the forefront of health care facilities, hospitals, and clinics. Staff, patients, and other visitors should be made aware of positive changes done for healthy living. Changes can include providing healthy food options and banning sugary drinks. This can show that the institution is serious about prevention and healthy behaviors.

Health care insurance plans should also be an area of focus in obesity prevention. Insurance plans should discuss prevention treatment to include and cover costs of programs aimed at reducing obesity. Programs and education can be aimed at promoting nutrition and exercise (Harvard School of Public Health, 2014c).

Another area of obesity prevention focus should be workplace. Most people spend as much as one-third of their lives at work. Obesity is a chronic condition in itself and can lead to other comorbid conditions. This can decrease workplace productivity, lead to more job-related injuries, and increase the number of sick days. It can also increase the number of insurance claims as well as decrease mobility on the job and morale.

As with school employees, the workplace can also provide employee wellness programs, and it can encourage healthier lifestyles through proper nutrition education and physical activity. Employers can also provide facilities for exercise as well as lockers or changing rooms. Workplace policies could also include reimbursement for exercise expenses or policies that provide healthier food options (Harvard School of Public Health, 2014j).

The food environment in the United States has been referred to as "toxic." Although the food itself is safe to eat, consumers have the tough choice of a healthy option or an unhealthy option. Many factors play a large part in the food environment, such as broad federal policies and local issues. These policies range from agricultural, revenue, and community policies to worksite permits and farmers' markets.

Agricultural policies can include growing and buying fresh fruits and vegetables. Increasing taxes on unhealthy food can be one aspect of revenue policy. Limiting fast-food restaurants in areas where large numbers already exist as well as bringing grocery stores to low-income neighborhoods are two means by which zoning regulations can help with obesity prevention. In addition, communication policies can aid in restricting unhealthy advertising (Harvard School of Public Health, 2014f).

The last section focuses on a healthy activity environment. This includes our surroundings in the communities we live in, such as encouraging sidewalks and/or bike lanes for travel. It also encourages more facilities to promote activity. This includes parks, gyms, or even community centers where people can exercise in a safe and comfortable environment. The following are possible strategies that can increase safety, accessibility, and affordability (Harvard School of Public Health, 2014e):

- Increase the number of parks, recreational areas, and athletic facilities in the community.
- Increase access to recreational facilities.
- Provide low or no-cost access to these facilities.

- Provide incentives to these facilities.
- Create and ensure a safe environment for physical activity.

Obesity prevention should be a top priority for all APNs. Cost and coverage for prevention programs, especially through insurance, is difficult to obtain; however, it could change the direction of this disease. Efforts should be made to make obesity prevention one of the forefronts of health care attention before this disease continues to damage our nation.

REFERENCES

August, G. P., Caprio, S., Fennoy, I., Freemark, M., Kaugman, F. R., Lustig, R. H., . . . Montori, V. M. (2008). Prevention and treatment of pediatric obesity: An endocrine society clinical practice guideline based on expert opinion. *Journal of Clinical Endocrinology & Metabolism, 93*(12), 4576–4599. Retrieved from http://press.endocrine .org/doi/10.1210/jc.2007-2458?url_ver=Z39.88-2003&rfr_id=ori:rid:crossref.org&rfr_ dat=cr_pub%3dpubmed

Harvard School of Public Health. (2014a). *Early child care.* Retrieved from http://www .hsph.harvard.edu/obesity-prevention-source/obesity-prevention/early-child-care

Harvard School of Public Health. (2014b). *Families.* Retrieved from http://www.hsph .harvard.edu/obesity-prevention-source/obesity-prevention/families

Harvard School of Public Health. (2014c). *Health care.* Retrieved from http://www.hsph .harvard.edu/obesity-prevention-source/obesity-prevention/healthcare

Harvard School of Public Health. (2014d). *Health education and school wellness.* Retrieved from http://www.hsph.harvard.edu/obesity-prevention-source/obesity- prevention/schools/health-education-and-school-wellness/#ref5

Harvard School of Public Health. (2014e). *Healthy activity environment.* Retrieved from http://www.hsph.harvard.edu/obesity-prevention-source/obesity-prevention/physical- activity-environment/

Harvard School of Public Health. (2014f). *Healthy food environment.* Retrieved from http://www.hsph.harvard.edu/obesity-prevention-source/obesity-prevention/food- environment/

Harvard School of Public Health. (2014g). *Obesity prevention strategies.* Retrieved from http://www.hsph.harvard.edu/obesity-prevention-source/obesity-prevention

Harvard School of Public Health. (2014h). *Schools.* Retrieved from http://www.hsph .harvard.edu/obesity-prevention-source/obesity-prevention/schools

Harvard School of Public Health. (2014i). *School obesity prevention recommendations: Complete list.* Retrieved from http://www.hsph.harvard.edu/obesity-prevention-source/ obesity-prevention/schools/school-obesity-prevention-recommendations-read-and-print

Harvard School of Public Health. (2014j). *Worksites.* Retrieved from http://www.hsph .harvard.edu/obesity-prevention-source/obesity-prevention/worksites

Weight Cycling

This chapter addresses weight cycling, also known as the "yo-yo dieting" pheno-menon. Difficulties in maintaining weight is often what fuels the repeated weight loss. These repeated attempts at weight loss are commonly referred to as weight cycling. Although a definition of *weight cycling* is hard to find, "basically, a single weight cycle refers to a loss followed by a gain" (Lahti-Koski et al., 2005, p. 333). As obesity is on the rise, so are the number of attempts for weight loss. Many of these attempts result in poor outcomes. Dieters do not have a certain set of charac-teristics. Men, women, young, old, overweight, obese, and even thin or normal weight people can be upset or even unsatisfied with their weight. Men, more often than women, do not feel that they may need to lose weight even if they are over-weight or obese (Lahti-Koski, Mannisto, Pietinen, & Vartiainen, 2005).

Weight cycling has a strong association with body mass index (BMI) (Montani, Viecelli, Prevot, & Dulloo, 2006). Repeated cycles of weight loss and regain are common not only in overweight or obese people but also in normal-weight people, especially young women (Montani et al., 2006; Strohacker, Carpenter, & McFarlin, 2009). Many people who have problems with weight cycling are also unhappy with their appearance and express unprecedented levels of body dissat-isfaction (Bacon & Aphramor, 2011; Montani et al., 2006). These individuals are often the ones who have repeated weight-loss attempts (Bacon & Aphramor, 2011). Weight cycling most often starts at a young age and continues into adult-hood (Montani et al., 2006).

Variable results have been observed in weight cycling. Weight fluctuations can be seen in unsuccessful dieters or even in athletes losing weight for a sport. One of the most common reasons for variable results is that there is no common definition of *weight cycling* (Montani et al., 2006). Strohacker et al. (2009) define *weight cycling* as "repeated periods of weight loss and regain that form a pattern" (p. 191). Lahti-Koski et al. (2005) define the terms *mild weight cycling* and *severe weight cycling*. *Mild weight cycling* is defined as a weight loss greater than or equal to 5 kg with weight regain once or twice. *Severe weight cycling* uses the same weight loss, greater than or equal to 5 kg with weight regain on at least three separate occasions.

The number of cycles or attempts at weight loss makes it hard to establish the condition's prevalence. The prevalence of weight cycling is assumed to be high, as the number of dieters is quite common and thus relapses are assumed to occur (Lahti-Koski et al., 2005). The prevalence of dieting has increased over the past 50 years. As the incidence of dieting has increased, this trend also lies parallel to the increase in obesity. From 1950 through 1966, an estimated 7% of men and

14% of women reported dieting or trying to lose weight. By the late 1980s, this trend had increased to as much as 25% of men and 40% of women. The mid-1990s showed another increase in weight-loss attempts. This number jumped to 29% in men and 44% in women (Montani et al., 2006).

Increased health risks were seen as a result of weight cycling reported in several studies in the early 1990s. Although these early studies show a direct correlation between weight cycling and morbidity and mortality, more recent studies have not been as consistent. Discrepancies exist between the early and latter weight cycling studies. Because of this, results are difficult to compare. One such example is the variability in weight cycling measures as well as the lack of discerning intentional versus unintentional weight loss (Field et al., 1999).

Intentional weight loss is defined as one or more episodes of weight loss that is either planned or deliberate (Field et al., 2004). The study by French et al. (1997) demonstrated equality between intentional and unintentional weight loss of at least 20 pounds at least once. "If unintentional weight loss carries a risk not associated with voluntary weight loss, a failure to account for the intentionality of the weight loss could potentially lead to drawing faulty inferences" (Field et al., 2004, p. 268). Unintentional weight loss was seen as a predictor of mortality, as those with unintentional weight loss had a 31% higher death rate. That same study also found that intentional weight loss had a strong association with lower risk of death (24% lower mortality rate) (Gregg, Gerzoff, Thompson, & Williamson, 2003). Both intentional and unintentional weight loss were seen as strong predictors of hypertension (HTN), coronary artery disease (CAD), and diabetes mellitus (DM) (French et al., 1997). In contrast, the First Cancer Prevention Study showed as much as a 21% to 28% reduction in diabetes in those with intentional weight loss (Will, Williamson, Ford, Calle, & Thun, 2002).

If intentional weight loss correlates with increased morbidity, focus should be on prevention of weight gain. However, if only unintentional weight loss is related to an increased risk of morbidity, current recommendations would hold for weight loss as well as to promote no further weight gain (Field et al., 2004).

COMMONALITIES IN WEIGHT CYCLING

Weight cycling is commonly associated with diet-induced weight loss. A majority of weight loss attempts are seen in overweight and obese people. Studies have shown that as many as 54% of overweight people and 77% of obese people have reported an attempt at weight loss at least once. At least two types of weight fluctuations are observed with weight loss: (1) mild fluctuations in weight related to slight deviations from healthy behavior or (2) larger, wider fluctuations related to weight relapse. Montani et al. (2006) reviewed a study in Denmark that showed approximately one-third of child participants gained more than 30% of the weight they lost after a 9-month period. Much of the weight gain was seen in the first 4 months (Montani et al., 2006).

Weight cycling is not only seen in the overweight or obese. It is also observed in younger individuals and those at a normal weight. Many of those who attempt weight loss are unsatisfied with their body image. Low self-esteem and the desire to "fit in" also drive people toward weight loss. Conforming to the idea that "slim is beautiful" and body dissatisfaction are driving forces for those of a normal weight working toward weight loss.

Some sports require weight loss to achieve lower or healthy body weights for competition. These sports could include wrestling, cycling, rowing, boxing, martial arts, or weightlifting. Ballerinas, models, or even entertainers maintain a professional advantage by keeping their weight down. Activities and sports are starting at an earlier age and becoming more competitive; thus, weight cycling is also starting earlier. Some sports even require athletes to gain weight. This can include football or wrestling (Montani et al., 2006). In any sport or activity scenario, weight cycling can be an issue.

Not all of these sports or activities use a classification system to regulate weight loss or weight gain. Although there are many positive benefits to lean body mass and lower fat mass levels, negative health effects are seen with excessive gain or loss of body mass. The current research and literature review led the National Athletic Trainers' Association (NATA) to suggest the following to all those participating in sports and physical activities. These are safe weight loss and weight maintenance strategies that are supported by scientific evidence levels using the Strength of Recommendation Taxonomy criterion scale. The letters A through C are used to describe the level of research and literature-supported scientific evidence:

A means there are well-designed experimental, clinical, or epidemiologic studies to support the recommendation; B means there are experimental, clinical, or epidemiologic studies that provide a strong theoretical rationale for the recommendation; and C means the recommendation is based largely on anecdotal evidence at this time. (Turocy et al., 2011, p. 323)

The following are the supported recommendations for *assessing body composition and weight* along with the evidence category (Turocy et al., 2011, p. 323):

1. Body composition assessments should be used to determine safe body weight and body composition goals. Evidence Category: B
2. Body composition data should be collected, managed, and used in the same manner as other personal and confidential medical information. Evidence Category: C
3. The body composition assessor should be appropriately trained and should use a valid and reliable body composition assessment technique. Evidence Category: C
4. Body weight should be determined in a hydrated state. Evidence Category: B
5. When determining goal weight, body weight should be assessed relative to body composition. This assessment should occur twice annually for most people, with no less than 2 to 3 months between measurements. Evidence Category: C
6. To track a person's progress toward a weight or body composition goal, private weigh-ins and body composition assessments should be scheduled at intervals that provide information to guide and refine progress, as well as to establish reinforcement and reassessment periods. Evidence Category: C
7. When hydration is a concern, regular or more frequent (or both) assessments of body weight are indicated. Evidence Category: C
8. Active clients and athletes in weight classification sports should not gain or lose excessive amounts of body weight at any point in their training cycles. Evidence Category: C
9. Management of body composition should include both diet and exercise. Evidence Category: B

10. Total caloric intake should be determined by calculating the basal metabolic rate (BMR) and the energy needs for activity. Evidence Category: B
11. Caloric intake should be based on the body weight goal. Evidence Category: C
12. A safe and healthy dietary plan that supplies sufficient energy and nutrients should be maintained throughout the year. Evidence Category: B
13. The U.S. Department of Agriculture's Food Pyramid Guide is one of the methods that can be used to ensure adequate nutrient intake. Evidence Category: C
14. The metabolic qualities of the activity should be considered when calculating the need for each energy-producing nutrient in the diet. Evidence Category: B
15. Safe and appropriate aerobic exercise will facilitate weight and body fat loss. Evidence Category: C
16. Body composition adjustments should be gradual, with no excessive restrictions or use of unsafe behaviors or products. Evidence Category: C
17. Combining weight management and body composition goals with physical conditioning periodization goals will assist athletes or clients in reaching weight goals. Evidence Category: C
18. Education on safe dietary and weight management practices should be communicated on a regular and planned basis. Evidence Category: C
19. Individual body composition or dietary needs should be discussed privately with appropriately trained nutrition and weight management experts. Evidence Category: C
20. Ergogenic and dietary aids should be ingested cautiously and under the advisement of those knowledgeable of the requirements of sports and other governing organizations. Evidence Category: C

NATA recommends that athletes review weight goals with a trainer and have individual monitoring plans. This should include body weight assessments both during the season and during the offseason. Weight fluctuations can occur secondary to sweat or dehydration. These too should be monitored closely. Weight maintenance should be encouraged when in competition as well as when not in competition (Turocy et al., 2011).

Weight fluctuations are also seen in those suffering from chronic diseases. Those at a higher risk include those suffering from cancer, gastrointestinal diseases, lung diseases, and alcoholism. Those living in developing countries are also at a higher risk of weight fluctuation (Montani et al., 2006).

HEALTH CONSEQUENCES OF WEIGHT CYCLING

Do negative health consequences exist with repeated cycles of weight loss and regain? Does this cycle pose a greater disease risk than that of obesity maintenance? These are the common questions that many seek to answer (Strohacker et al., 2009). Weight cycling can be the cause of many health consequences; this is not limited to only obesity. These can include disordered eating behaviors, numerous psychological disorders, cancer, bone fractures, type 2 diabetes mellitus (T2DM), and HTN. Many studies have shown increased risk for cardiovascular mortality. Although the direct cause of this is not understood completely, studies are currently ongoing. Several cardiovascular risk factors specifically associated with weight cycling are known. These include enhanced weight gain, total body and visceral fat accumulation, alteration in the composition of tissue lipids, insulin resistance and T2DM, dyslipidemia, and HTN.

Enhanced weight gain is commonly seen with weight cycling. Although weight gain has not been seen in all studies, it has been seen in a vast number of populations. Some of these subjects include obese women, young and middle-aged women, German nonsmoking people, middle-aged Japanese men, and elite athletes.

Total body and visceral fat is seen in excess in those who have repeated weight gain and weight loss. Body composition is changed, thus reducing lean body mass and therefore increasing both total body and visceral fat. Human data are not as convincing as animal data; even so, data still show body composition differences in those with normal weight or non-weight cyclers versus those who have repeatedly weight cycled. Stimulation of lipogenic enzymes located in white adipose tissue could cause preferential fat deposition. This has been observed in rats who underwent a change in feeding, such as starvation, limiting, and refeeding. Another change noted with weight cycling and a change in body fat may be the redistribution of fat to the central areas. This occurs without body composition changes. Obese women with a history of weight cycling are often found to have android or abdominal weight distribution. This type of weight distribution is found more commonly than the gluteal or gynoid type, which is why the measurement of waist-to-hip ratio is crucial. This measurement is often elevated in women who have a history of weight cycling.

An alteration in the composition of tissue lipids or a change in the fatty acid composition may also be found in weight cycling. Rats studied while submitting to weight cycling were found to have a progressive increase of saturated fatty acids and a decrease of essential polyunsaturated fatty acids such as linoleic acid and alpha-linolenic acid, which results in a decrease of the ratio of essential polyunsaturated to saturated fatty acids. Quick and rapid weight loss in humans, similar to that observed in rats, can lead to an enhanced reduction of alpha-linolenic acid. Lower levels of alpha-linolenic acid found in human tissue have a direct correlation with an increased risk of cardiovascular disease (CVD), especially CAD.

Insulin resistance and T2DM also have a strong association with weight cycling. However, weight cycling is not an independent predictor of T2DM. A Japanese study of overweight adults demonstrated a strong association with hyperinsulinemia. Positive weight fluctuations were seen over a 30-year period. Those with larger weight fluctuations had higher fluctuations of fasting blood glucose. A second Japanese study also validated a strong relationship between weight cycling and metabolic syndrome. Studies have also shown a higher correlation with weight cycling and insulin resistance even in normal-weight people (Montani et al., 2006).

Dyslipidemia is also found in those who have a history of weight cycling. Those with an increase in low-density lipoprotein (LDL) or a decrease in high-density lipoprotein (HDL) are also at an increased risk for CVD. Olson et al. (2000) completed a study of 485 women with risk factors for CAD. Twenty-seven percent of these women reported a history of weight cycling. (Weight cycling in this study was defined as a weight loss greater than or equal to 4.5 kg on at least three separate occasions.) This study concluded that women who weight cycled had 7% lower HDL levels. Participants who cycled more weight had a lower HDL weight than those who cycled less weight. Those with weight cycled greater than or equal to 50 pounds per cycle had 27% lower HDL levels in comparison to non-weight cyclers. This shows that a direct correlation exists between weight cycling and lower HDL levels, therefore increasing one's risk of CAD. Another study showed blood lipid alterations along with metabolic syndrome in those who had documented weight fluctuations and body weight variability. This was more evident in the group of men with a BMI less than 25 kg/m^2 in comparison with those with a BMI greater than or equal to 25 kg/m^2.

HTN is viewed as both a direct and an indirect outcome of weight cycling. The effects of weight cycling on blood pressure (BP) have also been evaluated in human and rat studies. HTN was found more commonly among male weight cyclers as well as among obese women with a history of weight cycling. The EPIC study demonstrated an increased risk for the development of HTN in the obese subjects; however, it did not show a significant risk in the nonobese subjects (Montani et al., 2006). Nonobese Japanese men with a history of weight cycling also demonstrated an increase in HTN. In addition, nonobese Japanese women also showed evidence of elevated systolic and diastolic BP at the end of a study. This voluntary study had a period of two cycles of weight loss and regain. The elevated BPs were seen in excess of 100 days post completion of the second weight cycle (Montani et al., 2006).

An indirect association between weight cycling and HTN was observed in the Nurses' Health Study II. This showed a positive association between body weight, body weight gain, and the development of HTN. Again, this was not viewed as a direct correlation; however, it was indirectly associated thorough its adverse effect on body weight (Montani et al., 2006). Similar findings were reported in women in the study by Graci et al. (2004). However, both genders with high frequency and magnitude of weight cycling were also associated with adverse effects on BP (Graci et al., 2004). These results are not too surprising, as a positive relationship exists between BMI and BP.

Growing evidence suggests the correlation between weight cycling and increased cardiovascular risk. Increased cardiovascular morbidity and mortality via weight fluctuations are seen either per se or indirectly with weight gain. As this was thought to affect only the overweight or obese, studies are showing the negative health consequences of weight cycling on even those of a normal weight. Again, concerns with weight cycling affecting younger age groups are also relevant, as the risk for CVD prevalence is evident (Montani et al., 2006).

Little information on weight cycling and its psychological impacts exists; however, studies are being done. Although weight cycling has not been linked directly to psychopathological conditions, it has been linked to lowered feelings of well-being. It has also been found to have a relationship with binge eating as well as with poorer perceived health status (Lahti-Koski, et al., 2005).

Fluctuations of risk parameters found in CVD should also be examined with weight cycling or times during increased food intake. Elevated levels of BP, heart rate, sympathetic activity, glucose, insulin, cholesterol, triglycerides, and glomerular hyperfiltration can be seen and are referred to as complications of the "repeated overshoot" theory. The *repeated overshoot theory* is defined as an "overshoot of some cardiovascular risk factors during the weight regain phase of weight cycling." It "may contribute to overall cardiovascular morbidity and mortality even when the average values are normal" (Montani et al., 2006, p. 563).

Weight cycling exists. One of the reasons that this condition may be so difficult to understand and treat is that there is no one established definition. Due to the many variables that exist with weight cycling, the outcomes are variable. It is also important to understand that effects of weight cycling are observed in different lean, overweight, and obese people. There is even variability in obese subjects, as those with morbid obesity have demonstrated different outcomes and have also been studied less (Graci et al., 2004). Advanced practice nurses (APNs) are at the forefront to stop weight cycling from continuing.

REFERENCES

Bacon, L., & Aphramor, L. (2011). Weight science: Evaluating the evidence for a paradigm shift. *Nutrition Journal, 10*(9). Retrieved from http://www.nutritionj.com/content/10/1/9

Field, A. E., Byers, T., Hunter, D. J., Laird, N. M., Manson, J. E., Williamson, D. F., . . . Colditz, G. A. (1999). Weight cycling, weight gain, and risk of hypertension in women. *American Journal of Epidemiology, 150*(6), 573–579.

Field, A. E., Manson, J. E., Laird, N., Williamson, D. F., Willett, W. C., & Colditz, G. A. (2004). Weight cycling and the risk of developing type 2 diabetes among adult women in the United States. *Obesity Research, 12*(2), 267–274.

French, S. A., Folsom, A. R., Jeffery, R. W., Zheng, W., Mink, P. J., & Baxter, J. E. (1997). Weight variability and incident disease in older women: The Iowa women's health study. *International Journal of Obesity and Related Metabolic Disorders, 21*(3), 217–223.

Graci, S., Izzo, G., Savino, S., Cattani, L., Lezzi, G., Berselli, M. E., . . . Petroni, M. L. (2004). Weight cycling and cardiovascular risk factor in obesity. *International Journal of Obesity, 28*, 65–71.

Gregg, E. W., Gerzoff, R. B., Thompson, T. J., & Williamson, D. F. (2003). Intentional weight loss and death in overweight and obese U.S. adults 35 years of age and older. *Annals of Internal Medicine, 138*(5), 383–389.

Lahti-Koski, M., Mannisto, S., Pietinen, P., & Vartiainen, E. (2005). Prevalence of weight cycling and its relation to health indicators in Finland. *Obesity: A Research Journal, 13*(2), 333–341. doi:10.1038/oby.2005.45

Montani, J. P., Viecelli, A. K., Prevot, A., & Dulloo, A. G. (2006). Weight cycling during growth and beyond as a risk factor for later cardiovascular diseases: The "repeated overshoot" theory. *International Journal of Obesity, 30*, S58–S66. Retrieved from http://www.nature.com/ijo/journal/v30/n4s/pdf/0803520a.pdf

Olson, M. B., Kelsey, S. F., Bittner, V., Reis, S. E., Reichek, N., Handberg, E. M., & Merz, C. N. (2000). Weight cycling and high-density lipoprotein cholesterol in women: Evidence of adverse effect: A report from the NHLBI-sponsored WISE study. Women's Ischemia Syndrome Evaluation Study Group. *Journal of the American College of Cardiology, 1*(36), 1565–1571.

Strohacker, K., Carpenter, K. C., & McFarlin, B. K. (2009). Consequence of weight cycling: An increase in disease risk. *International Journal of Exercise Science, 2*(3), 191–201. Retrieved from http://digitalcommons.wku.edu/cgi/viewcontent.cgi?article=1040&context=ijes

Turocy, P. S., DePalma, B. F., Horswill, C. A., Laquale, K. M., Martin, T. J., Perry, A. C., . . . Utter, A. C. (2011). National Athletic Trainers' Association position statement: Safe weight loss and maintenance practices in sport and exercise. *Journal of Athletic Training, 46*(3), 322–336.

Will, J. C., Williamson, D. F., Ford, E. S., Calle, E. E., & Thun, M. J. (2002). Intentional weight loss and 13-year diabetes incidence in overweight adults. *American Journal of Public Health, 92*(8), 1245–1248.

Case Study 4

This case study builds on disease management information found in Chapters 15 to 19.

- *Chapter 15: Disease Management and the Role of the Advanced Practice Nurse*
- *Chapter 16: Obesity-Related Diseases*
- *Chapter 17: Obesity-Related Diseases: A Pediatric Focus*
- *Chapter 18: Prevention*
- *Chapter 19: Weight Cycling*

Mr. Dundee is a pleasant 40-year-old man who presents to the clinic today. He follows up routinely for his hypertension (HTN) and type 2 diabetes mellitus (T2DM). He is on HCTZ 25 mg PO daily, lisinopril 20 mg PO daily, and metformin 1,000 mg PO BID. His blood pressure (BP) today is 150/88. After sitting 10 minutes, his BP is 144/86. He had labs drawn before his appointment. They are as follows:

HgA1c: 9.0

Basic Metabolic Panel (BMP)

Sodium: 140
Potassium: 3.7
Chloride: 101
CO_2: 25
Blood urea nitrogen (BUN): 24
Creatinine: 1.5
Glucose: 155

Fasting Lipid Panel

Total cholesterol: 250
Triglycerides: 300
High-density lipoprotein (HDL): 40
Low-density lipoprotein (LDL): 135

His other vitals are as follows:

Pulse: 65 bpm
Respirations: 12

Height: 5 feet, 11 inches
Weight: 275 pounds
Body mass index (BMI): 38.4 kg/m^2
Pulse oximetry: 95% on room air
Neck circumference: 17.5 inches

How would you address and treat his blood pressure?

What about his type 2 diabetes mellitus (T2DM)?

How would you address his weight?

What would be a good weight-loss goal for him?

How would you present him with a plan for weight loss? What would this include?

Would you make any additional referrals?

His physical examination shows the following:

General: Looks stated age, appropriate conversation, in no acute distress
Head, Eyes, Ears, Nose, Throat (HEENT): PERRLA, extraocular muscles intact. Conjunctiva normal, anicteric
Neck: Supple, no jugular vein distension (JVD)
Skin: Warm. Pink. Dry
Mucosa: No cyanosis, moist
Cardiovascular: Normal S1 and S2. No murmur
Lungs: Good bilateral air entry
Abdomen: Obese, soft, and nontender. Normal bowel sounds. No rebound pain or rigidity
Extremities: No edema, no cyanosis, no clubbing
Neurological: Alert and oriented ×3. No motor or sensory deficit

After talking with the patient further, he said that over the past 2 months when he has been exercising he has noticed more instances of shortness of breath. He also reports that he has occasional chest tightness. It is present with activity and resolved with sitting down and resting. At times, he also feels that his jaw is sore, but he does not know why. Reluctantly, he also mentions that his wife is worried about his snoring. He reports that she states it is so bad that sometimes she gets up and goes into another room to sleep. The patient admits to feeling more tired, but thinks it is due to the extra hours he is picking up at work. He also reports that he has been under more stress because of his long work hours. He reports that smoking is his stress relief. He is now smoking a half pack per day.

In reviewing his family history, one notices that his father is deceased secondary to sudden cardiac death at the age of 45.

Would you order any additional testing? If yes, what testing and why?

What dietary advice would you provide?

What lifestyle changes would you suggest?

What physical activity would you encourage? Please include mode/type, frequency, duration, and time.

Would you recommend stretching and strengthening activities? Please include mode/type, frequency, duration, and time.

Would you consider any additional medications? If yes, what?

Would you order any other laboratory work? If yes, what?

When would you repeat laboratory work?

When would you schedule his next follow-up appointment?

Would you involve any other advanced practice nurses (APNs) in his care?

What additional education, if any, would you provide?

Treatment

Treatment of Addiction and Eating Disorders

This chapter addresses the treatment of addiction and eating disorders from the perspective of the advanced practice nurse (APN). Treatment of addiction and eating disorders should be a multidisciplinary approach that includes referral as needed. For further definitions, facts, and screening tools used in addiction and eating disorders, please refer Chapter 8 and Chapter 14.

FOOD ADDICTION

The role of the APN in addiction is to identify any concerning behaviors, symptoms, or patterns that would indicate a possible food addiction. The APN should use screening tools to initially identify any possible addiction or eating disorder. If the APN identifies a food addiction, further workup should ensue. The APN should first recommend referral to a mental health provider such as a psychiatric mental health nurse practitioner (PMHNP) or counselor. Another appropriate and necessary referral would be to a registered dietitian (RD). Continued workup and treatment from a nursing standpoint can follow, but it is also important for continued treatment of weight loss with more experienced team members as stated earlier.

It is important to identify the triggers that cause the overeating. The APN should work with the patient to identify and make a list of the triggers. This list can then be used with all the health professionals and team members involved in the case. Another treatment idea would be to provide the patient with a list of support groups that work with food addicts. The following organizations are free to patients; however, it is important to offer suggestions, as each organization may not be in the treatment area:

- Compulsive Eaters Anonymous-HOW (CEA-HOW)
- Food Addicts Anonymous (FAA)
- Food Addicts in Recovery Anonymous (FA)
- Greysheeters Anonymous (GSA)
- Overeaters Anonymous (OA)
- Overcomers Outreach (OO)
- Recovery from Food Addiction (RFA)

BOX 20.1 ADDICTION RESOURCES

Compulsive Eaters Anonymous-HOW (CEA-HOW)
www.ceahow.org

Food Addicts Anonymous (FAA)
www.foodaddictsanonymous.org

Food Addicts in Recovery Anonymous (FA)
www.foodaddicts.org

Greysheeters Anonymous (GSA)
www.greysheet.org

Overeaters Anonymous (OA)
www.oa.org

Overcomers Outreach (OO)
www.overcomersoutreach.org

Recovery from Food Addiction (RFA)
www.recoveryfromfoodaddiction.org

OA is the largest and oldest organization of those listed earlier; however, it is important for each patient to find his or her best fit (Food Addiction Institute [FAI], 2015a; Box 20.1).

Most important in the treatment process, the APN needs to be able to educate the patient on the dangers of food addiction and obesity, provide continued support, and refer him or her to appropriate professionals. According to the FAI (2015b), the following principles of food addiction apply to all people. Treatment should be aimed at addressing the following issues (FAI, 2015b, n.p.):

- Food addicts need to abstain from their trigger foods and binge foods completely to eliminate cravings.
- Food addicts need to ask for and accept help to the degree they have lost control.
- Food addicts need varying levels of support for withdrawal and detoxification.
- Food addicts who are unable to achieve and maintain abstinence need higher levels of structure and support.
- Food addicts need a process for challenging and breaking their own food addiction denial.

Again, it should be known that most health professionals are unable to provide all the levels of care needed for food addicts within the time and practice constraints. Chronically active food addicts should be referred on for a specialized approach. There are thousands of clinical case studies and research articles available for review.

In making an appropriate referral, the following suggestions may be used to help identify health professionals who understand food addiction (FAI, 2015b, n.p.):

- Do they clearly understand the difference between obesity, eating disorders, and chemical dependency on food?
- Do they assess for different stages of food addiction and have stage-appropriate treatment?
- Do they treat food addiction as a substance use disorder, that is, complete elimination of major binge foods?
- Do they educate about the nature of addiction?
- Do they have a strategy for effectively confronting food addiction denial individually and in groups?
- Do they have a positive track record in terms of successfully working with food addicts?

Food addiction is difficult to treat. It should not be attempted alone. A multi-disciplinary approach with appropriate referrals and supportive patient care is the best way to achieve success.

EATING DISORDERS—ANOREXIA AND BULIMIA

The following eating disorders will be addressed in regards to treatment from the APN's standpoint. Anorexia and bulimia are difficult to treat. These diseases will require a multidisciplinary approach as well as referral to appropriate mental health professionals.

Treatment of anorexia starts with its appropriate diagnosis. There are many differentials for both anorexia and bulimia. They can include any of the following (Burns, Dunn, Brady, Starr, & Blosser, 2004):

- AIDS
- Central nervous system neoplasm
- Depression
- Diabetes
- Hyperthyroidism
- Inflammatory bowel disease
- Malignancy
- Pregnancy
- Substance abuse
- Systemic lupus erythematosus

Once these differentials are excluded, and anorexia is confirmed, treatment should ensue.

Laboratory studies should be ordered to assess for anorexia or bulimia and/or rule out any associated conditions. These can include the following:

- Thyroid-stimulating hormone (TSH)
- Iron studies—hemoglobin (Hb), hematocrit (Hct), and transferrin
- Basic metabolic panel (BMP)—assess serum glucose, albumin, electrolytes, and creatinine
- Liver function tests (LFTs)

Thyroid studies should be done and should assess for low thyroxine, a common finding found in anorexia or bulimia. A patient with anorexia or bulimia could have low iron levels. Abnormalities in a BMP could indicate hyponatremia or elevated creatinine. An EKG should also be ordered and reviewed for any abnormality.

Treatment of anorexia and/or bulimia is difficult. Oftentimes, these conditions are found in younger individuals, making the diagnosis and treatment very difficult. Many times, there is denial involved with these diseases from the patient, family, or even the provider. This can even cause a delay in diagnosis and treatment. Because these diseases are not associated with food, but sociopsychological factors, treatment is even more difficult. Treatment should focus on treating the psychological and physiological aspects of the diseases. This is where a multidisciplinary approach and appropriate referral are essential. Treatment modalities may vary depending on the age, stage, and complexity of the disease (Burns et al., 2004).

As with treatment of any disease, the APN should provide a comfortable environment for the patient. A trusting, safe environment will facilitate further discussion. Once the patient feels comfortable with the relationship, further education can follow (Kelly-Weeder, Phillips, Leonard, & Veroneau, 2014).

The APN should be responsible for the medical care and education of the patient with anorexia and bulimia. This could include hospital admission and management for the patient with severe electrolyte imbalance. Further hospitalization management could include fluid stabilization and working with the RD for caloric intake (Burns et al., 2004).

Nutritional rehabilitation is used for severely underweight patients to correct malnutrition and restore and normalize an eating pattern. Treatment with nutritional rehabilitation should be done with healthy weight goals while keeping both men and women in mind. The goal for a woman would be to restore ovulation and normal menstruation cycles, whereas the healthy weight goal for a man would be that of normal testicular function.

Refeeding programs are also used in the treatment of anorexia. Oral "normal" foods are used, but in smaller amounts. Both inpatient and outpatient refeeding programs exist. Targets for weight gain should be realistic in nature. Inpatient programs should aim at 2 to 3 pound weight gains per week. Outpatient programs have lower goal weight gains aimed at 0.5 to 1 pound per week. Initial total caloric intake is usually aimed at 1,000 to 1,600 calories per day or at 30 to 40 calories/kg per day with a goal as high as 70 to 100 calories/kg per day in some patients. Forced nasogastric or parenteral feedings are also used; in extreme cases, gastrostomy or jejunostomy tubes may be placed.

Weight maintenance programs are used to treat those with anorexia. Recommendations are made to add as much as 200 to 400 more calories than those of comparable age, weight, height, and sex. Those with severe anorexia also often have higher rates of hospital readmission.

Medication therapy is also used for the treatment of anorexia. Two classes of antidepressants have been used to treat anorexia. These include selective serotonin reuptake inhibitors (SSRIs, e.g., fluoxetine and citalopram) and tricyclic antidepressants (TCs; e.g., amitriptyline and cyproheptadine). Antipsychotics (olanzapine, quetiapine, and haloperidol) are also used to treat anorexia in certain patients. Antiepileptics (carbamazepine and valproate) are currently under further investigation in treatment of anorexia. Growth hormone (rGH), testosterone, and estrogen have also been studied in regards to the treatment of anorexia with no statistically significant results to report.

Fluoxetine is the only medication used in treatment of both anorexia and bulimia. However, several of the same medication classes are used. Antidepressants, including SSRIs (fluoxetine, fluvoxamine, sertraline, and trazodone), TCs (desipramine), and mono amine oxidase (MAO) inhibitors (brofaromine), are commonly used to treat bulimia. A 5-HT$_3$ antagonist, ondansetron, is used to help reduce the urge to binge or vomit. There have been many medications used experimentally in the treatment of bulimia, including fenfluramine (now off the market), lithium carbonate, naltrexone, topiramate, carbamazepine, and valproate (Chakraborty & Basu, 2010).

Other medications and supplements used in treatment of both anorexia and bulimia can include progesterone, folate, potassium, calcium, phosphate, zinc, magnesium, or iron. Referrals can also be made for additional nutritional coun-

seling, individual psychotherapy, group psychotherapy, family therapy, and asser-
tiveness training. Stress management and education about body relaxation is
also essential. A referral could also be made to an exercise specialist or personal
trainer for movement therapy (Burns et al., 2004).

Dialectic behavior therapy (DBT) and self-help trials have also been used in
treatment for bulimia. DBT therapy consists of a 20-week treatment program,
whereas self-help trials are self-guided for approximately 18 weeks. Some bulimic
patients have found professional support groups, similar to those listed earlier
for food addicts, helpful, although no data exist to support this. Guided imagery
therapy, light therapy, and crisis intervention are also additional interventions
that some patients have tried in the treatment of bulimia (Chakraborty & Basu,
2010).

APNs are in a unique position to screen for, diagnose, and treat addiction and
eating disorders. Continued education on these diseases is needed. A multidisciplinary approach is essential in treatment. The APN should consider referral of
any patient with any behavior or addiction disorder. Long-term goals with these
patients should include prevention of future health problems or complications.

REFERENCES

Burns, C. E., Dunn, A. M., Brady, M. A., Starr, N. B., & Blosser, C. G. (2004). *Pediatric primary care: A handbook for nurse practitioners* (3rd ed.). St. Louis, MO: Saunders.

Chakraborty, K., & Basu, D. (2010). Management of anorexia and bulimia nervosa: An evidence-based review. *Indian Journal of Psychiatry, 52*(2), 174–186. Retrieved from http://www.ncbi.nlm.nih.gov/pmc/articles/PMC2927890

Food Addiction Institute (FAI). (2015a). *Assess, treat and refer.* Retrieved from http://foodaddictioninstitute.org/for-professionals/assess-treat-and-refer

Food Addiction Institute (FAI). (2015b). *Doctors, dietitians and therapists.* Retrieved from http://foodaddictioninstitute.org/for-professionals/dear-doctors-dietitians-and-therapists

Kelly-Weeder, S., Phillips, K., Leonard, K., & Veroneau, M. (2014). Binge eating and weight loss behaviors of overweight and obese college students. *Journal of the American Association of Nurse Practitioners, 26*(8), 445–451.

Pharmacological Therapy

This chapter addresses pharmacological therapies associated with obesity. Pharmacological agents play an important part in the treatment of obesity. Although medications are not for everyone, they are beneficial to some patients. This chapter focuses on who will benefit from these medications, the different classes of antiobesity medications, and the benefits of weight loss.

Medical professionals have often been wary to prescribe medications to treat obesity. Historically, treatment has been aimed at lifestyle modifications; however, more recently, it has come to include medications as well as bariatric surgery. Concerns have arisen about the addictive or harmful nature of these drugs. There has been confusion over the short-term versus long-term safety and efficacy of these medications. Rapid expansion of obesity medications has come recently, secondary to the ongoing efforts of research in genetic and chemical studies on obesity (Rippe, 2013). Along with the Food and Drug Administration (FDA)-approved medications to treat obesity, this chapter also focuses on the off-label use, over-the-counter (OTC) medications, diet supplements, and the role of the FDA.

PHARMACOTHERAPY FOR OBESITY

Historically, medications for obesity have been around since the late 1950s. They have become increasingly more popular in the past 30 years. From 1996 to 1998, an estimated 4.6 million Americans used prescription weight-loss medications. According to the U.S. Department of Health and Human Services (HHS), an estimated 1.2 to 4.7 million used fenfluramines—either fenfluramine or dexfenfluramine—between 1995 and 1997. The use of nonprescription weight-loss products, including phenylpropanolamine and ephedra, was also popular during this time frame. Serious side effects were noted from these medications, and the FDA withdrew use of many medications (Hsu, Chu, Ku, Liou, & Chou, 2010).

Which patients should receive pharmacotherapy for treatment of obesity? Although there is no ideal pharmacotherapy or proven algorithm for the treatment of obesity, there are body mass index (BMI) guidelines that can help guide the advanced practice nurse (APN) to find an appropriate patient for treatment. These guidelines suggest that pharmacotherapy is appropriate for any of the following:

- Upper overweight BMI category (27–29.9 kg/m^2) with comorbidities
- Obese BMI category (≥30 kg/m^2) with or without associated comorbidities

Prior to prescribing pharmacotherapy, the APN should work with the patient on lifestyle changes. The patient should have either tried and failed or tried with limited benefit before being prescribed medication. Lifestyle changes could include, but are not limited to, behavior modification and dietary and/or exercise changes. Many times, the patient has tried some type of nonpharmacological weight loss before seeking professional help. This is due to the variety of self-help, television, and online programs that offer nonmedically supervised programs consisting of diet and/or exercise.

Prescribing the antiobesity medications comes with provider responsibility. APNs should have specific knowledge of the safety and efficacy of these medications as well as a general understanding of the pharmacology and side effects. Along with medication prescription, the APN should provide the patient with education, including behavior modification as well as lifestyle changes—diet and exercise. The APN also has the responsibility of determining how to use the FDA-approved agents in alignment with the guidelines or for treatment beyond the recommended guidelines. This "off-label" use is within the scope of practice, as it is not pro-hibited by the FDA. An example of this is using pharmacotherapy sooner rather than later for a patient whose obesity is limiting quality of life, while at the same time implementing lifestyle changes. Ultimately, the APN has the responsibility to do what is best and safest for the patient.

The timing and "the when" pharmacological agents for obesity should be discussed with the patient is ill-defined and therefore is left up to the individual APN's discretion. APNs who have a good and working relationship with the patient and address weight issues in a timely manner are more likely to have this conversation earlier than other providers. Education, experience, and medical expertise are likely to guide the APN to a conversation with the patient and match that patient's individual needs with the appropriate treatment course of action and pharmacological options. Treatment will vary depending on the patient's read-iness to lose weight. Compliance, willingness, and affordability for treatment must be assessed, which will help improve the APN's ability to successfully implement pharmacotherapy.

Assessing the patient's self-motivation is also important. Why does this patient want to take medication or pills to lose weight? Is it medically necessary? Does the patient have a related health condition that would be aided by weight loss? Does he or she want to lose weight for cosmetic reasons? Has he or she tried other means to lose weight and has been unsuccessful? Does he or she insist on medica-tion during the initial appointment? Has he or she been a yo-yo dieter? All these are important questions to consider when assessing patient motivation. Unfortu-nately, change in health status has not been seen as a patient motivator for weight loss; when used as the only argument by the APN, it may prove unsuccessful. Vanity, in contrast, may prove to be a significant motivating factor. Many times, the thought is to turn these patients away; however, if they qualify for treatment, they should not be turned away.

The APN should address the risks and benefits to pharmacotherapy. Caution should arise with the use of treatment in the patient older than 65 years. Although pharmacological therapy may prove a benefit, it is not a cure for obesity. A relapse of weight is possible after discontinuation of the medication. This is why it is important to incorporate lifestyle changes before, during, and after treatment with pharmacotherapy (Rippe, 2013).

FDA-APPROVED OBESITY MEDICATIONS

Currently, there are seven pharmacological therapies that are FDA approved for the treatment of obesity. This vast array of medications dates back as far as 1959 to as current as 2014. Many medications have been tried and have been unsuccessful in gaining FDA approval. For many years, only two FDA-approved prescription weight-loss medications were on the market—orlistat and sibutramine; however, sibutramine was later withdrawn (Hsu et al., 2010). More recent years have seen the addition of four new medications—Lorcaserin, Qsymia, Contrave, and Saxenda. This section reviews the general pharmacological information as well as the relevant literature data that will help guide the APN in prescription decision making.

Phentermine

Phentermine was first FDA approved for the treatment of obesity in 1959 and is still used today. It is approved for short-term use—up to 3 months. Phentermine is part of the β-phenethylamine family and is a centrally acting appetite suppressant agent. No randomized controlled trials (RCTs) have been completed on phentermine since 1999. The longest trial of 36 weeks was completed in 1968. Phentermine demonstrated a mean weight loss of 12.2 kg in comparison to the placebo with 4.8 kg. Another study, a meta-analysis of six RCTs, demonstrated an increase in weight loss of 3.6 kg with phentermine in comparison with the placebo (Kang & Park, 2012).

Phentermine is a controlled substance scheduled IV. Adverse effects associated with the use of phentermine are numerous and can include elevated blood pressure (BP), tachycardia, pulmonary hypertension (HTN), dizziness, dry mouth, constipation, diarrhea, hand tremor, restlessness, stimulation, and insomnia. This medication should not be used with other anorectic or antiobesity drugs. Phentermine should not be used with or within 14 days of monoamine oxidase inhibitors (MAOIs) because of increased risk of hypertensive crisis (Wong, Kaur, Ma, Patel, & Ringel, 2013). A few studies have shown the use of phentermine alone to cause primary pulmonary HTN. Addiction and drug abuse potential have been reported as minimal.

Phentermine is available in scored or nonscored tablets or capsule form. Maximum approved doses are 37.5 mg (scored tablet) and 30 mg (nonscored or tablet) (Rippe, 2013).

Diethylpropion (Tenuate)

Diethylpropion is a phenylethylamine ring compound that was initially FDA approved for its treatment in obesity in 1959 (Kang & Park, 2012). It has a similar action to phentermine and is structurally similar to bupropion (Rippe, 2013). It is a schedule IV drug. Side effects are similar to amphetamines (Kang & Park, 2012). These can include insomnia, sleepiness, palpitations, elevation in BP, as well as headache, dizziness, dry mouth, or rash (Kang & Park, 2012; Rippe, 2013). Other associated factors with sleep can include a delay in moving from rapid eye movement (REM) sleep to stage I sleep. This medication is not recommended for people with HTN, hyperthyroidism, glaucoma, or heart disease (Rippe, 2013).

A meta-analysis comprised 13 studies that demonstrated an additional 3.0 kg of weight was lost with diethylpropion in comparison to the placebo. These studies varied in length from 6 to 52 weeks, with most of the studies being less than 20 weeks in length. No RCTs have been done since 1983 (Kang & Park, 2012).

Diethylpropion has a recommended dose of 75 mg daily (Rippe, 2013).

Orlistat (Xenical)

Orlistat is a gastrointestinal lipase inhibitor that was approved for the treatment of obesity by the FDA in 1998. This medication blocks the absorption of fat in the gastrointestinal tract. With this decreased absorption, approximately one-third of dietary triglycerides are immediately excreted instead of readily absorbed (Crocker & Yanovski, 2009). With the immediate excretion, some unwanted side effects can be seen—oily stools, increased flatulence, abdominal bloating or pain, diarrhea, increased fecal urgency or incontinence, and uncontrollable anal leaking (Crocker & Yanovski, 2009; Rippe, 2013). Vitamins A, D, E, and K—the fat-soluble vitamins—are oftentimes diminished; therefore, it is recommended that a multivitamin be taken more than 2 hours after taking orlistat (Crocker & Yanovski, 2009).

Two 3-year studies were done with orlistat. One study involved 383 adults with abdominal obesity as well as comorbid conditions of impaired fasting glucose, diet-controlled type 2 diabetes mellitus (T2DM), and hyperlipidemia. The aim was to evaluate orlistat use in the prevention of weight gain. This was done after dietary implementation of a very-low-energy diet (VLED). The subjects who lost at least 5% of total body weight were then randomized to receive orlistat 120 mg PO three times daily (TID) versus a placebo for a total of 3 years. Both groups received additional lifestyle counseling. The orlistat group lost an average of an additional 2.4 kg in comparison to the placebo group. This orlistat group also reduced the occurrence of T2DM during the 3-year time period. Another 3-year study showed that orlistat increased dietary restraint and decreased binge eating (Rippe, 2013).

In February 2007, the FDA approved OTC orlistat—Alli for use. This lower dose still has side effects similar to orlistat. This medication should be used in combination with dietary and exercise choices.

Orlistat is approved for 120 mg capsules thrice daily. Alli is available in 60 mg capsules and should be taken thrice daily (Rippe, 2013).

Lorcaserin (Belviq)

Lorcaserin was initially rejected by the FDA in December 2010, but received FDA approval in June 2012 (Kang & Park, 2012). It is approved for chronic weight management in adult patients in addition to a reduced calorie diet and physical activity (Wong et al., 2013). This selective serotonin 2C (5-HT2C) receptor agonist works by reducing food intake, thus reducing body weight. This medication initially raised concern because of its similarity to 5-HT2B, which is associated with nonselective serotonergic agents—fenfluramine and dexfenfluramine—and the possibility of cardiac valvulopathy. Studies completed to date have not shown any evidence of this (Kang & Park, 2012). Side effects seen with lorcaserin can include nausea, headache, and dizziness (Kang & Park, 2012; Rippe, 2013).

A 2-year double-blind study with 3,182 patients examined the effects of lorcaserin. Those treated with lorcaserin 10 mg twice daily lost 3.6 kg more than the placebo group after 12 months. Those who continued the medication up to 24 months did better with weight maintenance in comparison to the placebo group at 67.9% and 50.3%, respectively. A similar design trial examined the effectiveness of lorcaserin in 4,008 patients. Lorcaserin 10 mg daily or 10 mg twice daily was compared against placebo. Both groups received a dietary and exercise program. Both lorcaserin groups showed a weight loss in comparison to placebo at the end of 12 months. The patients taking lorcaserin 10 mg twice daily lost an average of 5.9% of body weight, whereas the lorcaserin 10 mg daily group lost an average of 4.8% and the placebo group lost only 2.8% (Kang & Park, 2012).

Lorcaserin is prescribed as 10 mg daily (Kang & Park, 2012).

Phentermine/Topiramate (Qsymia)

Qsymia, a combination of a sympathomimetic amine anorectic drug and an antiepileptic drug, was FDA approved for the treatment of weight loss in July 2012. Approved for chronic weight management, it is a combination medication that has listed side effects of insomnia, dry mouth, constipation, dizziness, and paraesthesia (Shin & Gadde, 2013). It too should be used in addition to a reduced calorie diet and increased physical activity (Wong et al., 2013). It should not be used in pregnant women. If increased heart rate (HR), suicidal behavior, acute myopia and secondary angle closure glaucoma, mood or sleep disorders, or cognitive impairments occur, the use of these medications should be discontinued. Electrolytes and creatinine should be monitored on patients taking Qsymia. Glucose levels should also be monitored secondary to the effects of weight loss.

A Phase II, 24-week, randomized clinical trial consisting of 200 patients randomized patients to a placebo, phentermine 15 mg, topiramate 100 mg, or Qsymia. Doses of Qsymia were gradually increased to full dose by week 4. All were given education on diet and exercise. Body weight changes were seen in all groups: placebo –2.1%, phentermine –4.6%, topiramate –6.3%, and Qsymia –10.7% (Shin & Gadde, 2013).

All Phase III trials—OB-301, OB-302, and OB-303—were randomized trials that showed that mid-doses and full doses of Qsymia were more successful in achieving weight loss versus the placebo groups. OB-305, a 2-year extension of OB-303, continued treatment assigned in OB-303. Although all groups demonstrated weight regain, there was still a greater weight loss with the mid-doses and full doses of Qsymia (–9.3% and –10.5%, respectively) compared with placebo (–1.8%) (Shin & Gadde, 2013).

Qsymia is available in the following capsules (phentermine mg/topiramate mg extended release):

- 3.75/23 mg
- 7.5/46 mg
- 11.25/69 mg
- 15/92 mg

To begin a patient on this medication, 3.75/23 mg daily for 14 days should be started and then increased to 7.5/46 mg daily. After week 12 on the 7.5/46 mg dose, weight loss should be evaluated. If a 3% weight loss (baseline body weight) is not achieved in 12 weeks after the 7.5/46 mg dose, either it should be discontinued or the dose should be increased. To escalate the dose, it should be increased to 11.25/69 mg daily for 14 days and then increased to 15/92 mg daily. After 12 weeks on the maximum dose of 15/92 mg daily, if a 5% weight loss is not achieved, the medication should be discontinued gradually. To avoid the risk of a seizure, the patient should be advised to take one dose of the 15/92 mg capsules every other day for at least 1 week. Then, the medication may be discontinued altogether (Vivus, 2014).

Naltrexone HCl/Bupropion HCl (Contrave)

Contrave became FDA approved in September 2014 for the treatment of obesity. Contrave was initially approved by the FDA Advisory Committee in December 2010, but was turned down by the FDA in 2011. After more studies were completed, approval was granted. Initial concerns were related to the side effect of HTN. Other side effects of Contrave can include dry mouth, dizziness, headache, vomiting, and constipation (Rippe, 2013). Side effects can also include suicidal thoughts or ideations. This thought is secondary to the bupropion (Takeda Pharmaceuticals America, Inc., 2014).

The COR-I trial consisted of 1,742 participants who were randomized to double-blind treatment. This included naltrexone 32 mg plus bupropion, naltrexone 16 mg plus bupropion, or the placebo group. After 56 weeks of treatment, the naltrexone 32 mg plus bupropion demonstrated a mean change in body weight of −6.1%, the naltrexone 16 mg plus bupropion demonstrated a mean change in body weight of −5.0%, and the placebo demonstrated a lesser result of −1.3% (Greenway et al., 2010). These, along with the COR-II, COR-BMOD, and COR-Diabetes, were randomized to Contrave versus placebo along with a reduced caloric intake and increased physical activity. All these studies have demonstrated weight loss with the use of Contrave.

The dose of Contrave should be gradually increased. It is available in extended-release tablets: 8 mg naltrexone HCl/90 mg bupropion HCl. Contrave should be administered as shown in Table 21.1.

Liraglutide Injection (Saxenda)

Saxenda, the first injectable treatment for chronic weight management, was approved in December 2014. It is to be used along with a reduced-calorie diet in addition to activity. Saxenda, a glucagon-like peptide-1 (GLP-1) receptor agonist, is similar to Victoza. The two should not be confused, as Saxenda is not approved for the treatment of diabetes and vice versa. Side effects reported with the use of the medication include suicidal thoughts, renal impairment, pancreatitis, and gallbladder disease. HR should also be monitored and discontinued if a sustained resting HR occurs. Decreased appetite, nausea, vomiting, diarrhea, constipation, and low blood sugars were also seen during clinical trials.

TABLE 21.1

CONTRAVE DOSING	
Week 1	One tablet daily in the morning
Week 2	One tablet twice daily
Week 3	Two tablets daily in the morning, one tablet daily at night
Week 4—onward	Two tablets twice daily

Source: Takeda Pharmaceuticals America, Inc. (2014).

Saxenda also carries a black box warning of thyroid gland tumors (thyroid C-cell tumors) seen in rodent studies. Although it is unknown if this is seen in humans, those with a history of medullary thyroid carcinoma (MTC) or multiple endocrine neoplasia syndrome type 2 should not be given Saxenda.

Three clinical trials to date have been completed in approximately 4,800 patients. One 12-month trial, using patients who are not diabetic, demonstrated a 4.5% weight loss in comparison to the placebo group. Another trial involving diabetic patients also demonstrated a weight loss of 3.7% with use of Saxenda in comparison to the placebo group (U.S. Food and Drug Administration [FDA], 2014).

Postmarketing studies are under way. These have been requested and required by the FDA. They include the following (FDA, 2014):

- Studies in pediatric patients to include dosing, safety, and efficacy
- Rodent studies to include effects of growth and development and central nervous system (CNS) development
- A 15-year MTC case registry
- Potential risk of breast cancer related to the use of Saxenda
- Cardiovascular safety in relation to the use of Saxenda

Saxenda can be injected into the upper arm, thigh, or abdomen. The injection site, as well as the timing, can be changed at any time. The maximum dosage of Saxenda is 3 mg daily. Dosing should be initiated at 0.6 mg daily for 1 week. The dose should be increased at weekly intervals to the maximum dose of 3 mg daily (Novo Nordisk, 2015). After 16 weeks, the patient should undergo an evaluation to determine if the therapy has been successful. A weight loss of at least 4% of baseline body weight should be met; if not, the medication should be discontinued, as it is unlikely that the patient could achieve and/or sustain weight loss (FDA, 2014).

OFF-LABEL DRUG USE

Off-label use of medications is not illegal. The FDA defines the use of off-label and investigational use of marketed drugs as cited in Rippe (2013, p. 552):

Good medical practice and the best interests of the patient require that physicians use legally available drugs, biologics, and devices according to their best knowledge and judgment. If physicians use a product for an indication not in the approved labeling, they have the responsibility to be well informed about the product, to base its use of the firm scientific rationale and on sound medical evidence, and to maintain records of the product's use and effects. Use of a marketed product in this manner *when the intent is the "practice of medicine"* does not require the submission of an Investigational New Drug (IND) Application, Investigational Device Exemption (IDE), or review by an Institutional Review Board (IRB). However, the institution at which the product will be used may, under its own authority, require IRB review or other institutional oversight.

If the APN determines that an off-label use drug would be best for the patient, careful education and documentation should take place. The APN should carefully review the known side effects of the drug as well as review the potential risk versus added benefit to the patient of off-label use. The APN's rationale should be carefully documented in the patient's chart. The APN should also provide the patient with a rationale as to why this medication is prescribed. It is also recommended that a signed document by the patient accompanies his or her chart. Medications in the following classes are supported by clinical evidence: antidepressants, antidiabetic drugs, and antiseizure medications.

Antidepressants

Fluoxetine and bupropion are two antidepressants used for off-label use for obesity treatment.

Fluoxetine (Prozac)

Fluoxetine is a highly selective serotonin reuptake inhibitor (SSRI) FDA approved for the treatment of depression. However, it has also been investigated for its weight-loss effect. Weight loss has not been consistent in all trials. In fact, those who have lost weight within the first 6 months of trial tended to have weight regain. This was despite the fact that fluoxetine therapy was continued. In studies on fluoxetine in which behavior therapy accompanied medication, weight loss was found to be significant at 1 year (Rippe, 2013).

Side effects found with therapy include nervousness or anxiety, decreased appetite, decreased sexual desire, weakness, nausea, and diarrhea. Insomnia, dry mouth, dizziness, and flu-like symptoms have also been reported.

The dose of fluoxetine for treatment of obesity has ranged from 20 to 80 mg.

Bupropion (Wellbutrin)

Bupropion inhibits the reuptake of dopamine, serotonin, and norepinephrine. It is FDA approved for the treatment of depression and smoking cessation. Bupropion also demonstrated a range of weight-loss results. Studies ranged in length from 26 to 48 weeks. Similar to fluoxetine, weight loss was maintained in some trials for as much as 1 year. Side effects seen with this medication include weight loss, dry mouth, dizziness, headache, and tremors. Bradycardia, nausea, and constipation can also be seen (Rippe, 2013).

The dose of bupropion for treatment of obesity can vary from 300 to 400 mg daily.

Antidiabetic Drugs

Antidiabetic drugs have also demonstrated pharmacological success in the treatment of obesity. Metformin, exenatide, amylin, pramlintide, and acarbose have been studied for their off-label use of weight loss.

Metformin (Glucophage)

Metformin is FDA approved for the treatment of diabetes. Clinical trials involving metformin have shown two different results with regard to obesity—weight loss or weight neutral. Clinical trial authors have concluded that metformin can be used early in the treatment of diabetes mellitus in order to prevent weight gain or to aid in weight loss. Modest weight loss with metformin use was seen in children. Side effects seen with the use of metformin include fatigue, loose stools, or nausea (Rippe, 2013).

Metformin is available in 500, 750, and 1,000 mg tablets. A maximum dose of 2,000 mg is recommended.

Exenatide

Exenatide is a GLP-1 hormone, similar to Saxenda, produced in the ileum and colon. Glucagon secretion is inhibited with its use, whereas stimulation of insulin secretion after ingestion of carbohydrates is present, all of which aid in delayed gastric emptying, thus increasing satiety. Studies are ongoing in the treatment of obesity in nondiabetics (Rippe, 2013).

Amylin

Because amylin slows gastric emptying, satiety is felt directly after a meal and can lead to weight loss. Amylin is a peptide hormone that is part of the neurohormonal feedback system. Because it promotes satiety, amylin is thought to be a signal for adiposity. Studies done in rats and humans demonstrate that amylin levels in the blood may set homeostatic weight controls to a lower mass and contribute to weight constancy (Rippe, 2013).

Pramlintide

Pramlintide is the injectable form of the synthetic analog of amylin. It is FDA approved for the treatment of type 1 and type 2 diabetes. Pramlintide is oftentimes added to treatment in addition to insulin therapy. When added to pre-existing therapy, reduction in HgA1c is seen in addition to weight loss. Studies with combination therapy in nondiabetic patients receiving pramlintide and metreleptin (leptin) were more successful than those with either agent alone. Nausea has been reported as the main side effect. Further trials are ongoing (Rippe, 2013).

Acarbose (Precose)

Acarbose is an alpha-glucosidase inhibitor that is FDA approved for the treatment of diabetes. It blocks the digestion of complex carbohydrates. Small weight-loss changes have been seen in the treatment of obesity. Side effects can include abdominal pain, diarrhea, and flatulence. A National Institutes of Health (NIH) study deemed there was insufficient evidence to consider while prescribing this medication for obesity in nondiabetics (Rippe, 2013).

Antiseizure Medications

Three antiseizure medications have also shown success in off-label treatment of obesity. These medications are topiramate, zonisamide, and atomoxetine.

Topiramate (Topamax)

Topiramate is an antiepileptic drug that works by improving the neuroinhibition of γ–aminobutyric acid (GABA) and blocks sodium channels. Side effects associated with topiramate are often considered neurological side effects, such as difficulty with focus and concentration, memory problems, ataxia, and speech problems. Diplopia, nystagmus, dizziness, and headache can also be seen.

The weight loss associated with topiramate is found in several clinical trials. Success with topiramate can also be seen in clinical trials associated with Qysmia, as this includes topiramate in combination with phentermine. One study that used topiramate for the treatment of bipolar disorder and schizoaffective disease showed weight loss ranging from 8 to 56 pounds (Rippe, 2013).

Zonisamide (Zonegran)

Zonisamide was first FDA approved for the treatment of seizures, specifically atrial focal seizures found in adults with epilepsy. Side effects associated with the medication can include cognitive impairments, dizziness, and somnolence.

Zonisamide has been studied alone and in combination with bupropion; both demonstrated weight loss. One study with Zonisamide, in combination with a 500-calorie deficit, demonstrated a 9.2 kg weight loss in comparison to the placebo, which demonstrated 1.5 kg (Rippe, 2013).

Atomoxetine

FDA approved for the treatment of attention deficit hyperactivity disorder (ADHD), atomoxetine is a central norepinephrine uptake inhibitor that has also demonstrated weight-loss effects. Modest weight loss was associated in a small-participant, 12-week study. Decreased appetite was reported (Rippe, 2013).

NONPRESCRIPTION MEDICATIONS

Nonprescription medications can be used for the treatment of obesity. The APN should review the evidence for and against the following treatments. The patient's best interest should always be entertained.

Alli

Alli is the approved OTC version of orlistat. Details, studies, side effects, and doses can be found in the Orlistat (Xenical) entry under the *FDA Approved Obesity Medications* heading.

Laxatives

No data exist to support the use of laxatives for weight loss; however, there are patients who use these products to assist them in weight loss.

Dietary Supplements

Dietary supplements are also used by some to aid in weight loss. A *dietary supplement* is best defined as a product taken in order to fill a deficit or supply an ingredient that the body is missing. Vitamins, minerals, and herbs are some of these supplements. Amino acids, enzymes, metabolites, or even organ tissues may be other supplements used. Many forms of dietary supplements exist. These can include liquids, powders, tablets, or capsules. Many men and women have taken some form of supplement at some point and not reported its use with his or her other medications. This has been estimated in as many as 9.7% of men and 20.6% of women.

The FDA does not become involved in the process of dietary supplements until after there have been reported side effects. The FDA does not approve or analyze dietary supplements before they go to market and are sold to consumers. The only information that dietary supplements need to share are the ingredients. Product safety or claims made are monitored by the FDA's Center for Food Safety and Applied Nutrition (CFSAN).

The APN is responsible for the documentation and charting of any dietary supplements. The APN should provide education about the misconceptions of weight-loss supplements in a nonjudgmental manner. The safety and efficacy of dietary supplements should also be addressed with the patient.

Fat Substitutes

Fat substitutes were used by the commercial food industry as nonprescription food additives to provide a lower fat content to prepackaged foods. Olestra (Olean) is one of those products. Used to replace fat in such products as chips or crackers, it is made of a molecule too big to be both digested and/or absorbed. Unpleasant side effects can be seen with use of this product. This has included side effects similar to those seen with orlistat—abdominal bloating, diarrhea, loose stools, flatulence, and fecal incontinence leakage (Rippe, 2013).

FDA-WITHDRAWN MEDICATIONS

The FDA has withdrawn several medications that were previously approved for weight loss. These include fenfluramine, dexfenfluramine, and sibutramine (Meridia). Fenfluramine was originally approved by the FDA for weight loss in 1973. It was withdrawn from the market in 1997 secondary to valvulopathies (Crocker & Yanovski, 2009). Dexfenfluramine was FDA approved in 1996 and was withdrawn in 1997. Meridia (sibutramine) was FDA approved for the treatment of obesity in 1997 and was voluntarily withdrawn from the market in October 2010 secondary to a 16% increased risk of cardiovascular events (FDA, 2010). Rimonabant was approved by the European Union (EU) in 2006, but was never approved for use in the United States. It was withdrawn from the European market in January 2009 (Hsu et al., 2010).

Other medications that have been previously approved for weight loss and are now banned include dinitrophenol, amphetamines (dexamphetamine, methamphetamine), amphetamine-like analogues (phenylpropanolamine [PPA]), aminorex, and mazindol. Phentermine, although approved for short-term use in the United States, was banned in 2000 in the United Kingdom. The use of any dietary supplement containing ephedra was also banned in 2004. The use of ephedrine with caffeine and/or aspirin is also not recommended (Ioannides-Demos, Piccenna, & McNeil, 2011).

The APN must be familiar with antiobesity medications, pharmacotherapy, and side effects associated with these medications. Pharmacotherapy should be used only in addition to lifestyle modification. The APN has a responsibility to educate the patient and to base treatment individually.

REFERENCES

Crocker, M., & Yanovski, J. A. (2009). Pediatric obesity: Etiology and treatment. *Endocrinology and Metabolism Clinics in North America*, 38(3), 525–548. doi:10.1016/j.ecl.2009.06.007

Greenway, F. L., Fujioka, K., Plodkowski, R. A., Mudaliar, S., Guttadauria, M., Erickson, J., . . . Dunayevich, E. (2010). Effect of naltrexone plus bupropion on weight loss in overweight and obese adults (COR-I): A multicenter, randomized, double-blind, placebo-controlled, phase 3 trial. *Lancet, 376*(9741), 595–605. doi:http://dx.doi.org/10.1016/S0140-6736(10)60888-4

Hsu, Y. W., Chu, D. C., Ku, P. W., Liou, T. H., & Chou, P. (2010). Pharmacotherapy for obesity: Past, present and future. *Journal of Experimental and Clinical Medicine, 2*(3), 118–123.

Ioannides-Demos, L. L., Piccenna, L., & McNeil, J. J. (2011). Pharmacotherapies for obesity: Past, current, and future therapies. *Journal of Obesity, 2011,* 179674. doi:10.1155/2011/179674

Kang, J. G., & Park, C. Y. (2012). Anti-obesity drugs: A review about their effects and safety. *Diabetes Metabolic Journal, 36*(1), 13–25. doi:10.4093/dmj.2012.36.1.13

Novo Nordisk. (2015). *Saxenda: Highlights of prescribing information.* Retrieved from http://www.novo-pi.com/saxenda.pdf

Rippe, J. M. (Ed.). (2013). *Lifestyle medicine* (2nd ed.). Boca Raton, FL: CRC Press.

Shin, J. H., & Gadde, K. M. (2013). Clinic utility of phentermine/topiramate (Qsymia) combination for the treatment of obesity. *Diabetes, Metabolic Syndrome and Obesity: Targets and Therapy, 6,* 131–139. doi:10.2147/DMSO.S43403

Takeda Pharmaceuticals America, Inc. (2014). *Contrave: Highlights of prescribing information.* Retrieved from http://general.takedapharm.com/content/file.aspx?filetype code=CONTRAVEPI&CountryCode=US&LanguageCode=EN&cacheRandomizer= 39686d9f-b6f4-4e51-89ba-8beb87ee030b

Vivus. (2014). *Qsymia: Highlights of prescribing information.* Retrieved from https://qsymia.com/hcc/include/media/pdf/prescribing-information.pdf

U.S. Food and Drug Administration (FDA). (2010). *FDA drug safety communication: FDA recommends against the continued use of Meridia (sibutramine).* Retrieved from http://www.fda.gov/Drugs/DrugSafety/ucm228746.htm

U.S. Food and Drug Administration (FDA). (2014). *FDA approves weight-management drug Saxenda.* Retrieved from http://www.fda.gov/NewsEvents/Newsroom/Press Announcements/ucm427913.htm

Wong, E., Kaur, N., Ma, N., Patel, K., & Ringel, M. (2013). Obesity: A focus on pharmacotherapy. *Journal for Nurse Practitioners, 9*(6), 387–395.

Surgical Therapy

This chapter addresses the indications and options with regard to bariatric surgery. Referring a patient for bariatric surgery can be one of the easiest as well as one of the toughest decisions for the advanced practice nurse (APN). It is difficult to initiate the subject of weight loss, let alone telling the patient that he or she needs surgery to fix the problem. This chapter defines the candidates for bariatric surgery as well as addresses the different surgical procedures available.

CANDIDATES FOR BARIATRIC SURGERY

Bariatric surgery is not for everybody. Bariatric surgery is indicated for those with a body mass index (BMI) greater than or equal to 40 kg/m², with or without comorbid conditions. Bariatric surgery is also indicated for those with a BMI greater than or equal to 35 kg/m² with comorbid conditions related to obesity. A BMI greater than or equal to 35 kg/m² must be accompanied by one or more severe obesity-related conditions (Brethauer, Kashyap, & Schauer, 2013; Mechanick et al., 2013). These can include type 2 diabetes mellitus (T2DM), hypertension (HTN), hyperlipidemia, obstructive sleep apnea (OSA), obesity-hypoventilation syndrome (OHS), nonalcoholic fatty liver disease (NAFLD) or nonalcoholic steatohepatitis (NASH), pseudotumor cerebri, gastroesophageal reflux disease (GERD), asthma, venous stasis disease, debilitating arthritis, severe urinary incontinence, or considerably impaired quality of life. For patients with a BMI of 30 to 34.9 kg/m² and diabetes mellitus (DM) or metabolic syndrome, bariatric surgery may be considered; however, current evidence is limited on the benefits. Bariatric surgery has demonstrated insufficient evidence for the following alone: lipid lowering, glycemic control, or cardiovascular risk reduction (Mechanick et al., 2013).

Appropriate candidates for bariatric surgery are also within the ages of 18 to 60 years. Data in more recent years have shown evidence that bariatric surgery may be safe and effective for some adolescents and patients older than age 60 under certain conditions (Brethauer et al., 2013; Mechanick et al., 2013). Candidates should also be deemed acceptable surgical patients and present optimal operative risk. Patients should be motivated for surgery and have family support. A good candidate should be psychologically stable, have no signs of "uncontrolled psychotic or depressive disorder," and abstain from active alcohol and/or substance abuse. The bariatric candidate must also have documented failure of a previous medical/nonsurgical weight-loss program (Brethauer et al., 2013), as well as understand the risks, benefits, and alternatives to the procedure as well as complete routine follow-up and blood work. Patients must also agree to take daily vitamins and supplements, as well as be committed to self-monitoring. Finally, the patient must agree to exercise daily (Goritz & Duff, 2014).

There are also contraindications for bariatric surgery. These include those who cannot tolerate general anesthesia. Those with a history of cardiac, pulmonary, or hepatic problems should be screened by an anesthesiologist prior to surgery (Brethauer et al., 2013).

MEDICAL CLEARANCE FOR BARIATRIC SURGERY

Twenty recommendations comprise the elements of medical clearance for bariatric surgery. They are as follows (Mechanick et al., 2013):

1. Glycemic control. Blood sugars should be optimized prior to surgery using a combination of nutrition, activity, and medications. A glycosylated hemoglobin (HgAlc) level of 6.5% to 7.0% or less should be the goal preoperatively with fasting blood glucose levels less than or equal to 110 mg/dL.
2. Hypothyroidism. Those at risk for or with concerns of thyroid disease should have a thyroid-stimulating hormone (TSH) level drawn. A patient with a thyroid abnormality should be treated with L-thyroxine therapy.
3. Lipid panel. A fasting lipid panel should be drawn, and abnormal levels should be treated according to the National Cholesterol Education Program Adult Treatment Panel III guidelines.
4. Pregnancy. Pregnancy should be avoided 12 months prior to surgery and for the 18 months after surgery. Appropriate contraceptive counseling should be provided to all women.
5. Estrogen therapy. Oral contraceptives should be avoided for one cycle prior to bariatric surgery. Hormone replacements in postmenopausal women should be avoided for at least 3 weeks after surgery.
6. Polycystic ovary syndrome (PCOS). Women should be counseled about fertility status improvement after surgery.
7. Rare causes of obesity. Screening may be done for rare causes of obesity should the APN see fit to do so.
8. Noninvasive cardiac testing. An electrocardiogram (ECG) should be completed prior to surgery. Those with cardiovascular disease (CVD) may require a formal cardiology evaluation.
9. Chest radiography and screening for OSA. Consideration should be given for a chest X-ray and screening of OSA. Those with "intrinsic lung disease or disordered sleep patterns should have a formal pulmonary evaluation, including arterial blood gas measurement, when knowledge of the results would alter patient care" (Mechanick et al., 2013, p. 9).
10. Tobacco use. Tobacco abuse should be avoided for 6 weeks prior to surgery. The APN should also stress tobacco cessation postoperatively, as this raises concerns for poor wound healing.
11. Deep venous thrombosis (DVT) and cor pulmonale. Patients with a history of either of these conditions should be screened preoperatively.
12. Gastrointestinal symptoms. Imaging studies should be used for those with severe gastrointestinal symptoms.
13. Abdominal ultrasound. Those with symptomatic liver disease or with elevation of liver function tests (LFTs) should undergo an abdominal ultrasound.

14. *Helicobacter pylori*. Screening can be considered in high-prevalence areas.
15. Gout. Prophylactic treatment can be given for patients with gout.
16. Bone mineral density (BMD) screening. There is insufficient evidence for BMD screening prior to surgery.
17. Psychosocial-behavioral evaluation.

> A psychosocial-behavioral evaluation, which assesses environmental, familial, and behavioral factors, should be required to be done for all patients before bariatric surgery. Any patient considered for bariatric surgery with a known or suspected psychiatric illness, substance abuse, or dependence should undergo a formal mental healthy evaluation before performance of the surgical procedure. (p. 9)

18. Nutritional and behavioral evaluation. Before and after surgery, patients should undergo evaluation and counseling of nutritional and behavioral changes.
19. Nutritional evaluation. Patients should receive a nutritional evaluation before surgery.
20. Primary care provider and cancer screening. Patients should have a primary care provider. They should also undergo appropriate cancer screening prior to surgery.

The APN plays a big role in assisting the bariatric care team prior to surgery. Encouragement should continue to be aimed at weight loss. Any weight loss prior to surgery can help reduce operating time and decrease the length of hospital stay. This may also help reduce the liver size, thus reducing mesenteric fat deposits in the abdominal wall (Goritz & Duff, 2014). Dietary restrictions and diets immediately prior to surgery should be determined by the bariatric surgeon.

SURGICAL PROCEDURES

Several surgical options exist for those requesting surgery for weight loss. At this time, there is no significant evidence to favor one bariatric surgery over another (Mechanick et al., 2013). Generally, laparoscopic bariatric procedures are preferred more than open surgeries; however, these are not for everyone. Surgical options can include laparoscopic adjustable gastric banding (LAGB), laparoscopic sleeve gastrectomy (LSG), laparoscopic Roux-en-Y gastric bypass (RYGB), laparoscopic biliopancreatic diversion (BPD), and BPD/duodenal switch (BPD-DS).

Laparoscopic Adjustable Gastric Banding

The LAGB was approved for use in the United States in 2001. This procedure uses a silicone band placed around the upper portion of the stomach and an inflatable collar used for restriction. The device is controlled by injecting saline through a port placed in the subcutaneous tissue in the abdominal wall. The band is adjusted by the bariatric professional either by adding or removing saline, depending on the patient's hunger, satiety, or weight loss. Mortality risk is lower than in comparison for RYGB. Weight loss with the LAGB is usually a more gradual process.

Risks and benefits exist with any surgery. Risks of bariatric surgery include bowel perforation, band slippage, band leakage, band erosion, and/or a tube or port malfunction. Band slippage or leakage presents the highest risk at 2% to 25%. There are many benefits of LAGB. This can include a 40% to 60% excess weight loss (EWL) and a 55% resolution of DM. Improvements of hyperlipidemia as well as resolutions of HTN and OSA are also seen at 60%, 45%, and 95% resolution, respectively (Brethauer et al., 2013).

Laparoscopic Sleeve Gastrectomy

LSG has been used for more than 10 years. The body and fundus of the stomach are removed through a vertical resection during this operation. This leaves "a tubular gastric lumen from the gastroesophageal junction to the antrum. The pylorus is left intact and there is no device or bypass associated with this procedure" (Brethauer et al., 2013, n.p.). This procedure was initially used as a stepping stone for patients with extremely high BMI. Once desired weight was achieved with LSG, patients were considered candidates for further surgery—either RYGB or a duodenal switch.

This operation also includes a consideration of risks versus benefits. Initial complications can include leaking or bleeding at the gastric staple line. Other complications can include narrowing or gastric incisura strictures. A high incidence (20%–30%) of long-term GERD can also be seen along with a 5% reoperation rate. A 50% to 60% EWL is one significant benefit of the operation. This EWL has been seen in patients 5 years postsurgery. Remission of OSA (75%), HTN (60%–75%), and DM (50%–60%) is also seen (Brethauer et al., 2013).

Roux-En-Y Gastric Bypass

RYGB is the most common bariatric surgery performed in the United States; 80% of all bariatric surgeries use this method (Brethauer et al., 2013). RYGB can be done as an open or laparoscopic procedure. However, the laparoscopic procedure is most commonly used (Johns Hopkins Medicine, n.d.). The RYGB is popular when done laparoscopically, as it combines both a restrictive component and an intestinal bypass, resulting in "superior" weight loss. This procedure is named after the "roux" limb that connects a small, sectioned-off portion of the stomach to the small intestine by bypassing the duodenum and proximal jejunum. The gastric pouch made holds about 15 to 30 mL in order to restrict the amount of intake. The length of the roux limb is approximately 150 cm.

Similar to the previous procedures, RYGB has both risks and benefits. The highest risk is the anastomotic stricture rate at 2% to 10%. Other risks include anastomotic leak, anastomotic ulcer, or late bowel obstruction (Brethauer et al., 2013). Infection, DVT, pulmonary embolism (PE), and respiratory problems can also be seen. Long-term complications can include malnutrition, iron and calcium deficiencies, vital and protein deficiencies, gastric dumping, or internal hernias. Finally, failure can be seen in lack of weight loss, especially if the patient does not comply with the recommended dietary and exercise prescriptions (Johns Hopkins Medicine, n.d.). Benefits include its superiority in long-term weight loss with an estimated EWL of 50% to 55% even 10 years postsurgery. EWL immediately postsurgery is 65% to 80%. Resolutions in DM, OSA, and HTN are seen at 84%, 78%, and 68%, respectively. A 97% improvement is seen in hyperlipidemia. Unique effects that are weight loss independent are produced by gut hormones and glucose homeostasis and have shown rapid improvement in DM secondary to these incretin effects (Brethauer et al., 2013).

Biliopancreatic Diversion

BPD is performed by less than 3% of U.S. bariatric surgeons. More often an open procedure rather than a laparoscopic surgery, it is a malabsorptive procedure in which the lower two-thirds of the stomach is removed. The remaining portion of the stomach attached to the distal lower small intestine (the ilium) bypasses the duodenum and jejunum, thus limiting the available area for absorption. This surgery also requires removal of the gallbladder secondary to the high risk of gallstones (Brethauer et al., 2013).

Advantages and disadvantages exist for this procedure. The major advantage is the high success weight-loss rate both preoperatively and 10 years postoperatively. This is estimated by as much as 75% to 80% EWL in 10 years. Weight loss is also seen continuing as long as 18 to 24 months postoperatively. Reductions in HTN, DM, and OSA are also seen. However, risks are numerous with this procedure; the rate of death is estimated to be 1 in 200 surgeries. Recovery time is also longer in comparison to the other bariatric surgeries; it is typically estimated at 6 to 8 weeks. Because obesity is a malabsorptive disease, it requires long-term supplementation of fat-soluble vitamins (A, D, E, K), B_{12}, calcium, and iron. Dumping syndrome (DS), increased number of stools, and foul flatulence are also observed. Damage to adjacent organs and strictures of the opening of the stomach and small intestine are other seen. Abdominal hernias, bleeding ulcers, and kidney stones are other complications seen with BPD (Your Practice Online, n.d.).

POSTOPERATIVE COMPLICATIONS

Individual postoperative conditions are listed earlier under each specific bariatric surgery. However, DS and nutritional deficiencies need to be further defined so that the APN is more aware of these conditions. DS results from malabsorptive surgeries and is triggered by ingestion of simple carbohydrate foods or liquids. These contents rush into the stomach and leave the intestine too quickly, causing symptoms of "dumping." These symptoms can include cramping, nausea, vomiting, diarrhea, sweating, flushing, salivation, dizziness, or even tachycardia. Dumping symptoms can last up to 2 hours and can be very scary for patients. The APN should encourage dietary adherence and also to avoid large portions as well as drinking with meals.

Nutritional deficiencies are common after bariatric surgery, especially malabsorptive procedures. Routine laboratory values should be monitored according to symptoms or as the APN sees fit. Routine nutritional monitoring laboratories include the following:

- Complete blood count (CBC)
- Basic metabolic panel (BMP)
- LFTs
- Albumin
- Iron
- Ferritin
- Vitamin B_{12}
- 25-Dihydroxyvitamin D
- Vitamin A
- Folate

- Zinc
- Parathyroid hormone

Common deficiencies after any of the bariatric procedures can include the following (Goritz & Duff, 2014):

- Protein malnutrition
- Iron deficiency anemia
- Macrocytic anemia
- Hypocalcemia
- Low vitamin A levels
- Low vitamin D levels

The APN can also monitor for and treat the following nutritional deficiencies, especially those seen after RYGB. These recommendations are according to the American Society for Metabolic and Bariatric Surgery (ASMBS). Vitamin D deficiency and hypocalcemia should be treated with calcium citrate in combination with vitamin D. A dose of 1,200 mg of calcium citrate with 400 to 800 IU of vitamin D is recommended. A multivitamin containing at least 200% of the recommended daily value is also recommended for all patients postsurgery. Vitamin B_{12} is also recommended to aid in reducing bone fractures. Although there is iron found in the multivitamin supplement, some weight-loss patients may require as much as 50 to 100 mg of additional elemental iron, especially teenagers and menstruating women. Vitamin C is also recommended to help with iron absorption.

Postsurgery may cause a number of problems for the patient, including changes to the skin and hair, such as dry skin and thinning or loss of hair. Mood changes may also be seen; this is essential for the APN to address, to avoid any complications related to possible depression. Tiredness and feelings of cold may also be present after surgery. It is important to educate the patient on these immediate side effects and also to inform the patient that as weight stabilizes, these symptoms should resolve (Johns Hopkins Medicine, n.d.).

Immediate referral to the bariatric surgeon and cause for concern are when a patient presents with any vomiting or new onset of abdominal pain. Onset of concern consists of a time frame of months to years. Any complaints of GERD should also be referred back to the surgeon. Any of these symptoms could be a concern, from an anastomotic ulcer or stricture to even bowel obstruction. A patient with a history of LAGB who presents with GERD or dysphagia should also raise red flags as to a possible gastric prolapse through the band; immediate referral should be made to the bariatric surgeon (Brethauer et al., 2013).

LONG-TERM FOLLOW-UP

Lifetime follow-up is recommended for patients who have undergone bariatric surgery. The Endocrine Society provides a summary of recommendations of the postbariatric surgery to include the following:

1. Prevention and treatment of weight regain (WR)
2. Postoperative nutritional management
3. Management of DM and lipids
4. Bone health and gout
5. Gastroenterological and eating behavior considerations

Prevention and treatment of WR is a very important issue for the APN to address and to continue to monitor. A surgical team, medical support team, as well as dietary support are recommended immediately postoperatively as well as available for long-term follow-up. A multidisciplinary approach should be used to provide nutrition advice, exercise therapy, behavior modification, and pharmacological management. If severe postoperative weight gain exists, the APN should refer to the surgical team for further help.

Postoperative nutrition management should include an average of 60 to 120 g of protein daily, long-term vitamin and mineral supplementation, and biochemical monitoring for any nutrition deficiencies.

Postoperative management of DM is also an important issue for the APN to address: a postoperative HgA1c goal less than or equal to 7%, a fasting glucose greater than or equal to 110 mg/dL, and postprandial glucose greater than or equal to 180 mg/dL. Inpatient APNs should be familiar with the recommended glycemic targets and protocols. Type 1 diabetic patients should receive scheduled insulin while hospitalized. Lipid abnormalities should be treated according to the recommended guidelines.

It is recommended that patients who have undergone malabsorptive [i.e. RYGB, gastric sleeve (GS), BPD] obesity surgical procedures should have vitamin D, calcium, phosphorus, PTH [parathyroid hormone], and alkaline phosphatase levels followed every 6 months and have a dual-energy x-ray absorptiometry for bone density performed yearly until stable. (Heber et al., 2010, p. 4)

Vitamin D and calcium should be monitored and adjusted as needed. Gout sufferers should receive prophylactic therapy.

Patients are recommended to sip liquids in the immediate postoperative period. Gradual progression of food consistency is recommended to minimize vomiting. Patients should avoid simple carbohydrate-dense foods and drinks. This will help minimize DS. If patients present with postprandial symptoms, further testing should be done to evaluate for the possibility of insulin-mediated hypoglycemia (Heber et al., 2010).

Mechanick et al. (2013) provide 21 recommendations for optimal follow-up after bariatric surgery. These range from adherence in follow-up visits to revisions in surgery and are as follows:

- Educate on adherence of follow-up visits
- Monitor postprandial hypoglycemia to avoid noninsulinoma pancreatogenous hypoglycemia syndrome (NIPHS)
- Educate on physical activity
- Encourage support groups
- Recommend calcium and vitamin D supplementation
- Monitor BMD
- Manage dehydration to avoid hyperoxaluria
- Monitor anemia resulting from deficiencies in vitamin B_{12}, folate, protein, copper, selenium, and zinc
- Recommend copper supplementation
- Recommend thiamine supplementation
- Monitor lipid levels
- Evaluate the need for antihypertensives
- Monitor gastrointestitional symptoms

- Recommend avoidance of nonsteroidal anti-inflammatory drug (NSAID) use
- Consider endoscopy for chronic abdominal pain
- Consider revisional surgery for problems with nonpartitioned stomach
- Consider referral to bariatric surgery if symptoms of nausea and acid reflux persist after LAGB
- Use of ultrasound to assess for gallstones
- Consider bacterial overgrowth and treat empirically after BPD
- Consider surgical referral for hernia repair as needed
- Consider body-contouring procedures 12–18 months post surgery

Consider hospital readmission if any of the following occur:

- Severe malnutrition
- Failure of medical management of surgical complications for revision of bariatric surgery
- Failure of medical and surgical management for reversal of bariatric surgery

Not all of these recommendations are geared toward the APN–patient relationship; some are clearly between the surgeon and patient. The APN should review these guidelines and address the pertinent issues. Encouragement should be given for routine follow-up with the APN and the bariatric surgeon. Greater excess body weight (EBW) was seen with routine follow-up (missing less than 25% of appointments). This statistic is true for LAGB but has not been seen in RYGB. The APN should monitor for hypoglycemia postsurgery, especially with an accelerated weight loss. The APN should encourage routine physical activity pre- and postsurgery; for example, a combination of cardiovascular activity and strengthening activities. Positive relationships have been seen in those patients post-RYGB and post-LAGB who participate in support groups. BMD should be monitored as the incidence of osteoporosis and risk of fracture is higher after surgery (Mechanick et al., 2013).

According to the Merriam-Webster Medical Dictionary (2015), *hyperoxaluria* is defined as "the presence of excess oxalic acid or oxalates in the urine—called also oxaluria" (n.p.). RYGB and BPD patients should be given calcium supplementation as well as encouraged to limit dietary oxalate and dietary fats. Patients should also be encouraged to increase hydration status. Vitamin B_{12} levels, zinc, copper, and thiamine levels, as well as a lipid panel, should be monitored after surgery. The APN should be aware that chronic nausea and emesis could be directly associated with low thiamine levels. Reductions in both systolic and diastolic BP can continue up to a year postsurgery; the APN should be aware and make medication adjustments as needed. Loose stools and malodorous flatus are common after RYGB, BPD, and LAGB. Gastric and marginal ulcers may be observed, and NSAID use should be avoided. Rifaximin and probiotics are safe for use in IBS in the postoperative patient. Ultrasound is a safe way to assess if the APN is suspicious of gallstone postsurgery. Endoscopy, revisional surgeries, reversal surgeries, body-contouring procedures, and decisions on hernia repair are best left to the bariatric surgeon. The surgeon will also track hospital readmission rates within 30 days after discharge (Mechanick et al., 2013).

The APN plays an essential role in the treatment and care of the bariatric surgical patient. Again, a multidisciplinary approach is recommended pre- and postoperatively to help the patient achieve optimum weight loss. The APN should continue to monitor and encourage further weight loss and help avoid WR.

REFERENCES

Brethauer, S., Kashyap, S., & Schauer, P. (2013). *Obesity*. Cleveland Clinic. Retrieved from http://www.clevelandclinicmeded.com/medicalpubs/diseasemanagement/endocrinology/obesity

Goritz, T., & Duff, E. (2014). Bariatric surgery: Comprehensive strategies for management in primary care. *Journal for Nurse Practitioners, 10*(9), 687–693.

Heber, D., Greenway, F. L., Kaplan, L. M., Livingston, E., Salvador, J., & Still, C. (2010). Endocrine and nutritional management of the post-bariatric surgery patient: An endocrine society clinical practice guideline. *Journal of Clinical Endocrinology & Metabolism*, 1–30.

Johns Hopkins Medicine. (n.d.). *Roux-en-Y gastric bypass weight-loss surgery*. Retrieved from http://www.hopkinsmedicine.org/healthlibrary/test_procedures/gastroenterology/roux-en-y_gastric_bypass_weight-loss_surgery_135,65

Mechanick, J. I., Youdim, A., Jones, D. B., Garvey, W. T., Hurley, D. L., McMahon, M. M., . . . Brethauer, S. (2013). Clinical practice guidelines for the perioperative nutritional, metabolic, and nonsurgical support of the bariatric surgery patient—2013 update: Cosponsored by American Association of Clinical Endocrinologists, the Obesity Society, and American Society for Metabolic & Bariatric Surgery. *Endocrine Practice, 19*(2), 337–372.

Merriam-Webster Medical Dictionary. (2015). *Definition of hyperoxaluria*. Retrieved from http://www.merriam-webster.com/medical/hyperoxaluria

Your Practice Online. (n.d.). *Biliopancreatic diversion surgery*. Retrieved from http://www.ifso.com/wp-content/themes/ypo-theme/pdfs/bpd.pdf

Costs Associated With Obesity Treatment and Insurance Coverage

This chapter addresses the costs associated with obesity treatment and insurance coverage. These areas continue to be "hot topics," especially as the obesity epidemic continues to grow higher in terms of the body mass index (BMI) and cost. Insurance coverage is also being discussed.

COSTS ASSOCIATED WITH OBESITY

It is estimated that treatment of obesity and the associated conditions costs billions of dollars per year (The State of Obesity, 2015). Many different estimates in obesity costs exist. These are determined by the type of method used in calculating total costs. Estimates have ranged from $86 billion to $190 billion in 2005 and 2006 alone. This is up from the estimated cost of obesity in 1986 ($39 billion). The lower estimates are based on data compiled from the U.S. Medical Expenditure Panel Survey (MEPS). The MEPS does not include people who live in institutions. Another method used MEPS as well as a method called "instrumental variable approach." Other authors considered the National Health Expenditure Accounts dataset as the "gold-standard" source of health care spending. With any method used, the costs of obesity are increasing exponentially and need to be addressed. Researchers have estimated the costs of obesity alone to rise by as much as $48 billion to $66 billion per year.

The costs associated with obesity can be divided into two groups: direct costs and indirect costs. *Direct costs* are defined as costs associated with health care services. These can be inpatient or outpatient services provided, surgeries, medications or therapies, radiology or diagnostic testing, and/or laboratory studies. An indirect cost can consist of missed work days, wages, and/or insurance (Harvard School of Public Health, 2014a). *Indirect costs* are defined as "resources forgone as a result of a health condition" (Harvard School of Public Health, 2014a, n.p.). Although there is no price tag to define the value of lost work, missed days, wages, and work undone or unable to be completed, all fall under the definition. Presenteeism (lower productivity at work), sick days, absent days, long-term disability, and premature death occur more commonly in obese people compared with the nonobese. Lower total household incomes, lower wages, higher insurance premiums, and higher life insurance premiums are also linked with obesity.

Expenses in 2005 were estimated at $190 billion in the United States alone (Harvard School of Public Health, 2014a). A 2006 estimate of the direct medical costs of obesity ranged between $147 billion and $210 billion a year. As much as an additional 42% is spent on obese people in comparison to those of normal weight, with the cost of childhood obesity being as much as $14.1 billion. Obese people also spend more on health care, sometimes as high as 42% more. Because obese people also spend more, so do insurance companies. Insurance companies, including Medicare and Medicaid, are affected by the rise of obesity. The 2006 statistics show that Medicare and Medicaid alone paid a total of $61.8 billion for obese people. Without the costs of obesity, Medicare rates are estimated to be 8.5% lower, whereas Medicaid rates would be 11.8% lower in the absence of the disease. Insurance costs are also higher in obese children in comparison to nonobese children. Medicaid spent a total of $6,730 annually on the treatment of obese children, whereas an average annual amount for a nonobese child was $4,284 less. Private insurance is also affected by obesity. An average child's health expenses were approximately $1,100, whereas an obese child's cost was greater than $3,700 annually.

As with the other increased costs of health care, the cost of hospitalization is also on the rise. The cost of hospitalization for obese children in 1999 was nearly $126 million. In 2005, this cost was nearly double.

Decreased worker productivity can be measured in dollars. For example, increased job absenteeism and presenteeism are seen in obese individuals. Job absenteeism costs as much as $4.3 billion annually, whereas presenteeism costs employers a little more than $500 per worker annually. As BMI increases, so do the number of workers' compensation claims. Medical claims were also more than $43,500 higher in obese people in comparison with those of normal weight.

Costs to health and emergency responders and hospitals are also increased with obesity. An ambulance to transport and care for a patient weighing up to 1,000 pounds can cost as much as $40,000 more than an ambulance outfitted for up to 400 pounds. A bariatric setup within the hospital can also have higher costs. On average, a standard hospital bed can hold up to 500 pounds, whereas a bariatric bed holds up to 1,000 pounds. The cost for a bariatric bed is up to four times more at approximately $4,000 (The State of Obesity, 2015).

INSURANCE COVERAGE

Medical coverage of obesity is inconsistent, even with evidence of prevention and cost savings. Clinic visits, medications, and surgical options often struggle with reimbursement options. Oftentimes, obesity is not categorized as a disease; therefore, the comorbid conditions are most often reported as the reason for the provided service.

Throughout the years, obesity coverage has been an issue. Many medical providers often argue bias and discrimination with regard to coverage. The Internal Revenue Service (IRS) eliminated weight-loss programs as a medical deduction in 1998, even when they were medically prescribed. After much debate and petitions against this change, the IRS changed its policy in 2000 to allow for medical deductions for weight-loss treatment when under a specific medical prescription. The Social Security Administration has also eliminated obesity as a diagnosis for disability (Puhl & Brownell, 2001).

Both Frezza and Wachtel (2008) and Fujioka and Bakhru (2010) stress the importance of understanding what insurance companies will reimburse in terms of office visits and treatment options.

Oftentimes, the most challenging aspect of practicing obesity medicine is obtaining insurance coverage for treatment options. However, there are situations where insurance coverage can be successfully attained in many obese patients. To find these situations, one should treat obesity similar to any other medical condition and define the comorbid conditions. (Fujioka & Bakhru, 2010, p. 470)

Comorbid conditions, including diabetes, are readily used in combination with an obesity International Classification of Diseases (ICD-9) code.

Inadequate reimbursement continues to be a barrier for providing weight-related services and/or counseling. On November 29, 2011, the Centers for Medicare and Medicaid Services (CMS) announced coverage for obesity counseling and screening. This was done as part of their preventive service. These services are covered in primary care settings under primary care providers. This includes a nurse practitioner (NP), clinical nurse specialist, physician, and/or physician assistant. Services covered are limited to obesity screening, diet assessment, behavioral counseling, and diet and exercise therapy. Medications or meal replacements used for weight loss are not covered under the CMS preventive coverage; however, the previous services are free to beneficiaries (excluding deductible and co-pay). A summary of CMS coverage of intensive behavioral counseling for obesity as a preventive service can be found in Chapter 26 along with the recommended coverage time frames (Dennison Himmelfarb, 2012).

Diagnostic Codes Effective for claims with dates of service on or after November 29, 2011, Medicare will recognize HCPCS [Healthcare Common Procedure Coding System] code G0447, Face-to-Face Behavioral Counseling for Obesity, 15 minutes. G0447 must be billed along with 1 of the ICD-9 codes for BMI 30.0 and higher (V85.30–V85.39, V85.41–V85.45). The type of service (ToS) for G0447 is 1 (ICD-10 codes will be Z68.30–Z68.39, Z68.41–Z68.45). Effective for claims with dates of service on or after November 29, 2011, Medicare contractors will deny claims for HCPCS G0447 that are not submitted with the appropriate diagnostic code (V85.30–V85.39, V85.41–V85.45). (Department of Health and Human Services, Centers for Medicare and Medicaid Services [CMS], 2012)

The following are the ICD-9 codes and their description (CMS, n.d.a):

- V85.30—BMI 30.0–30.9, adult
- V85.31—BMI 31.0–31.9, adult
- V85.32—BMI 32.0–32.9, adult
- V85.33—BMI 33.0–33.9, adult
- V85.34—BMI 34.0–34.9, adult
- V85.35—BMI 35.0–35.9, adult
- V85.36—BMI 36.0–36.9, adult
- V85.37—BMI 37.0–37.9, adult
- V85.38—BMI 38.0–38.9, adult
- V85.39—BMI 39.0–39.9, adult

- V85.41—BMI 40.0–44.9, adult
- V85.42—BMI 45.0–49.9, adult
- V85.43—BMI 50.0–59.9, adult
- V85.44—BMI 60.0–69.9, adult
- V85.45—BMI 70 and higher, adult

As of October 1, 2015, ICD-10 replaces ICD-9. The following codes are to be used for billing after this date (CMS, n.d.b):

- Z68.30—BMI 30.0–30.9, adult
- Z68.31—BMI 31.0–31.9, adult
- Z68.32—BMI 32.0–32.9, adult
- Z68.33—BMI 33.0–33.9, adult
- Z68.34—BMI 34.0–34.9, adult
- Z68.35—BMI 35.0–35.9, adult
- Z68.36—BMI 36.0–36.9, adult
- Z68.37—BMI 37.0–37.9, adult
- Z68.38—BMI 38.0–38.9, adult
- Z68.39—BMI 39.0–39.9, adult
- Z68.41—BMI 40.0–44.9, adult
- Z68.42—BMI 45.0–49.9, adult
- Z68.43—BMI 50.0–59.9, adult
- Z68.44—BMI 60.0–69.9, adult
- Z68.45—BMI 70 or greater, adult

It should be noted that an *adult* is defined as an individual aged 15 to 124 years inclusive.

CMS updates to the initial 2012 intensive behavioral therapy (IBT) include the addition of a new HCPCS code: G0473 (face-to-face behavioral counseling for obesity, group [2–10], 30 minutes). This code is not to be billed alone, but should be billed with one of the previous ICD-9 codes (V85.30–V85.39, V85.41–V85.45) or the new ICD-10 codes (Z68.30–Z68.39, Z68.41–Z68.45).

For payment, codes G0447 or G0473 must include the provider specialty:

- 01—General Practice
- 08—Family Practice
- 11—Internal Medicine
- 16—Obstetrics/Gynecology
- 37—Pediatric Medicine
- 38—Geriatric Medicine
- 50—NP
- 89—Certified Clinical Nurse Specialist
- 97—Physician Assistant

The places of services (POS) must also be listed to payment:

- 11—Physician's Office
- 22—Outpatient Hospital
- 49—Independent Clinic
- 71—State or Local Public Health Clinic

Medicare will deny payments if the codes G0447 or G0473 are billed more than 22 times during a 12-month period (Department of Health and Human Services, CMS, 2015).

The American Academy of Pediatrics (AAP), the Institute of Medicine (IOM), America's Health Insurance Plans, The White House, The Obesity Society (TOS), Childhood Obesity Action Network, and the National Committee for Quality Assurance comprise a summary of health care obesity prevention recommendations aimed at health insurance providers. These recommendations are to (Harvard School of Public Health, 2014b, n.p.):

- Cover obesity-related services such as assessment, prevention, evaluation, treatment, and follow-up, and streamline reimbursement procedures.
- Provide subscribers with incentives for maintaining healthy body weight or adopting health behaviors, such as charting regular physical activity.
- Measure and track progress in BMI screening, through Health care Effectiveness Data and Information Set (HEDIS) data collection.
- Fund obesity prevention efforts in the community and/or participate in community obesity prevention coalitions.

As the cost of obesity is projected to continue with an upward trend, this area needs aggressive attention. Both costs and insurance continue to be under scrutiny with no real solution. Solutions aimed at prevention services and cost containment could be areas of future research.

REFERENCES

Centers for Medicare and Medicaid. (n.d.a). *ICD-9 code lookup*. Retrieved from http://www.cms.gov/medicare-coverage-database/staticpages/icd-9-code-lookup.aspx?KeyWord=mass&

Centers for Medicare and Medicaid. (n.d.b). *ICD-10 code lookup*. Retrieved from http://www.cms.gov/medicare-coverage-database/staticpages/icd-10-code-lookup.aspx

Dennison Himmelfarb, C. R. (2012). New evidence and policy support primary care-based weight loss interventions. *Journal of Cardiovascular Nursing, 27*(5), 379–381.

Department of Health and Human Services. Centers for Medicare and Medicaid Services. (2012). *Intensive behavioral therapy (IBT) for obesity*. Retrieved from http://www.cms.gov/Outreach-and-Education/Medicare-Learning-Network-MLN/MLNMattersArticles/downloads/MM7641.pdf

Department of Health and Human Services. Centers for Medicare and Medicaid Services. (2015). *Preventive and screening services—Update—intensive behavioral therapy for obesity, screening digital tomosynthesis mammography, and anesthesia associated with screening colonoscopy*. Retrieved from https://www.codemap.com/file/R3160CP.pdf

Frezza, E. E., & Wachtel, M. S. (2008). A successful model of setting up a bariatric practice. *Obesity Surgery, 18*, 877–881. doi:10.1007/s1169-007-9377-7

Fujioka, D., & Bakhru, N. (2010). Office-based management of obesity. *Mount Sinai Journal of Medicine, 77*, 466–471. doi: 10.1002/msj.20201

Harvard School of Public Health. (2014a). *Economic costs*. Retrieved from http://www.hsph.harvard.edu/obesity-prevention-source/obesity-consequences/economic

Harvard School of Public Health. (2014b). *Health insurance providers*. Retrieved from http://www.hsph.harvard.edu/obesity-prevention-source/obesity-prevention/healthcare/health-insurance-providers-obesity-prevention

Puhl, R., & Brownell, K. D. (2001). Bias, discrimination, and obesity. *Obesity Research*, 9(12), 788–805.

The State of Obesity. (2015). *Fast facts: Economic costs of obesity*. Retrieved from http://stateofobesity.org/facts-economic-costs-of-obesity

Treatment of the Obese Pediatric Patient

This chapter addresses the treatment of the obese pediatric patient. Concepts described in Chapter 26 can also be applied to the pediatric patient. Special consideration on how to measure weight should be reviewed from Chapter 4. Treatment can include medical therapy, pharmacotherapy, or even surgical therapy.

MEDICAL TREATMENT

Medical treatment is slightly different for a growing child in comparison to an adult, especially if the child is overweight or even mildly obese. If no other health concerns exist, the goal may not be weight loss, but rather weight maintenance. This should be discussed with the patient and family, especially if the child is expected to grow in height. Over time, the body mass index (BMI) may drop to a healthier ratio (Mayo Clinic, 2015). Again, this is age and patient specific.

The same treatment end goals apply to both the obese pediatric and adult patient—sustained weight loss. However, there are different methods to get to the end goal. An outline similar to that of the sample clinic found in Chapter 26 may also be used and tailored to the pediatric patient. The parent or family member can provide help, as needed, throughout the treatment.

A body composition scale may be helpful for certain pediatric patients, as the graphs may help better explain the information about the makeup of the entire weight number. Pediatric percentiles should be used, and graphs should be shown and explained to the patient and family. Blood pressure (BP), heart rate, respirations, and height (inches) should be measured. Neck circumference (NC), waist circumference (WC), and hip circumference (HC) should also be measured and recorded. Pediatric patients should also be screened for depression as well as sleep apnea, and referrals initiated for further counseling or testing, as needed. If baseline laboratory work has not been completed, the following laboratory values could be ordered and reviewed: complete blood count (CBC), comprehensive metabolic panel (CMP), thyroid-stimulating hormone (TSH), Free T3, Free T4, lipid panel, glycosylated hemoglobin (HbA1c), and vitamin D. The patient and family should also be introduced to a registered dietitian (RD) and exercise specialist, as needed, for each individualized program.

The 5 A's as well as two to three reasonable goals should be discussed with the patient. A next appointment should also be arranged with the patient and family. The second and subsequent visits should be structured in the same way to record vitals and discuss weight. Depending on the individualized plan, the patient and family should have one-on-one time with the RD and exercise specialist, as needed. Handouts should be available and given as needed.

Recommendations for subsequent visits should be discussed. Evidence has shown that weight loss is more successful with frequent follow-up and planned education and counseling (Chao et al., 2000; Institute for Clinical Systems Improvement [ICSI], 2011; National Heart, Lung, and Blood Institute [NHLBI], 2000; Rejeski, Focht, & Messier, 2002; Tuomilehto et al., 2001). Again, weight loss should be individualized; however, suggested monitoring is as follows: "weekly follow-up for the first three months and gradually decreasing to month for the next six months to four years can produce successful weight loss and maintenance" (Fitch et al., 2003, p. 87). Intensive intervention with regular or weekly contact for the first 3 months, with continued support up to 4 years, has a proven significance of 5% to 10% weight loss (ICSI, 2011).

Depending on the child's situation and associated medical conditions, the patient should be recommended to lose weight at a slow and steady pace. This can be anywhere from 1 pound a month up to 2 pounds per week. Weight loss for children less than 6 years of age is not typically recommended unless there are significant associated comorbid conditions that would warrant weight loss. Treatment and weight maintenance methods are similar in that they both recommend and encourage a healthy diet and appropriate physical activity (Mayo Clinic, 2015).

Encouraging parents to eat healthy is a large part of healthy eating for children. The Endocrine Society made dietary recommendations in the updated *Prevention and Treatment of Pediatric Obesity: An Endocrine Society Clinical Practice Guideline Based on Expert Opinion*. The first recommendation is with regard to promotion and support of healthy eating habits. The second recommendation is to discuss caloric intakes, reduction in saturated fat, increase of dietary fiber, and timely meals. The recommendations suggest guidance of caloric intake and portion control through the American Academy of Pediatrics (AAP). More information can be found at http://pediatrics.aappublications.org/cgi/reprint/117/2/544 (August et al., 2013).

Dietary fiber should be increased through fruits and vegetables. Fruits and vegetables should be readily available in the home for meals and snacks. Prepackaged foods, meals, and snacks should be avoided whenever possible. These convenience foods are often high in sugar and/or fat content. Any sweetened beverages should also be limited, as they often provide little nutritional value. Many times, these drinks also provide extra calories and may even make the child feel too full for nutritional foods. Appropriate (child-size) portions are recommended. Children should be encouraged to eat until they are full—sometimes, this means leaving food on the plate. With the obesity epidemic, the "clean plate club" is no longer recommended. Home-prepared meals are best; therefore, limiting the number of times that the child eats out is important, especially at fast-food restaurants. Finally, encouraging the family to eat together is important. During this time, the focus should be on conversation and the food, not the television, computer, or video game (Mayo Clinic, 2015).

Although many diets exist for weight loss, there is insufficient evidence to recommend one specific diet for children. In some cases, low-carbohydrate diets may be used; these demonstrated a moderate weight loss in a 6-month period, but the effects were generally not seen after 12 months. Hypocaloric diets may be dangerous, as some may lack essential vitamins and minerals needed for pediatric growth and development (August et al., 2013).

Physical activity is also important for children. When physical activity is encouraged and started while young, children are more apt to continue these healthy habits into adulthood (Mayo Clinic, 2015). The Endocrine Society encourages moderate to vigorous activity at least 1 hour daily. Decreased screen time is also encouraged (August et al., 2013). Recreational television, computer, video games, and/or phone time should be limited to no more than 2 hours per day. The focus of physical activity should be on the activity, not exercise. Free play time should be encouraged; the child's imagination should be allowed to go wild! To keep a child's interest and defer boredom, the type of activity should be varied; children should also help choose activities. Again, children often do best when they have positive parental examples—parents should be encouraged to be active (Mayo Clinic, 2015).

PHARMACOLOGICAL THERAPY

Prescription weight-loss medications are not often recommended for children or adolescents, as long-term side effects of many prescription medications are unknown (Mayo Clinic, 2015). Only one weight-loss medication is approved in the United States for children younger than the age of 16—orlistat (Crocker & Yanovski, 2009). Orlistat (Xenical) is approved for adolescents older than age 12. Patients and families should be reminded that medications do not replace healthy eating or physical activity; these should be encouraged in addition to prescription medication (Mayo Clinic, 2015).

There are different opinions with regard to medication use in the pediatric patient. The Endocrine Society recommends limited use of weight-loss medications. These medications should be reserved for those with a greater than 95th percentile BMI who have shown failed dietary and lifestyle interventions. The Endocrine Society also recommends limited use in those with a greater than 85th percentile and severe comorbidities. Other groups have suggested use only in pediatric patients with a greater than 95th percentile with associated comorbid conditions.

Sibutramine, an anorexigenic agent, was previously used as an appetite suppressant (Crocker & Yanovski, 2009). Sibutramine was approved for adolescents aged 16 years and older, but the Food and Drug Administration (FDA) recommended that it be taken off the market in November 2009 and January 2010 (U.S. Food and Drug Administration [FDA], 2010). Orlistat, the gastrointestinal lipase inhibitor, is also approved for adolescent use in patients as young as 12 years of age. The largest study with orlistat was a randomized study that included 539 patients aged 12 to 16. This study had a 35% drop-out rate after 1 year. Results were statistically significant with the BMI in the orlistat group falling by 0.55 kg/m^2, whereas the placebo group increased by 0.31 kg/m^2 (Crocker & Yanovski, 2009).

Metformin is used for the treatment of type 2 diabetes mellitus (T2DM), but has been evaluated for treatment of pediatric obesity in patients aged 10 and older. This medication is not FDA approved for obesity. Three randomized trials have evaluated T2DM; results have differed, indicating an average loss of 3.15 kg in one trial and a small, nonsignificant change in another (Crocker & Yanovski, 2009).

There are several other medications that have been studied with regard to the treatment of pediatric obesity. Although these medications are not FDA approved for the treatment of obesity, they are discussed by the Endocrine Society in the guidelines. Growth hormone (GH) is also not FDA approved for pediatric obesity.

It has been seen as a benefit to children with the Prader–Willi syndrome and has been shown to decrease fat mass while increasing lean mass. Best results were seen when GH was started before 18 months of age. Octreotide, a GH inhibitor, decreases the insulin response to glucose. Although it has demonstrated weight loss in adults, studies have not assessed pediatric weight loss. Those with leptin gene mutations (seen as early as 6 months of age) that have received leptin therapy have demonstrated significant weight and fat mass loss. Topiramate, an anticonvulsant used in children, has a direct effect on adipocytes, thus producing anorexia and weight loss in 10% to 40% of children (August et al., 2013).

BARIATRIC SURGERY

Bariatric surgery is oftentimes a last resort with pediatric or adolescent patients, although the number of surgeries is increasing. Bariatric surgery is not for everyone. In the case of pediatric patients, it is reserved for the extremely obese with associated comorbid diseases. The concept of "early" intervention in certain adolescent patients has also demonstrated success in weight loss. Roux-en-Y gastric bypass (RYGB) and laparoscopic adjustable gastric banding (LAGB) are the two most common procedures currently used in pediatric bariatric surgery.

Although pediatric qualifications are different because they do not have BMI to define surgical criteria, they do have percentiles that can correlate with BMI. Patient selection is very specific with regard to surgical patients. BMI for age, as well as a greater than or equal to 99th BMI percentile, has demonstrated increased risk for cardiovascular disease (CVD). A fixed BMI cutoff has been considered a more accurate estimate of BMI in adolescents.

Because all adolescent boys and most adolescent girls <18 years old with a BMI of 35 kg/m^2 are greater than the 99th BMI percentile, the BMI thresholds used for adult selection criterion appear to be appropriate for adolescents, with some modification with regard to associated co-morbid disease thresholds. (Michalsky, Reichard, Inge, Pratt, & Lenders, 2012, p. 3)

The selection criteria for adolescent bariatric surgery is a BMI greater than or equal to 35 kg/m^2 accompanied by "major" comorbid conditions or a BMI greater than or equal to 40 kg/m^2 with "other" comorbid conditions. Major comorbid conditions include T2DM, obstructive sleep apnea (OSA) with an apnea–hypopnea index (AHI) greater than 15, pseudotumor cerebri, or severe nonalcoholic steatohepatitis (NASH). Other comorbid conditions that may accompany a BMI greater than or equal to 40 kg/m^2 include glucose intolerance, insulin resistance, hypertension (HTN), dyslipidemia, mild OSA (AHI greater than five), and impaired tolerance of daily living or quality of life (QOL) (Michalsky et al., 2012).

Crocker and Yanovski (2009) also address guidelines for bariatric surgery in pediatric patients. These guidelines are stricter than those listed earlier. These authors recommend a BMI greater than 50 kg/m^2 or a BMI greater than 40 kg/m^2 with associated comorbid conditions. These authors also recommend surgery only after failure (greater than 6 months) of lifestyle changes in a defined program. Because of the possible impact that surgery may have on growth and development, recommendations are made about Tanner staging and bone age. The patient should be evaluated, and documentation should be made such that the Tanner IV staging as well as a bone age of 95% of final height has been reached (Crocker & Yanovski, 2009).

Along with Tanner staging, BMI recommendations, and failure of a formal lifestyle program, the Endocrine Society has three more recommendations with regard to bariatric surgery. A psychological evaluation is essential. This helps determine the stability of the child as well as the family unit. The guidelines also recommend surgery by an experienced surgeon and medical team. A multidisciplinary surgical team should include additional medical expertise in endocrine, gastrointestinal, pulmonary, cardiovascular, nutritional, psychological, and otolaryngological areas. Long-term follow-up with the surgical team as well as shared data is also recommended. Postoperative care should focus on growth and development. Attention to appropriate nutritional care as well as adequate vitamin and mineral intake is also important. Finally, patient adherence of healthy dietary and exercise patterns is recommended.

Bariatric surgery is not recommended for adolescents who are pregnant or breastfeeding or those who wish to become pregnant up to 2 years after surgery. Surgery is also not recommended for those who have an untreated psychiatric disorder, including an eating disorder. Children who are unable to demonstrate healthy dietary and exercise habits should not be considered for surgery. Finally, those with the Prader–Willi syndrome are also not recommended for surgery (August et al., 2013).

Treating childhood obesity is critical in preventing obesity and comorbid conditions in adults. There is no one right way to treat childhood obesity, but guidelines focus on patient and family education as well as on lifestyle, pharmacological, and surgical treatment options. Environmental factors as well as behavioral changes need to be addressed to help provide further weight-loss recommendations.

REFERENCES

August, G. P., Caprio, S., Fennoy, I., Freemark, M., Kaugman, F. R., Lustig, R. H., . . . Montori, V.M. (2013). Prevention and treatment of pediatric obesity: An endocrine society clinical practice guideline based on expert opinion. *Journal of Clinical Endocrinology & Metabolism*, 93(12). Retrieved from http://press.endocrine.org/doi/full/10.1210/jc.2007–2458

Chao, D., Espeland, M. A., Farmer, D., Register, T. C., Lenchik, L., Applegate, W. B., & Ettinger, W. H. (2000). Effect of voluntary weight loss on bone mineral density in older overweight women. *Journal of American Geriatric Society*, 48(7), 753–759.

Crocker, M., & Yanovski, J. A. (2009). Pediatric obesity: Etiology and treatment. *Endocrinology and Metabolism Clinics in North America*, 38(3), 525–548. doi:10.1016/j.ecl.2009.06.007

Fitch, A., Everling, L., Fox, C., Goldberg, J., Heim, C., Johnson, K., . . . Webb, B. (2013). *Institute for clinical systems improvement. Prevention and management of obesity for adults.* Retrieved from https://www.icsi.org/_asset/s935hy/Obesity-Interactive0411.pdf

Institute for Clinical Systems Improvement (ICSI). (2011). *Health care guideline: Prevention and management of obesity (Mature Adolescents and Adults).* Retrieved from http://www.obesitycast.com/guidelinecasts/ICSI_Obesity.pdf

Mayo Clinic. (2015). *Diseases and conditions: Childhood obesity. Treatment and drugs*. Retrieved from http://www.mayoclinic.org/diseases-conditions/childhood-obesity/basics/treatment/con-20027428

Michalsky, M., Reichard, K., Inge, T., Pratt, J., & Lenders, C. (2012). ASMBS pediatric committee best practice guidelines. *Surgery for Obesity and Related Diseases, 8*, 1–7. Retrieved from https://asmbs.org/wp/uploads/2011/09/PediatricBestPracticeGuide lines-January2012.pdf

National Heart, Lung, and Blood Institute. (2000). *The practical guide: Identification, evaluation, and treatment of overweight and obesity in adults*. NIH Publication Number 00-4084. Retrieved from http://www.nhlbi.nih.gov/files/docs/guidelines/prctgd_c.pdf

Rejeski, W. J., Focht, B. C., & Messier, S. P. (2002). Obese, older adults with knee osteoarthritis: Weight loss, exercise, and quality of life. *Health Psychology*, (21), 419–426. Retrieved from http://pediatrics.aappublications.org/content/120/Supplement_4/S254.full.pdf+html

Tuomilehto, J., Lindstrom, J., Eriksson, J. G., Valle, T. T., Hämäläinen, H., Ilanne-Parikka, P., . . . Uusitupa, M. (2001). Prevention of type 2 diabetes by changes in lifestyle among subjects with impaired glucose tolerance. *New England Journal of Medicine, 344*(18), 1343–1350.

U.S. Food and Drug Administration. (2010). *FDA drug safety communication: FDA recommends against the continued use of Meridia (sibutramine)*. Retrieved from http://www.fda.gov/Drugs/DrugSafety/ucm228746.htm

What Is Lifestyle Medicine?

> *Lifestyle practices and health habits are among the nation's most impor-*
> *tant health determinants. Changing unhealthy behaviors is foundational*
> *to medical care, disease prevention, and health promotion.*
> —American College of Lifestyle Medicine (ACLM; 2011a)

This chapter addresses the concept and practice of lifestyle medicine (LM). The role of advanced practice nurses (APNs) in LM is essential to everyday practice, prevention, and treatment. As the obesity epidemic continues and this treatment method continues to gain popularity along with it, more patients may inquire about this concept.

LM is the idea of using lifestyle changes or modifications in the prevention and treatment of chronic disease. Interventions used in LM can include healthy dietary changes, exercise therapy, stress management, smoking cessation, and even reduction in alcohol consumption. Many chronic diseases, such as obesity, will benefit from the practice of LM. Other diseases in which lifestyle intervention has proved beneficial include type 2 diabetes mellitus (T2DM), metabolic syndrome, coronary artery disease (CAD), hypertension (HTN), osteoporosis, and even some types of cancer.

LM can benefit a number of patients—all without the unwanted side effects that often develop from other medications. Although the goal of LM focuses on treatment through lifestyle modification, medication knowledge is essential. Medications may need to be reduced or even re-titrated as the patient incorporates the lifestyle changes into daily life. LM is often something that most APNs do on routine office visits, but they tend to be brief in nature. The goal of LM is to spend more quality time addressing these lifestyle goals. Most often, these interventions can be best provided through outpatient services. This also provides an opportunity for group sessions on each topic. These group sessions can address the basics of each topic; however, individual appointments will be needed for specific planning, treatment, and continued follow-up and management (ACLM, 2011a).

The American College of Lifestyle Medicine (ACLM) established standards in the field of LM that were published in the July 2010 issue of *The Journal of the American Medical Association (JAMA)*. The publication, titled "Physician Competencies for Prescribing Lifestyle Medicine," has set a precedence in this growing field by providing guidelines for those serving in primary care settings. Leadership, knowledge, assessment and management skills, and the use of office and community support are vital ingredients for the APN to be successful in LM.

Leadership encourages the promotion and practice of healthy behaviors. This is the focus of the care provided in the clinic; it also provides and supports healthy behavior practices in the community. Healthy environments should be encouraged in all aspects of life—school, work, and home.

Knowledge allows the APN to demonstrate effective changes with LM through patient education as well as the creation of a positive experience and effect on the patient's health. Positive health outcomes are recognized by the patient and family. Knowledge is passed on from the patients to others around them.

Assessment skills are the third skill set needed. A thorough assessment allows the APN to determine a patient's social and psychological status, as well as his or her biological predisposition. Understanding the patient's history, as well as health and mental status, allows the APN to provide thorough and more accurate care. Assessment also includes recognizing the readiness or lack of readiness to make the recommended lifestyle changes. A complete physical examination is also recommended with particular attention spent on the lifestyle-related health status. The lifestyle-related health status can include, but is not limited to, the assessment of body mass index (BMI), stress level, mental well-being, sleep habits, tobacco and/or alcohol use, nutritional status, and exercise or activity. The final piece of assessment skills includes the ordering and interpretation of basic tests to continue to monitor and manage chronic disease.

Management skills include the use of nationally recognized practice guidelines, as needed, to advance treatment of chronic diseases. Creating effective patient and family relationships as well as use of team collaboration to achieve specific, measurable, attainable, relevant, and timely (SMART) goals is also essential. Finally, sustaining healthy styles is of utmost importance.

The use of office and community support includes the use of a multidisciplinary team to support individualized and group patient care. Encouragement of office-wide healthy practices is also essential. Finding and using appropriate community resources that support healthy lifestyle practices will aid in efficiency of the program and patient outcomes (ACLM, 2011b).

Harvard Medical School also supports the research and practice of LM. The Institute of Lifestyle Medicine (ILM) was founded in 2007; its goal is to support and engage clinician involvement in LM through education, research, and advocacy organization. This organization aims at reducing modifiable behaviors, as these modifiable behaviors are driving forces in increased health care costs as well as in decreased disease rates and death. The ILM offers many beneficial services that can be used not only to increase awareness of LM but also to provide ongoing resources and consulting services for APNs, corporations, medical practices, health and wellness providers, and fitness facilities (Institute of Lifestyle Medicine [ILM], 2014).

There are many articles that support the use and demonstrate scientific evidence of LM. These articles show success with the Dietary Approaches to Stop Hypertension (DASH)—a diet low in sodium that consists of low-fat dairy, reduced saturated and total fat, and rich in fruits and vegetables. The Mediterranean diet, a diet low in cholesterol, and a vegetarian diet are also healthy LM approaches to eating. Other LM interventions—aerobic exercise, stress management training, smoking cessation, and group psychosocial support—also show overall disease risk reduction. Regression of CAD, lower blood pressure (BP), and lower cholesterol levels are also shown.

Many articles have demonstrated success with LM. Articles also support school curriculum classes in LM. These articles support the growing concept that daily habits and actions affect quality of life (QOL). The study of prevention is on the rise. These programs would prove beneficial for recognition of the treatment of obesity.

Rippe (2013, p. xxiii) states the following:

> The key consideration now will be for those of us in the health care community to apply these understandings to the modern practice of medicine. This is, in my view, the single greatest opportunity that we have to improve health outcomes and lower costs. This is crucial to bringing additional value to the practice of medicine. It is, in essence, both the challenge and opportunity for the future of lifestyle medicine.

The concept of LM has been around for a while; however, it does not have the popularity that treatments with medications do. Some of this deals with the lack of insurance payment, whereas others may argue that treatment with LM takes too much time. Nonetheless, this concept is important and must continue to be investigated.

REFERENCES

American College of Lifestyle Medicine [ACLM]. (2011a). *What is lifestyle medicine?* Retrieved from http://www.lifestylemedicine.org/define

American College of Lifestyle Medicine [ACLM]. (2011b). *Core competencies.* Retrieved from http://www.lifestylemedicine.org/core

Institute of Lifestyle Medicine [ILM]. (2014). *About the ILM.* Retrieved from http://www.instituteoflifestylemedicine.org/home/about-the-ilm/

Rippe, J. M. (Ed.). (2013). *Lifestyle medicine* (2nd ed.). Boca Raton, FL: CRC Press, Taylor & Francis Group.

Clinic Establishment, Medical Therapy, and a Multidisciplinary Approach

In the gradual division of labor, by which civilization has emerged from barbarism, the doctor and nurse have been evolved.
—Sir William Osler (1891; Wagner, 2000)

The following is an example of how a weight-loss clinic was implemented from the initial idea to the treatment of patients. For the sake of this chapter and definition purposes, the name of this clinic will be "The Center for Lifestyle Medicine" (CLM). Clinic establishment, action plan, risk analysis, time frame budget, treatment approach, evaluation, and challenges faced are addressed. The following is to be used as a guideline. It was used as a model for treatment in overweight and obese patients with either cardiovascular disease (CVD) or cardiovascular risk factors. Again, the following is not a guarantee of patient success. Each plan and treatment option should be tailored to fit each patient and each practice situation.

CLINIC ESTABLISHMENT

Financial savvy and business experience are stated as two indispensable skills needed to establish a clinic or practice (Frezza & Wachtel, 2008). Along with business expertise, a team approach, counseling, and flexibility are key aspects in establishing a successful weight-loss or obesity clinic (Frezza & Wachtel, 2008; Fujioka & Bakhru, 2010). Campbell (2014) states twelve golden rules for the success of a project. These rules can guide the process and serve as an outline for clinical establishments. A summary of these rules is as follows: Project outcomes should be established with the support of the entire team. The team itself should consist of a collaboration of the best people for the project. A plan and a time line should be developed and followed—these should be realistic. Upper management and stakeholders should be kept informed so that they remains on board while the plan moves forward. Change is inevitable—embrace it. Keep all involved in the project up to date. Lastly, be a leader (Campbell, 2014).

A positive attitude is also essential when treating obese patients. Many patients feel providers are discriminatory about weight and pass prior judgment when treating obesity (Chang, Asch, & Werner, 2010; Ferrante, Piasecki,

Ohman-Strickland, & Crabtree, 2009; Wadden et al., 2000). Increasing the number of patient referrals is crucial for further productivity (Frezza & Wachtel, 2008).

Development of a formal business plan is essential when establishing, promoting, and sustaining a business or product. A formal business plan may include the description, mission, vision, goals, and objectives of the business. The business philosophy and target market are also acknowledged. Core strengths and the competitive advantage are described, as is a literature review. Principal owners, provider description, and a legal form of ownership, along with products and services, are also discussed. In addition, a budget needs to be addressed. Because each budget will be different, an example is not provided. A strengths, weaknesses, opportunities, and threats (SWOT) analysis is included. A sample copy of a formal business plan is available for review (see Center for Lifestyle Medicine Sample Business Plan in the Appendix section).

Research and further investigation of the topic with a literature review are also essential. A literature review must be thorough and include recent inquiries on the proposed topic. Such articles are compiled to provide the necessary information to support the preparation, intervention, and project.

The identification of stakeholders is also essential in further project development. "A stakeholder is defined as any person or group who has an interest in the project being evaluated or in the results of the evaluation" (W. K. Kellogg Foundation, *Evaluation Handbook*, 2004a, p. 48). Key stakeholders can include coworkers (including nursing staff), the program director, administrative staff and administrative board, and billing and coding staff. Supporting staff, a dietitian, an exercise specialist, and a counselor are also stakeholders. In addition, referring providers and potential patients are crucial stakeholders.

ACTION PLAN

An implementation or action plan for this project began with the identification of the need for weight-loss education and services. Further meetings followed. Then, the development of a formal business template as well as a SWOT analysis were completed (Appendix A). The SWOT can provide organization and overview for a risk management matrix, budget, and further project development.

Initial assumptions, found in the Implementation Plan/Theory Outcomes Model (Appendix B) and Timeline (Appendix C), for development of a formal business plan could include, but are not limited to, the following:

- Obesity is undertreated and misunderstood by many medical professionals.
- Obesity is the No. 1 killer in America.
- Establishing a formal business plan will lead to the development of a medical weight-loss clinic.
- Establishing a weight-loss clinic will improve a patient's overall quality of life (QOL).
- There is a lack of nonpharmacological medical treatment of obesity.

These were identified as possible threats and challenges to further development. These assumptions were the foundation of the logic outcome model. Coronary artery disease (CAD), type 2 diabetes mellitus (T2DM), hypertension (HTN), hyperlipidemia, and obstructive sleep apnea (OSA) are listed as comorbidities of obesity. These comorbidities are reasons that obesity should be viewed as a life-threatening disease requiring more immediate attention. Recognition and further promotion of prevention and treatment will help achieve the ultimate goal of sustained weight loss.

The impact or desired outcomes of the CLM included the following:

- Establishing a medical weight-loss clinic
- Achieving patient weight loss of 10% in 6 months
- Sustaining patient weight loss at 1 year

The establishment of a medical weight-loss clinic will address these vital health care issues. These are further discussed in the Evaluation Plan section.

RISK ANALYSIS

According to Zwikael and Ahn (2011), "The global business environment involves high levels of risk and complexity, which is a necessary condition for future growth and development" (p. 25). Most companies have formal plans in place to assess and provide risk management (Zwikael & Ahn). Understanding the concept of risk management allows one to plan for the probability that a problem will occur and to manage it appropriately. Evaluating the impact if the problem arises and having solutions prepared in advance allows for continued development of the project or business. These risks should be identified and kept at an acceptable level. The following steps are suggested to analyze risk (Campbell, 2014):

- Identify the risks
  - List and describe potential impact
- Analyze the probability that risk will occur
  - Analyze potential impact of risk
- Determine overall severity of risk
- Determine risk importance and further action
- Document response plan for risk
  - Accept risk
  - Avoid risk
  - Monitor risk and develop a contingency plan for imminent risk
  - Transfer risk

Identification and analysis of risk aided in formatting the SWOT analysis. As stated earlier, the SWOT analysis provided further definitions and assessment of five types of risks. These risks are identified in a Risk Management Matrix (Appendix D). Five risks and analyses—*markets, liquidity, operational, legal, and reputational*—provide insight for initial problem solving.

A geographic review of clinics within the area of the start-up clinic should be a priority. A rival clinic can be seen as a market risk. The start-up clinic should promote a specific niche for ongoing success. The sample clinic provides a specific target population focusing on weight loss for people with cardiac disease and risk factors for cardiac disease. This clinic promotes a team approach, collaborative care, a new clinic, and testing located within one facility. According to Frezza and Wachtel (2008), a team approach, counseling, and flexibility are also key aspects in establishing a successful obesity clinic. These authors also state that increasing the number of patient referrals is crucial for productivity (Frezza & Wachtel,

2008). Therefore, it is important to increase internal patient referrals, if needed, to fill open slots or schedules.

Advertising will also play a key role in the clinic's success. Initial strategies for marketing the sample clinic will involve word of mouth, newspaper advertisement, a formal letter to patients and area providers (Appendices E–G), and meeting with area providers and hospital staff. Marketing tools will include information and brochures highlighting important facts and clinic features.

The development of a formal business plan provides for an easier implementation and establishment of a clinic. The CLM provides individualized weight-loss counseling, dietary advice, and exercise strategies without the use of any medications or supplements. The target of this clinic was to educate and treat overweight and obese patients.

Emphasizing strengths is vital for success. A natural approach to weight loss, the ease and availability of cardiac testing and exercise equipment, structured nutrition advice provided by a registered dietitian (RD), exercise advice provided by an exercise specialist, and a new facility continue to be key strengths. Another benefit is the one-on-one guidance by an advanced practice nurse (APN).

The second threat, liquidity and questionable funding/billing, arose due to the lack of funding and billing codes accepted for preventative care and treatment. Existing cuts to primary care and specialty practices and testing constitute another threat that has and will continue to affect the funding and billing. The length of time per visit spent on one-on-one weight counseling should be included in formal dictation, supporting higher billable levels.

As stated earlier, both Fujioka and Bakhru (2010) and Frezza and Wachtel (2008) highlight and discuss the importance of reimbursement. International Classification of Diseases (ICD-9) codes, including diabetes (790.1), essential HTN (401), hyperlipidemia (272.0), and CAD (414.0), are appropriate diagnostic codes for medical treatment of weight loss and obesity (Fujioka & Bakhru). These ICD-9 codes are essential to bill, in addition to obesity (278.00).

Private payment plans can and should be arranged for each service offered. This can eliminate the concern with insurance billing.

An operational risk—inadequate training—is the third threat listed in the matrix. This may place the clinic's reputation and/or the patients in jeopardy. A detailed plan for staff education is found in Appendix H.

The fourth risk, legal or appropriate certification or accreditation, argues on behalf of the credibility of the practice. Formal staff training and education is one method of managing this risk and is included next. Another way to protect this risk is through licensure, liability coverage, and timely and proper documentation with the patient.

The fifth risk is reputational. This low risk is manageable with word of mouth and advertising. Promoting current patient satisfaction also proves to be essential.

Although several risks were defined, these were addressed in the Risk Management Matrix. Each clinic should discuss the risk and benefits before proceeding with further establishment. Recognizing and understanding these risks is of critical importance.

TIME FRAME

A logic model allows for visualization of the project's sequencing. Development of this model allows stakeholders and those involved in project management to conceptualize events. According to the W. K. Kellogg Foundation (2004b), a logic model and timeline provide clear ideas "as well as an organized approach to capturing, documenting, and disseminating program results—enhance the case for investment in your program" (p. 6). Establishing a timeline and target dates provides organization and specifies an ultimate cutoff date. A project schedule may be beneficial, as this shows the project or network path.

If properly sequenced, a network diagram is also beneficial in establishing a time line. This helps in establishing the sequence of events as well as the relationships that are important in reaching these milestones. A work breakdown structure (WBS) hierarchy is also helpful in organizing various activities. Lastly, the time line should consist of smaller phases that reduce uncertainty, as these help in breaking down larger tasks (Campbell, 2014).

BUDGET

After establishing an initial budget, it is important to know that it is a difficult process to change. That is why it is so important to take time to accurately estimate the budget. It is essential to note the basis of the estimate, assumptions made in establishing the budget, budget constraints, and the confidence level in developing the budget. Three types of estimates can be used during the project: a ballpark estimate, rough order of magnitude/parametric estimate, and/or a detailed estimate. Direct and indirect costs also affect a budget. *Direct costs* are defined as those specifically or "directly" related to the project. *Indirect costs* are defined as those "indirectly" related to the project or those that can be shared among several projects. Direct costs can include any of the following: labor, supplies or raw materials, equipment, travel, legal fees, training, and marketing or advertising. Indirect costs could include, but are not limited to, facilities, site-specific requirements, and/or management and administrative overhead.

Working capital is crucial to any new or start-up business. Along with working capital, good cash flow management is essential to any successful business. Understanding cash flow projections is necessary to develop the required capital to meet and sustain business needs. It is also important to understand and recognize when additional monetary resources are needed and how they can be attained. Many businesses fail without sufficient start-up and ongoing cash assets. As with start-up costs, bad debt should also be included in the budget planning. Building a budget is not easy; it may take weeks or months. One should never be afraid to seek input from the experts (Campbell, 2014).

TREATMENT APPROACH

The strong guidance of a leader is essential to any execution. Campbell (2014) suggests eight tips to be an effective leader:

- Listen
- Be dependable
- Be observant
- Be humble
- Be available

- Be decisive
- Learn to delegate
- Don't micromanage

These small tips for leadership can make a big impact in project management and long-term success.

The following is an example of operations from the sample clinic. New patients were accepted through either internal or external referrals. Patients with known cardiac disease and risk factors for cardiac disease were also readily accepted. Clinic staff included those working at the front desk; a certified medical assistant (CMA); a doctorate-prepared, board-certified nurse practitioner (NP); an RD; an exercise specialist; and a board-certified cardiologist. Prior to arrival at the first appointment, patients were mailed a questionnaire (a sample is included in Chapter 10) and asked to bring in a 3-day food diary.

Upon arrival to the first visit, the patient should be checked in by a CMA or nurse and asked a series of questions (a sample is included in Chapter 10). After this, the patient should be weighed. Many weight clinics may use more than a regular scale. A body composition scale, which figures total body fat, total body water, fat-free mass, daily calorie burn rates, and body mass index (BMI), provides added benefit and gives the patient more information. Then, blood pressure (BP), heart rate (HR), respirations, and height (inches) should be recorded. Body measurements, including neck circumference (NC), waist circumference (WC), and hip circumference (HC), are to be measured in inches and recorded. BMI, basal metabolic rate (BMR), and the Harris–Benedict Formula should also be calculated. A baseline resting EKG is also beneficial to ensure there is no underlying cardiac abnormality. A depression screening tool and the Epworth Sleepiness Scale should be administered to the patient. There are mixed reviews about the relationship between obesity and depression; however, higher rates of depression are identified in severely obese people (Institute for Clinical Systems Improvement [ICSI], 2011). "Patients with documented sleep apnea need to be encouraged to be compliant with their treatment plan in order to improve their ability to lose weight" (p. 17).

The APN will complete a head-to-toe physical assessment and review the patient's vitals, measurements, initial paperwork, questions, EKG, and the Beck Depression Inventory and the Epworth Sleepiness Scale. If the EKG shows an abnormality and/or chest pain or anginal symptoms are present, the patient records will be further reviewed and a baseline Treadmill Stress Test will be set up prior to any physical activity recommendations. A referral to cardiology would also be appropriate. The results of the depression screening tool should be computed and placed in the proper risk category. Referral to a counselor and/or mental health professional/psychiatric mental health nurse practitioner (PMHNP) will take place as per the APN's discretion. Also, pending the results of the Epworth Sleepiness Scale, the patient may be referred on for further polysomnography.

The APN should also screen for a possible eating disorder. Questions for screening for an eating disorder can include the following:

Do you eat a large amount of food in a short period—such as eating more food than another person may eat in, say, a 2-hour period? Do you ever feel like you cannot stop eating even after you feel full? When you overeat, what do you do? (ICSI, 2011, p. 16)

The APN should also review medications and screen for medication use that could contribute to weight gain. During this examination and review of findings, the RD and the exercise specialist should also be present to address questions as they arise.

Before goals are set, the 5 A's —*ask, advise, assess, assist, and arrange*—should be addressed with the patient. *Asking* involves discussing the patient's measurements, including weight and BMI. Education about accompanying risk factors and status should take place. This should be addressed at any routine office visit. The next step is to *advise* on weight maintenance or weight loss, as appropriate. Research has shown that patients who have received recommendations with regard to weight loss are more likely to initiate attempts. The third step involved in the 5 A's is *assess*. Assessing for readiness of change is a vital step in the weight-loss process. Using the rating scale is a great way to initiate conversation with regard to motivation of weight loss. "How interested are you in losing weight at this time? Please rate on a scale from 0 to 10, with 0 indicating no importance and 10 being a top priority or of high importance." The APN should then follow up by assessing the patient's confidence:

> Also, on a scale of 0 to 10, with 0 being not confident and 10 being very confident, how confident are you that you can lose weight? . . . On a scale of 0 to 10, with 0 being not interested and 10 being very interested, how interested are you in losing weight at this time? (Fitch et al., 2013, p. 86)

The next step is *assisting* with the weight loss. Again, this step should involve reassessing the patient's readiness for weight loss as well as providing the applicable tools for success. The fifth A stands for *arrange*. This can include arranging follow-up appointments as well as continued visits with the RD, exercise specialist, and counselor, as needed (Fitch et al., 2013).

Goals, both short term and long term, should be set and realistic expectations should be discussed. One goal should discuss the implementation and continuation of a dietary and exercise journal (Appendix I; a sample is also provided in Chapter 13). A second goal should focus on a safe and realistic weight loss of 1 to 2 pounds per week and a 10% weight loss in 6 months. The third goal, an exercise-based goal, will be set in collaboration with the APN and exercise specialist. The fourth goal, a nutrition-based goal, should be set in collaboration with the APN and RD. The RD and exercise specialist should each give brief presentations. The sample allowed time for 5-minute presentations. Questions should be answered and preparation for the second visit should take place. A short explanation of the baseline fitness assessment should also be addressed. Baseline laboratories—complete blood count (CBC), comprehensive metabolic panel (CMP), thyroid-stimulating hormone (TSH), Free T3, Free T4, lipid panel, glycosylated hemoglobin (HgA1c), and vitamin D—can be discussed and should be encouraged to be drawn prior to the second visit.

The patient's second visit should be scheduled within a 2- to 3-week time frame after the initial visit, during which baseline weight, vitals, measurements, and calculations should be taken. The APN should review these findings and also check for any weight loss. A full head-to-toe physical examination again takes place. Health coaching, assessment, and discussion of goals will also be addressed. After this portion is completed, the patient should complete a baseline physical assessment (Appendix J). This portion is led by the exercise specialist with the APN. The RD should be available for assistance, as needed. The level of fatigue and shortness of breath should be assessed with the BORG Scale (Appendix K) prior to and after the 6-Minute Walk Test and again once the entire assessment is completed to determine the patient's tolerance. A baseline physical assessment should consist of a combination of cardiorespiratory endurance, muscular endurance, muscular strength, flexibility, and agility exercises. These tests are used as a baseline to assess the current fitness level and aid in providing further exercise recommendations and goals. At the end of this test, vitals such as BP, HR, respirations, and oxygenation saturation should again be measured. The exercise specialist can then take time to instruct the patient on stretching and demonstrate the proper use of resistance bands and exercise machines. Handouts with pictures of the stretches and bands are encouraged (a sample can be seen in Chapter 12). The RD will also be available for questions at the end of this session. New goals should be set with a next meeting plan established for the following 2 to 3 weeks.

The third visit should begin in the same manner. Baseline weight, vitals, measurements, and calculations should take place. The APN again reviews findings and any weight loss and performs a full head-to-toe physical examination. Health coaching, assessment, and discussion of goals should be addressed. A majority of the third visit can be one-on-one time with the RD. Dietary and nutrition needs will be individually assessed. The APN and exercise specialist are available for questions and consultation, as needed. The patient should meet with all the team members at the end of the third visit to discuss goals, ask questions, and establish a plan of action for the weeks ahead.

The timing for the fourth and consecutive visits should be determined by the patient and team members. Some patients may wish to continue on a 2-week regimen, whereas others may wish to schedule a return visit for 4 weeks. As cited by the ICSI (2011, p. 19), "Weight loss requires frequent follow-up (initially weekly) with planned education/counseling by health care providers to be most effective (i.e., improve adherence)." Similar recommendations in regards to follow-up care are cited by many sources (Chao et al., 2000; National Heart, Lung, and Blood Institute [NHLBI], 2000; Rejeski, Focht, & Messier, 2002; Tuomilehto et al., 2001). Again, weight loss should be individualized; however, suggested monitoring is as follows: "weekly follow-up for the first three months and gradually decreasing to month for the next six months to four years can produce successful weight loss and maintenance" (Fitch et al., 2013, p. 87). "The purpose of these visits would be to measure weight, BMI, WC, BP and HR to assess any adverse effects, and to conduct laboratory tests and answer questions" (ICSI, 2011, p. 29). Regular monitoring of weight is the key for long-term success and weight maintenance. Intensive intervention with regular or weekly contact for the first 3 months with continued support up to 4 years has a proven significance of 5% to 10% weight loss (ICSI, 2011).

An added benefit to any specialty clinic is having an exercise room available for patient use under direct supervision of the exercise specialist during appointment time. Additional exercise sessions and times should be available for patients, but will most likely not be covered under insurance. A pricing list should be provided to patients. Samples can be found in Appendixes L to N.

EVALUATION

Patients should be weighed and assessed as stated earlier at the initial and following appointments to determine weight and inches lost. Patient weight loss should be documented in individual patient charts with a goal of achieving a 10% weight loss in 6 months. Therapy is considered successful once this goal is reached. If the weight loss goal has not been reached, further lifestyle modifications need to be considered at this point. These could include the addition of medication therapy, further caloric reduction, or recommendations for increased physical activity (ICSI, 2011).

Clinic success can be measured through sustained patient weight loss. It is recommended that sustained patient weight loss be tracked through each patient's chart on a yearly basis.

> Regular monitoring of weight is also a predictor of successful weight control. Evidence from the National Weight Control Registry (NWCR), which was created to compile data on individuals who were successful at losing at least 13.6 kg [30 pounds] and at maintaining that loss for one year or more, shows that more than 75% of these successful weight-loss maintainers report weighing themselves at least once a week. (ICSI, 2011, p. 27)

Success can also be measured by overall patient satisfaction, retention rates of current patients, and clinic and financial growth. This success can be tracked by patient satisfaction surveys, the number of patients, and the number of new referrals. Financial growth, another evaluation of success, should be evaluated monthly and yearly by the chief financial officer in relation to the clinic's total profit.

PRIMARY CARE WEIGHT-LOSS COUNSELING

Screening for obesity is recommended at all office appointments; however, it is stated that less than half the providers in primary care record BMI, let alone provide guidance on weight loss, diet, or exercise. Only one-fifth of primary care providers systematically track weight, and less than 10% of primary care providers refer patients on for weight management (Dennison Himmelfarb, 2012).

On November 29, 2011, the Centers for Medicare and Medicaid (CMS) announced that they would cover "Intensive Behavioral Therapy (IBT) for Obesity" for benefits with Medicare Part A and Part B. "In 2003, the USPSTF [United States Preventive Services Task Force] found good evidence that BMI 'is reliable and valid for identifying adults at increased risk for mortality and morbidity due to overweight and obesity'" (Department of Health and Human Services [HHS], Centers for Medicare and Medicaid Services [CMS], 2012). A "B" recommendation of good to fair evidence also found that a BMI greater than or equal to 30 kg/m², or an obese adult, benefited most from high-intensity counseling with behavioral intervention. This type of high-intensity counseling and behavioral intervention produced "modest, sustained weight loss" (HHS, CMS, 2012, n.p.). Specific recommendations are covered for services provided by two subtypes of APNs—an NP or a certified clinical nurse specialist. Other provider specialties include family practice, internal medicine, obstetrics/gynecology, pediatric medicine, geriatric medicine, or a physician assistant. Claims are payable only in the following places of service (POS): physician's office, outpatient hospital, independent clinic, or a state or local public health clinic.

Those suitable for IBT are eligible for the following time-sensitive visits:

- One face-to-face visit every week for the first month
- One face-to-face visit every other week for months 2 to 6
- One face-to-face visit every month for months 7 to 12, if the beneficiary meets the 3 kg (6.6 pounds) weight-loss requirement during the first 6 months, as discussed next.

> At the 6-month visit, a reassessment of obesity and a determination of the amount of weight loss should be performed. To be eligible for additional face-to-face visits occurring once a month for months 7 to 12, beneficiaries must have achieved a reduction in weight of at least 3 kg (6.6 pounds), over the course of the first 6 months of intensive therapy. This determination must be documented in the physician office records for applicable beneficiaries consistent with usual practice. For beneficiaries who do not achieve a weight loss of at least 3 kg (6.6 pounds) during the first 6 months of intensive therapy, a reassessment of their readiness to change and BMI is appropriate after an additional 6-month period. (HHS, CMS, 2012, n.p.)

CMS are also very specific about what IBT for obesity should cover. This includes screening for obesity and calculating BMI, a nutrition or dietary assessment, and "intensive behavioral counseling" that may include high-intensity dietary and exercise interventions. The guidelines also suggest the use of and consistency of the 5 A's framework: assess, advise, agree, assist, and arrange, as described earlier (HHS, CMS, 2012).

The long-term sustainability of IBT is questionable, especially if continued attendance is required for face-to-face counseling. Trials by Appel et al. (2011) and Wadden et al. (2011), who used face-to-face visits, had a 50% drop in attendance over a 24-month period. Appel et al. (2011) increased from a 5.0% drop-out rate at 6 months to a 13.0% drop-out rate at 24 months. Wadden et al. (2011) demonstrated a decline from year 1 (81.7% + 14.9%) to year 2 (61.0% + 39.2%). Appel et al. (2011) also provided remote counseling through use of a study website. Remote support attendance also decreased over time from 8.7% at 6 months to 15.9% at 24 months. It appears that fewer barriers are seen in remote monitoring, including patient flexibility, less travel time, and possible decreased cost (including travel costs); these steps might help increase attendance and long-term sustainability (Dennison Himmelfarb, 2012). The two studies—face-to-face method and remote counseling method—had similar patient outcomes over a 24-month period (Appel et al., 2011).

Currently, CMS do not provide coverage for remote programs aimed at IBT. Would a program combining both face-to-face and remote offerings have a higher sustainability of weight loss? This question certainly leaves room for future studies and demonstrates the need for further research.

2013 AHA/ACC/TOS GUIDELINE FOR THE MANAGEMENT OF OVERWEIGHT AND OBESITY IN ADULTS

The American College of Cardiology (ACC), the American Heart Association (AHA), and the National Heart, Lung, and Blood Institute (NHLBI) collaborated to form a set of four guidelines to reduce cardiovascular risk. These organizations, along with the Obesity Society (TOS), collaborated to provide help for the *Guideline for the Management of Overweight and Obesity in Adults.* "Recommendations were derived from randomized trials, meta-analyses, and observational studies evaluated for quality, and were not formulated when sufficient evidence was not available" (Jensen et al., 2013, p. 5). Critical questions (CQs) and evidence statements (ESs) as well as the NHLBI grading format to the ACC/AHA Class of Recommendation/Level of Evidence (COR/LOE) construct are used throughout the guidelines. Applying COR/LOE requires the size of treatment effect (Class I, Class IIa, Class IIb, Class III No Benefit, and Class III No Harm) and the estimate of certainty (precision) of treatment effect (Level A, Level B, and Level C). The NHLBI has also developed two tables, (1) the NHLBI grading the strength of recommendations and (2) the quality rating the strength of evidence. The NHLBI grading the strength of recommendations is as follows:

- Grade A: strong recommendation
- Grade B: moderate recommendation
- Grade C: weak recommendation
- Grade D: recommendation against
- Grade E: expert opinion
- Grade N: no recommendation for or against

The quality rating the strength of evidence uses a high, moderate, or low rating to explain the type of evidence.

The guidelines came up with five CQs to make further recommendations for obesity. For the purpose of this chapter, further content will include the NHLBI Grade only. These guidelines and their NHLBI Grade are listed as follows (Jensen et al., 2013):

- Identifying Patients Who Need to Lose Weight (BMI and WC)
  1a Document weight, height and calculate BMI at least annually.
  Grade: E
  1b Use the following BMI markers for overweight (BMI greater than 25.0 to 29.9 kg/m²) and obesity (BMI greater than or equal to 30 kg/m²) to identify risk for CVD and all-cause mortality.
  Grade: A
  1c Discuss the comorbid diseases and associated risk (CVD, T2DM, and mortality) with overweight, obesity, and comorbid conditions.
  Grade: A
  1d Document WC at least annually. Discuss the increased risk of CVD, T2DM, and mortality associated with increased WC.
  Grade: E

- Matching Treatments With Risk Profiles (Reduction in Body Weight Effect of CVD Risk Factors, Events, Morbidity, and Mortality)
  2 Advise those with cardiovascular risk (CV) risk factors that even a 3% to 5% sustained weight loss achieved through lifestyle changes produces health benefits.
    2a Reduction in triglycerides, blood glucose, HgA1c, and risk of developing T2DM can be achieved with a long-term weight loss of 3% to 5%.

2b Greater weight loss can lower blood pressure (BP) and medications needed to reduce BP, reduce blood glucose and lipids (reduce low-density lipoprotein [LDL]-C and triglycerides and improve high-density lipoprotein [HDL]-C) as well as medication needed to control glucose and lipid management.

Grade: A

- Diets for Weight Loss (Dietary Strategies for Weight Loss)
  3a Recommend a reduced calorie diet to achieve weight loss. Reduce calorie intake with the following options:
  a. Women: 1,200 to 1,500 kcal/day; men: 1,500 to 1,800 kcal/day (levels to be adjusted according to each individual's weight).
  b. Aim for a 500 kcal or 750 kcal daily deficit.
  c. Recommend one of the evidence-based diets—one that is low in carbohydrates or fat or high in fiber.

Grade: A

  3b Recommend a diet that is "built" and individualized for the patient based on personal preferences and is appropriate in calories. Refer to a nutrition professional or RD for more counseling.

Grade: A

- Lifestyle Intervention and Counseling (Comprehensive Lifestyle Intervention)
  4a Recommend a greater than or equal to 6-month comprehensive lifestyle intervention that consists of weight loss through proper dietary choices and physical activity with the use of behavioral strategies.

Grade: A

  4b Recommend a high-intensity weight-loss program in either individual or group sessions. This is to be greater than or equal to 14 sessions in a 6-month period and should be led by a trained professional.

Grade: A

  4c Recommend an electronic or telephone weight-loss program instructed by a trained professional. Because it is not delivered in person, it may produce less weight loss.

Grade: B

  4d Consider a commercial-based weight-loss program if there is published evidence of its safety.

Grade: B

  4e Prescribe use of a very low-calorie diet (less than 800 kcal daily) only when absolutely needed and instructed by a trained professional. Supervision is needed, as weight loss can be very rapid and may even expose the patient to potential health problems.

Grade: A

  4f Recommend participation in a long-term (greater than or equal to 1 year) comprehensive weight-loss program aimed at those who have been successful with initial weight loss.

Grade: A

  4g Weight-loss maintenance is also recommended. This can be delivered face to face or by telephone. A trained professional should conduct at least monthly meetings, discuss diet and physical activity, and advise monthly weigh-ins.

Grade: A

- Selecting Patients for Bariatric Surgical Treatment for Obesity (Bariatric Surgical Treatment for Obesity)

  5a Patients with a BMI greater than or equal to 40 should be recommended for bariatric surgery and referred to an experienced bariatric surgeon. Those with a BMI greater than or equal to 35 with accompanying comorbid conditions who have failed behavioral or pharmacological therapies and/or are not motivated to lose weight should be referred to an experienced bariatric surgeon.

  Grade: A

  5b There is no recommendation for obese individuals with a BMI less than 35 to have bariatric surgery.

  Grade: N

  5c The surgeon and surgical staff should advise patients on and about the different surgical options and explain the risks, benefits, and alternatives to surgical therapy. Patient risk factors, including age and BMI, as well as behavioral and psychosocial factors should be discussed with the patient.

  Grade: E

For further bariatric surgery discussion, please refer to Chapter 22. In the five CQs previously mentioned, a nutritional professional is usually an RD; a *trained interventionist* can be defined as a variety of health professionals, such as an RD, exercise specialist, health counselor, psychologist, or those who adhere to formal lifestyle or weight management protocols.

The five CQs cover a substantial amount of information; however, they "did not cover the entire scope of evaluation, prevention, and management of overweight/obesity, the panelists provided advice based upon other guidelines and expert opinion to give providers a more comprehensive approach to their patients with weight-related issues" (Jensen et al., 2013, p. 17). This was the reason for the development of the Treatment Algorithm—The Chronic Disease Management Model for Primary Care of Patients With Overweight and Obesity. The algorithm consists of 19 boxes that advise providers and APNs on the treatment of overweight and obese patients. The following list of recommendations is followed by a summation of the algorithm:

1. Patient encounter
2. Calculation of BMI
3. BMI categories
4. Assessment and treatment of CVD risk factors
5. Assessment of weight history
6. Assessment of weight-loss need
7. Instructions on avoidance of weight gain/regain
8. Assessment of willingness to change and barriers
9. Setting health and weight-loss goals
10. Discussing weight-loss options
11. Offering lifestyle intervention options
12. Discussing pharmacotherapies
13. Discussing referral to bariatric surgery
14. Weight-loss goals and health improvement
15. Weight maintenance
16. Inability to lose weight

17. More frequent weight follow-up
18. Reassessment of weight-loss goals and health improvement
19. Assessment and treatment of CVD risk factors

Upon the initial appointment, the APN should assess height and weight in order to calculate BMI. This allows the APN to categorize the patient into the correct BMI class and can lead to further weight discussion. This can help the APN initiate further discussion of comorbid conditions associated with overweight and/or obesity, especially CVD or diabetes. A risk assessment of the overweight or obese patient should be thorough and include baseline laboratories, vitals, patient history, and a physical examination. A review of weight and lifestyle history should then be discussed and reviewed with the patient. The patient's history should include weight loss or gain over time. The type and number of attempts to lose weight and the patient's dietary and physical activity habits should be addressed. Family history of weight gain and other medical conditions should also be reviewed. Finally, medications and other pertinent history should be discussed.

The patient with a BMI greater than 30 or a BMI between 25 and 30 with comorbid conditions should be advised to lose weight. If the patient has a normal weight or a BMI 25 less than 30 without additional risk, the patient should be advised to maintain his or her current weight and avoid any further weight gain. Overweight and obese patients should be assessed periodically for their readiness to lose weight and should always be advised of the need to reduce or treat CVD risk factors. The APN can use the following suggested question: "How prepared are you to make changes in your diet, to be more physical active, and to use behavior change strategies such as recording your weight and food intake?" (Jensen et al., 2013, p. 20). Recommendations for weight loss should be realistic. The Panel recommends an initial weight-loss goal of 5% to 10% in the first 6 months. Although a weight loss of 3% to 6% can be beneficial and reduce risk factors, larger amounts of weight loss can increase risk reduction and ill health effects. A dietary intake of 1,200 to 1,500 kcal/day is recommended for women, whereas an intake of 1,500 to 1,800 kcal/day is recommended for men. At this point, a referral to an RD should be considered, especially if the patient has multiple medical conditions. Comprehensive lifestyle intervention should be offered to all patients regardless of whether they have received any type of prior weight-loss counseling. Pharmacotherapy and/or bariatric surgery may be considered as an adjunct to comprehensive lifestyle intervention. These options may be considered if the patient's BMI is greater than or equal to 30 (or greater than or equal to 27 with comorbidities), and if he or she has been unsuccessful with comprehensive lifestyle intervention. Determination of what therapy to use and when or if to refer to a bariatric surgery program is up to the APN.

High-intensity comprehensive weight-loss intervention is considered the most successful behavioral treatment. This consists of greater than or equal to 14 sessions within a 6-month period; all of these visits are conducted in person. High-intensity programs include a combination of reduction in calories, physical activity, and behavioral strategies aimed at reducing weight on an average of 5% to 10% or 8 kg. If delivery of the comprehensive weight-loss intervention cannot be done in person, electronic interventions can be delivered through the Internet or telephone. Commercial-based programs using meal replacements can also be an option.

Although the panel did not review comprehensive pharmacotherapy for weight loss, they suggest it may be used as an adjunct, as deemed appropriate by the

APN. Bariatric surgery consultation and evaluation was also suggested for those with a BMI greater than or equal to 40 or a BMI greater than or equal to 35 with existing comorbidities.

The panelists reported a weight loss of 5% to 10% as successful and considered it enough weight to reduce risk factors for CVD. Weight-loss maintenance should be addressed with patients who have achieved weight loss. Flexibility in using different approaches is recommended as well as encouraging the patient to engage in weekly self-weighing, reduced caloric intake, and increased physical activity.

If the patient is unable to achieve weight loss with the current treatment regimen, other options should be considered. These may include an additional referral to a high-intensity program, medications, an alternative diet plan, referral to an RD, or a bariatric surgery referral. The patient's weight and BMI should be documented at least annually; for those with difficulty losing weight or maintaining weight loss, it should be monitored more frequently. After re-evaluating the patient, weight-loss success should be determined as previously discussed (a weight loss greater than or equal to 5% of initial body weight and a reduction in CVD risk). The earlier listed high-intensity therapy options should be continued, as well as work toward reduction of CVD risk. Periodic assessment of weight as well as continued follow-up of weight management options should be reviewed with the patient on a scheduled basis (Jensen et al., 2013).

CHALLENGES

The transition from current health care practice to a prevention focus will have a tremendous effect on health care. Addressing current health practices before it is too late is essential. Total medical costs associated with obesity were estimated at $147 billion in 2006, whereas medical costs for an obese person are estimated at $1,429 higher than for a nonobese individual. The costs associated with obesity continue to climb, and so do patients' fears of seeking help and treating obesity. The ICSI (2011) states that patients become overwhelmed when thinking about losing weight. "It is discouraging if they think they have to quit eating all of their favorite foods and/or do hours of grueling exercise. It is even more challenging if they have a high level of stress in their lives" (p. 17). Providers must be aware of these fears and address them appropriately. Patients as well as providers must realize that in today's culture it is difficult to eat less and engage in more physical activity.

Clinics providing education, evaluation, assessment, and treatment of obesity need to be aware of the challenges with preventative treatment. A thorough review of treatment and payment options and the use of multidisciplinary teams is essential. Providing patient education and promoting a safe and friendly environment is the key.

REFERENCES

Appel, L. J., Clark, J. M., Yeh, H. C., Wang, N. Y., Coughlin, J. W., Daumit, G., . . . Brancati, F. L. (2011). Comparative effectiveness of weight-loss interventions in clinical practice. *New England Journal of Medicine, 365*(21), 1959–1968.

Campbell, G. M. (2014). *Idiot's guide: Project management* (6th ed.). New York, NY: Alpha Books.

Chang, V. W., Asch, D. A., & Werner, R. M. (2010). Quality of care among obese patients. *Journal of the American Medical Association, 303*(13), 1274–1281. doi:10.1001/jama.2010.339

Chao, D., Espeland, M. A., Farmer, D., Register, T. C., Lenchik, L., Applegate, W. B., & Ettinger, W. H. (2000). Effect of voluntary weight loss on bone mineral density in older overweight women. *Journal of American Geriatric Society, 48*(7), 753–759.

Dennison Himmelfarb, C. R. (2012). New evidence and policy support primary care-based weight loss interventions. *Journal of Cardiovascular Nursing, 27*(5), 379–381.

Department of Health and Human Services, Centers for Medicare and Medicaid Services. (2012). *Intensive behavioral therapy (IBT) for obesity.* Retrieved from http://www.cms.gov/Outreach-and-Education/Medicare-Learning-Network-MLN/MLNMattersArticles/downloads/MM7641.pdf

Ferrante, J. M., Piasecki, A. K., Ohman-Strickland, P. A., & Crabtree, B. F. (2009). Family physicians' practices and attitudes regarding care of extremely obese patients. *Obesity, 17,* 1710–1716. doi:10.1038/oby.2009.62

Fitch, A., Everling, L., Fox, C., Goldberg, J., Heim, C., Johnson, K., . . . Webb, B. (2013). Institute for clinical systems improvement. *Prevention and management of obesity for adults.* Retrieved from https://www.icsi.org/_asset/s935hy/Obesity-Interactive0411.pdf

Frezza, E. E., & Wachtel, M. S. (2008). A successful model of setting up a bariatric practice. *Obesity Surgery, 18,* 877–881. doi:10.1007/s1169-007-9377-7

Fujioka, D., & Bakhru, N. (2010). Office-based management of obesity. *Mount Sinai Journal of Medicine, 77,* 466–471. doi:10.1002/msj.20201

Institute for Clinical Systems Improvement (ICSI). (2011). *Health care guideline: Prevention and management of obesity (Mature Adolescents and Adults).* Retrieved from http://www.obesitycast.com/guidelinecasts/ICSI_Obesity.pdf

Jensen, M. D., Ryan, D. H., Apovian, C. M., Ard, J. D., Comuzzie, A. G., Donato, K. A., . . . Yanovski, S. Z. (2013). 2013 AHA/ACC/TOS Guideline for the management of overweight and obesity in adults. Circulation published online November 12, 2013. doi:10.1161/01.cir.0000437739.71477.ee

National Heart, Lung, and Blood Institute. (2000). The practical guide: Identification, evaluation, and treatment of overweight and obesity in adults. NIH Publication Number 00-4084. Retrieved from http://www.nhlbi.nih.gov/files/docs/guidelines/prctgd_c.pdf

Rejeski, W. J., Focht, B. C., & Messier, S. P. (2002). Obese, older adults with knee osteoarthritis: Weight loss, exercise, and quality of life. *Health Psychology, 21,* 419–426.

Tuomilehto, J., Lindstrom, J., Eriksson, J. G., Valle, T. T., Hämäläinen, H., Ilanne-Parikka, P., . . . Uusitupa, M. (2001). Prevention of type 2 diabetes by changes in lifestyle among subjects with impaired glucose tolerance. *New England Journal of Medicine, 344*(18), 1343–1350.

Wadden, T. A., Anderson, D. W., Foster, G. D., Bennett, A., Steinberg, C., & Sarwer, D. B. (2000). Obese women's perceptions of their physicians' weight management attitudes and practices. *Archives of Family Medicine, 9,* 854–860. Retrieved from http://archfammed.com

Wadden, T. A., Volger, S., Sarwer, D. B., Vetter, M. L., Tsai, A. G., Berkowitz, R. I., . . . Moore, R. H. (2011). A two-year randomized trial of obesity treatment in primary care practice. *New England Journal of Medicine, 365*(21), 1969–1979.

Wagner, E. H. (2000). The role of patient care teams in chronic disease management. *British Medical Journal, 320*(7234), 569–572.

W. K. Kellogg Foundation. (2004a). *Evaluation handbook*. Battle Creek, MI: Author.

W. K. Kellogg Foundation. (2004b). *Using logic models to bring together planning, evaluation, and action logic model development guide* (1209). Battle Creek, MI: Author.

Zwikael, O., & Ahn, M. (2011). The effectiveness of risk management: An analysis of project risk planning across industries and countries. *Risk Analysis, 31*(1), 25–37. doi:10.1111/j.1539-6924.2010.01470.x

Case Study 5

This case study builds on information presented in Chapters 20 to 26, treatment of obesity.

- *Chapter 20: Treatment of Addiction and Eating Disorders*
- *Chapter 21: Pharmacological Therapy*
- *Chapter 22: Surgical Therapy*
- *Chapter 23: Costs Associated With Obesity Treatment and Insurance Coverage*
- *Chapter 24: Treatment of the Obese Pediatric Patient*
- *Chapter 25: What Is Lifestyle Medicine?*
- *Chapter 26: Clinic Establishment, Medical Therapy, and a Multidisciplinary Approach*

Mr. Jones is a 35-year-old man who presents today with concerns of weight gain. He just moved from out of state to start a new job. He reports that previously he was following with an advanced practice nurse (APN) and was taking Phentermine 37.5 mg once daily. He reports that he lost about 50 pounds with this medication and was doing great; however, now he has gained this back plus more. He blames his recent weight gain on stress. He is recently divorced and has moved from out of town. He is wondering if he could try medication again or if there are any other solutions to help him. He reports that he is currently using continuous positive airway pressure (CPAP) therapy for his obstructive sleep apnea (OSA). He also reports that he had been previously taking medication for high blood pressure (BP), but was taken off this with his previous 50-pound weight loss.

His vitals are as follows:

Blood pressure: 142/90
Pulse: 70 bpm
Respirations: 12
Height: 6 feet, 2 inches
Weight: 344 pounds
Body mass index (BMI): 44.2 kg/m^2
Pulse oximetry: 96% on room air
Neck circumference: 17.5 inches

His physical examination is as follows:

General: Looks stated age, appropriate conversation, in no acute distress
Head, Eyes, Ears, Nose, Throat (HEENT): PERRLA, extraocular muscles intact.
  Conjunctiva normal, anicteric
Neck: Supple, no jugular vein distension (JVD)
Skin: Warm. Pink. Dry
Mucosa: No cyanosis, moist
Cardiovascular: Normal S1 and S2. No murmur
Lungs: Good bilateral air entry
Abdomen: Obese, soft, and nontender. Normal bowel sounds. No rebound pain
  or rigidity
Extremities: No edema, no cyanosis, or clubbing
Neurological: Alert and oriented ×3. No motor or sensory deficit

Is he overweight or obese? What category does his BMI fall into?

How would you address his weight?

Is he a candidate for weight loss?

Would you consider medication for weight loss?

Would you restart Phentermine or try a new medication?

How would you present him with a plan for weight loss? What would this include?

What about his blood pressure (BP)? How would you treat this?

With his recent stress, you decide to suggest stress management and medical treatment. Since it is your first time of meeting him, you want to give him a chance to try and lose weight without medication and devise a treatment plan together. This includes a healthy diet and routine exercise. A referral to a registered dietitian (RD) was offered, but he declined. You give him a weight-loss goal of 10 pounds in 1 month. You decide to see if weight loss helps control his BP and hold off on any medication at this point. A follow-up appointment is set up for 1 month.

He comes back 1 month later and tells you that he did well with the changes for about a week, but then "fell apart." He reports that with his new job, he is trying to work extra and just did not have the time to continue "all of these changes."

His vitals today are as follows:

Blood pressure: 150/90
Pulse: 66 bpm

Respirations: 12
Height: 6 feet, 2 inches
Weight: 364 pounds
Body mass index (BMI): 46.7 kg/m^2
Pulse oximetry: 96% on room air
Neck circumference: 18 inches

His physical examination is within normal limits (WNL).

You also have fasting laboratories drawn before his appointment today. They are as follows:

Basic Metabolic Panel (BMP)

Sodium: 139
Potassium: 3.7
Chloride: 101
CO_2: 25
Blood urea nitrogen (BUN): 18
Creatinine: 0.7
Glucose: 110

Complete Blood Count (CBC)

White blood cells: 6.5
Hemoglobin (Hb): 14.7
Hematocrit (Hct): 44.5
Platelets: 180

Thyroid-stimulating hormone (TSH): 2.7

Fasting Lipid Panel

Total cholesterol: 200
Triglycerides: 250
High-density lipoprotein (HDL): 36
Low-density lipoprotein (LDL): 130

How would you address his weight?

Would you consider medication at this time for weight loss?

Would you restart Phentermine or try a new medication?

How would you present him with a plan for weight loss? What would this include?

What about his BP? How would you treat this?

What would you do about his cholesterol?

Would you make any additional referrals?

Would you order any testing? If yes, what testing and why?

What dietary advice would you provide?

What lifestyle changes would you suggest?

What physical activity would you encourage? Please include mode/type, frequency, duration, and time.

Would you recommend stretching and strengthening activities? Please include mode/type, frequency, duration, and time.

Would you consider any additional medications? If yes, what?

Would you order any other laboratory work? If yes, what?

When would you repeat laboratory work?

When would you schedule his next follow-up appointment?

Would you involve any other advanced practice nurses (APNs) in his care?

You decide to try him on Phentermine 37.5 mg PO daily, as he told you this had worked well for him. You set him up for a return appointment in 1 month. You also start him on low-dose hydrochlorothiazide (HCTZ) 12.5 mg PO daily for his BP. You repeat a fasting glucose test at his next appointment.

He presents 1 month later for his follow-up appointment and is very happy. He is down 20 pounds and reports that he is trying to make better choices.

His vitals today are as follows:

Blood pressure: 130/84
Pulse: 68 bpm

Respirations: 12
Height: 6 feet, 2 inches
Weight: 344 pounds
Body mass index (BMI): 44.2 kg/m^2
Pulse oximetry: 96% on room air
Neck circumference: 17.5 inches

His physical examination is WNL.
His fasting glucose is 100.

What would you suggest next for this patient? Would you continue medication? For how long?

When would you want to set up his next appointment?

　　You continue his Phentermine for a total of 3 months. He is followed up monthly in the clinic. After the 3-month period, he has a weight loss of 45 pounds. You discontinue his Phentermine at that time and advise good dietary and exercise choices. You scheduled his next appointment, but he called to cancel. You do not see him again for 6 months. When he presents again, his weight is at an all-time high, 380 pounds, and BMI is 48.8 kg/m^2. He reports that he ran out of HCTZ a month ago and his BP is elevated today at 152/96.

How would you treat this patient?

Would you discuss or consider referral to a bariatric surgeon? Why or why not?

What referrals would you suggest?

What other education would you provide at this time?

Comprehensive Case Study

Mrs. Anderson is a 54-year-old Caucasian woman who presents to the clinic for the first time today. She says that she desperately needs to lose weight. She wants to feel better, be less short of breath, and "just enjoy life more." She had a history of weight-loss surgery 10 years ago, but states that "it was something new at the time and it just didn't work for me." She has also tried fen-phen when it was popular in the 1990s and reports that it worked well for her but then it was taken off the market. She also reports that she has tried about any and every "fad diet"—her latest is the cookie diet. She read about this diet in a magazine and reports that "all the stars in Hollywood are doing this to lose weight." She has several pieces of exercise equipment at home: a treadmill, stationary bike, and elliptical. She also has an ab roller, step, and yoga mat. She reports that she has also tried going to the gymnasium and has participated in several group classes. She reports that she likes going to the classes for about a week, but then finds that they take up too much of her time and she either loses interest or gets too busy.

She has a husband and two children at home. Her husband is obese and she says that her children are "heavy." She wants to set a good example for her children, but is worried she is too late.

She works part-time at a flower shop and volunteers at the local food bank in her spare time. She reports that she used to smoke cigarettes, but quit about 5 years ago. She was previously smoking anywhere from one to two packs per day from the age of 18 onward, except during her two pregnancies. She reports drinking alcohol on the weekends (about four beers and two mixed drinks, with regular pop). She also drinks a cup of coffee right away in the morning. She then drinks coke the rest of the day (about five cans) and says that if she is really tired that she has to have an energy drink around lunchtime.

Her past medical history includes hypertension (HTN), hyperlipidemia, type 2 diabetes mellitus (T2DM), gastroesophageal reflux disease (GERD), and obstructive sleep apnea (OSA). She also has complaints of back pain and right knee pain. Her previous surgeries include tonsillectomy, wisdom teeth removal, and one cesarean section.

She reports having gone through menopause "about five years ago." She thinks she had her first menstrual period around age 14. She reports three pregnancies with two births. She also says that "about a year ago, I had some spotting, but it just quit on its own."

She has a family history of obesity in her mother, father, sister, and maternal grandparents. Her mother also has HTN, T2DM, and high cholesterol. Her father has HTN, T2DM, high cholesterol, and coronary artery disease (CAD) with previous coronary artery bypass grafting surgery (CABG). Her sister also has T2DM. Her maternal grandparents were both diabetic and had high cholesterol.

Her medication list includes the following:

- HCTZ 25 mg PO daily
- Lisinopril 40 mg PO daily
- Amlodipine 10 mg PO daily
- Crestor 40 mg PO HS
- Metformin 1,000 mg PO BID
- Glipizide 5 mg PO BID
- Omeprazole 20 mg PO daily
- Ibuprofen (IBU) 800 mg PO BID
- Aspirin 81 mg PO daily

Today, her vitals are as follows:

Blood pressure (BP): 142/86
Pulse: 85 bpm
Respirations: 14
Height: 5 feet, 1 inch
Weight: 262 pounds
Body mass index (BMI): 49.5 kg/m^2
Pulse oximetry: 92% on room air
Neck circumference (NC): 16.5 inches
Laboratory data drawn 1 week ago (fasting):
Basic metabolic panel (BMP):
    Sodium: 136
    Potassium: 4.0
    Chloride: 101
    CO_2: 25
    Blood urea nitrogen (BUN): 22
    Creatinine: 0.7
    Glucose: 164
Complete blood count (CBC):
    White blood cells (WBCs): 7.0
    Hemoglobin (Hb): 13.2
    Hematocrit (Hct): 39.5
    Platelets: 225
Thyroid-stimulating hormone (TSH): 4.0
Fasting lipid panel:
    Total cholesterol: 246
    Triglycerides: 300
    High-density lipoprotein (HDL): 32
    Low-density lipoprotein (LDL): 154
Glycosylated hemoglobin (HgA1c): 6.9

A SOAP (subjective, objective, assessment, plan) note outline can be utilized on the aforementioned patient. This can be used for practice and learning purposes. The following is a template that can be used to structure proper SOAP note formation:

(S) Subjective: (Chief Complaint, History of Presenting Illness) (Onset, Location, Duration, Character, Aggravating Factors, Relieving Factors, Treatment—OLD CART).

- Allergies
- Medications
- Past medical history
- Past surgical history
- Family history
- Social history
- Review of systems

(O) Objective:

- Vitals
- Physical examination

Results:

- Laboratory data
- Tests

(A) Assessment: (Differential Diagnosis).

(P) Plan: (Include Education, Dietary Recommendations, Exercise Recommendations, Referrals, Treatment Plan, Medication Changes/Additions, and Suggested Follow-Up).

SAMPLE SOAP NOTE

CHIEF COMPLAINT: "I desperately want to lose weight."

HISTORY: Mrs. Anderson is a 54-year-old Caucasian woman who presents to the clinic for the first time today. She wants to feel better, be less short of breath, and "just enjoy life more." She has a history of weight-loss surgery 10 years ago, but states that "it was something new at the time and it just didn't work for me." She has also tried fen-phen when it was popular in the 1990s and reports that it worked well for her, but then, it was taken off the market. She also reports that she has tried about any and every "fad diet"—her latest is the cookie diet. She read about this diet in a magazine and reports that "all the stars in Hollywood are doing this to lose weight." She has several pieces of exercise equipment at home: a treadmill, stationary bike, and elliptical. She also has an ab roller, step, and yoga mat. She reports that she has also tried going to the gymnasium and has participated in several group classes. She reports that she likes going to the classes for about a week, but then finds that they take up too much of her time and she either loses interest or gets too busy.

She has a husband and two children at home. Her husband is obese and she says that her children are "heavy." She wants to set a good example for her children, but is worried she is too late.

She works part-time at a flower shop and volunteers at the local food bank in her spare time.

Her past medical history includes hypertension (HTN), hyperlipidemia, type 2 diabetes mellitus (T2DM), gastroesophageal reflux disease (GERD), and obstructive sleep apnea (OSA). She also has complaints of back pain and right knee pain, which are especially noted with activity.

She denies any complaints of chest pain, pressure, or heaviness. There is no radiation of any pain to the arm, neck, jaw, or back. She notices significant shortness of breath. She blames this on the fact that she is not too active and reports that she is "too heavy." She experiences no PND or orthopnea. Her shortness of breath is clearly related to any activity or exertion. She denies any palpitations, dizziness, lightheadedness, syncope, fevers, or chills. She has lower-extremity edema. She also reports significant arthritic pain when she gets up and moves around and because of this is not too active.

Allergies

No reported medication allergies.

Current Medications

HCTZ 25 mg PO daily
Lisinopril 40 mg PO daily
Amlodipine 10 mg PO daily
Crestor 40 mg PO HS
Metformin 1,000 mg PO BID
Glipizide 5 mg PO BID
Omeprazole 20 mg PO daily
IBU 800 mg PO BID
Aspirin 81 mg PO daily

Past Medical History (PMH)

HTN
Hyperlipidemia
T2DM
GERD
OSA
Back pain
Right knee pain

Past Surgical History (PSH)

Tonsillectomy
Wisdom teeth removal
Cesarean section × 1

Gynecological History

Age of first menstrual cycle: 14
Age of menopause: 49
Number of pregnancies: 3
Number of births: 2
Any history of abnormal vaginal bleeding? Yes

Family History

Mother: Obesity, HTN, T2DM, and high cholesterol
Father: Obesity, HTN, T2DM, high cholesterol, and coronary artery disease (CAD) with coronary artery bypass grafting surgery (CABG)
Sister: Obesity, T2DM
Maternal grandparents: Obesity, T2DM, and high cholesterol

Personal History

History of smoking/tobacco use: One to two packs of cigarettes per day × 31 years; quit 5 years ago
Caffeine use: One cup coffee daily, five regular cokes, and energy drinks
Alcohol use: Weekends, four beers daily, and two mixed drinks with regular pop

Review of Systems (ROS)

Constitutional: No weight loss, fever, chills, weakness, or fatigue
Head, Eyes, Ears, Nose, Throat (HEENT): Eyes: No visual loss, blurred vision, double vision, or yellow sclera. Ears, nose, and throat: No hearing loss, sneezing, congestion, runny nose, or sore throat
Skin: No rash or itching
Cardiovascular: No chest pain, pressure, or discomfort. No palpitations or edema
Respiratory: No shortness of breath. No cough or sputum
Gastrointestinal: No anorexia, nausea, vomiting, or diarrhea. No abdominal pain or blood
Genitourinary: No burning on urination. Last menstrual period: Age 49 years
Neurological: No headache, dizziness, syncope, paralysis, ataxia, numbness, or tingling in the extremities. No change in bowel or bladder control
Musculoskeletal: No muscle pain. Positive back pain. Positive right knee pain. No joint stiffness
Hematological: No anemia, bleeding, or bruising
Lymphatics: No enlarged nodes. No history of splenectomy
Psychiatric: No history of depression or anxiety
Endocrinological: No reports of sweating, cold, or heat intolerance. No polyuria or polydipsia
Allergies: No history of asthma, hives, eczema, or rhinitis

Vital Signs

Blood pressure (BP): 142/86
Pulse: 85 bpm
Respirations: 14
Height: 5 feet, 1 inch
Weight: 262 pounds
Body mass index (BMI): 49.5 kg/m^2
Pulse oximetry: 92% on room air
Neck circumference: 16.5 inches

Physical Examination

HEENT: PERRLA, extraocular muscles were intact. Conjunctiva normal, anicteric
Neck: Supple, no jugular vein distension (JVD). No thyromegaly or masses
Skin: Warm and moist
Mucosa: No cyanosis
Cardiovascular: Normal palpation, percussion. Normal S1 and S2. No murmur. No clicks or gallops
Lungs: Normal palpation, percussion. Good bilateral air entry. No rales, rhonchi, or crepitation
Abdomen: Soft, nontender. Large and obese. Normal bowel sounds. No rebound or rigidity
Extremities: Trace bilateral edema, no cyanosis or clubbing
Neurological: Alert and oriented × 3. No motor or sensory deficit

Results

Laboratory data:
Basic metabolic panel (BMP):
  Sodium: 136
  Potassium: 4.0
  Chloride: 101
  CO_2: 25
  Blood urea nitrogen (BUN): 22
  Creatinine: 0.7
  Glucose: 164
Complete blood count (CBC):
  White blood cells (WBCs): 7.0
  Hemoglobin (Hb): 13.2
  Hematocrit (Hct): 39.5
  Platelets: 225
Thyroid-stimulating hormone (TSH): 4.0
Fasting lipid panel:
  Total cholesterol: 246
  Triglycerides: 300
  High-density lipoprotein (HDL): 32
  Low-density lipoprotein (LDL): 154
Glycosylated hemoglobin (HgA1c): 6.9

Health Management Plan

Basal Metabolic Rate (BMR)

Women: BMR = 655 + (4.35 × weight in pounds) + (4.7 × height in inches) − (4.7 × age in years)
BMR = 655 + (4.35 × 262 pounds) + (4.7 × 61 inches) − (4.7 × 54 years)
BMR = 655 + (1,139.7) + (286.7) − (253.8)
    = **1,827.6**

Harris–Benedict Formula:
Sedentary (little or no exercise)

Calorie-calculation = BMR × 1.2
1,827.6 × 1.2 = 2,193.12

Exercise

Walking, biking (indoor or outdoor), and elliptical. Perform 5 to 7 days per week, starting out with 15 minutes at a time, progressing to 30 to 60 minutes 5 to 7 days per week lifelong.

Stretches

- Triceps stretch
- Biceps stretch
- Chest stretch
- Shoulder stretch
- Side stretch
- Hamstring stretch
- Quadriceps stretch
- Groin stretch
- Calf stretch

Stretches should be done daily. Each stretch should be held at least 10 to 30 seconds and repeated on both sides of the body as needed.

Strengthening

- Chest press
- Triceps kickback
- Bent-over row
- Biceps curl
- Wall push-ups
- Seated leg extension
- Standing hamstring curl
- Hip adduction
- Hip abduction
- Hip extension
- Heel raises (calf raises)
- Squats

Strengthening activities should be done at least 3 days per week. The patient should be encouraged to start with 10 repetitions, progressing up to 15. Each strengthening activity should be repeated for a total of three sets.

Goals

- Keep a dietary and exercise journal daily
- Lose weight of 1 to 2 pounds per week
- Aim for 1,600 to 1,700 calories daily
- Consume three to five servings of fruits and vegetables daily
- Consume 64 ounces of fluid daily

Assessment (Differential Diagnoses)

1. Obesity
2. HTN
3. T2DM
4. Hyperlipidemia

5. OSA
6. GERD
7. Back pain
8. Knee pain
9. Edema
10. Alcohol use
11. Caffeine use
12. Sedentary lifestyle

Impression/Plan

1. Obesity: Her weight and BMI are elevated today. I discussed her weight and need for weight loss for her overall health and to reduce her risk factors related to her current disease processes. During today's visit, I addressed the 5 A's—asking, advising, assessing, assisting, and arranging—for weight-loss follow-up. I clearly think she needs risk factor modification as well as a cardiac workup before her baseline prior to beginning exercise. I will order at least a resting EKG and treadmill stress test prior to her next appointment. I outlined her plan for exercise, but advised her to wait until cardiac testing is found normal before beginning. I also discussed her caloric needs with regard to BMR and Harris–Benedict Formula. I recommended between 1,600 and 1,700 calories daily for a 1- to 2-pound weight loss. I also helped set appropriate goals for the patient. I will follow up with her in the next 1 to 2 weeks. I advised her to contact me with any further questions and/or concerns.

2. HTN: According to the latest Joint National Committee (JNC) HTN Guidelines, her BP is elevated. Unfortunately, she is on three medications already at the maximum recommended doses—hydrochlorothiazide (HCTZ), lisinopril, and amlodipine. I will hold off on adding an additional medication and recheck this at her next appointment. I recommended nightly use of her Pap machine and strict treatment of her OSA. I also recommended a low-sodium diet. If BP is still elevated according to the guidelines at her next appointment, I would consider an additional medication, most likely hydralazine. I would also consider ordering an ultrasound of the renal arteries to rule out any underlying renal artery stenosis.

3. T2DM: HgA1c is 6.9. I would recommend continued current medication treatment of metformin and glipizide. I would also recommend monitoring her total carbohydrates. I would consider referral to a registered dietitian (RD) as needed.

4. Hyperlipidemia: Her total cholesterol, triglycerides, and LDL cholesterol levels are elevated. Her 10-year atherosclerotic cardiovascular disease (ASCVD) risk score is elevated at 12.1% with a lifetime ASCVD risk of 50%. She is already on high-intensity statin therapy. I will change statin therapy from Crestor 40 mg PO daily to atorvastatin 80 mg PO daily to see if she responds better to this statin compared with the other. I will order a fasting lipid and liver panel to be repeated in 8 weeks. If cholesterol is still elevated, I would consider adding Zetia to her medication regimen.

5. OSA: I recommended continued nightly treatment with Pap therapy.

6. GERD: I recommended to continue omeprazole.

7. Joint pain (back and right knee): I will not make any changes at this time, but will continue to monitor her. I could order X-rays if needed, especially if her pain continues or worsens. I would recommend IBU/Tylenol use as needed

for pain. I counseled the patient regarding the importance against overuse. Her joint pain may get better with weight loss.

8. Edema: This is only traced bilaterally. I could consider discontinuing her amlodipine to see if this is the cause; however, because of her uncontrolled HTN, I will hold off on any medication changes as she reports that edema is not a major problem for her.

9. Alcohol use: I recommended cutting down on her alcohol use. According to the *Dietary Guidelines for Americans, moderate alcohol consumption* is defined as having up to one drink per day for women. I recommended that she choose a light beer or a mixed drink with water or diet cola instead of a regular cola.

10. Caffeine use: I recommended her to decrease caffeine use.

11. Sedentary lifestyle: I will wait for results from EKG and treadmill stress test before further exercise prescription, but did recommend increased movement and activity throughout the day.

Follow-Up: I will follow-up in 1 to 2 weeks. She will repeat fasting lipid panel and liver panel in 8 weeks. I would also recommend screening for depression if not done within the past few months.

Recommended Answers to Cases

CASE STUDY 1

Is she overweight or obese? What category does her BMI fall into?
Obese. Category Obesity, Class III.

How would you address her BMI?
Mrs. A., let's talk about your weight. Your BMI, which is a combination of your height and weight, puts you at risk for increased health problems. Your weight is also dangerous because of your family history of hypertension (HTN) and coronary artery disease (CAD). Have you thought about weight loss? What can we work on today to get you started on a plan to lose weight? How can I best help you lose weight?

Would you address her family history?
Yes, she has a strong family history of medical problems that need to be addressed. These problems put her at increased risk of medical problems too.

What cardiovascular risk factors does she have?
Elevated BMI—obesity
Sedentary lifestyle
Elevated blood pressure (BP)
Family history of CAD

What has led to her obesity?
Her sedentary lifestyle (both in her career and at home), probable depression, and lack of motivation.

Is she a candidate for weight loss?
Yes! Now is the time to address this issue, as she is still young and has significant risk factors.

How would you present her with a plan for weight loss? What would this include?
I would approach the subject carefully so as to not offend her. I would suggest keeping a daily dietary and activity journal to keep track of what she is eating and how much activity she is doing. I would recommend starting with cardiovascular exercise, 15 minutes daily. This could be done in a form of activity she enjoys (walking, biking, or even swimming). I would also recommend a weight-loss goal

of 1 to 2 pounds per week with a 6-month weight loss of 10% of her body weight. I would schedule close follow-up to review the journal and set any additional goals. Before finishing the appointment, I would address any further goals that she may have.

What would you do about her BP? What treatment options would you present to her?
Because she is presenting as a new patient, I would hold off on starting medication at this point. I would recommend an at-home BP monitoring device to check her BP daily at random times. I would recommend weight loss as well as low-sodium foods. I would see her for a return visit in 4 weeks to recheck her BP. I would also talk to her about medications, but tell her that I would like to hold off on medication if possible. If BP continues to be elevated, other secondary causes need to be ruled out (obstructive sleep apnea [OSA] or renal artery stenosis).

Would you make any additional referrals?
Yes, I would recommend a referral to a registered dietitian (RD) and/or exercise specialist.

Would you consider any medications for this patient? If yes, what medications and why?
I would recommend an 81 mg aspirin daily because of her risk factors for CAD. I would continue to monitor her BP and screen for any possible depression.

Would you order any testing? If yes, what testing and why?
Yes, with her known family history of CAD and sedentary lifestyle, I would consider a treadmill stress test prior to prescription exercise. I would also order baseline laboratories, including a basic metabolic panel (BMP), complete blood count (CBC), thyroid-stimulating hormone (TSH), and lipid panel.

What dietary advice would you provide?
I would use the basal metabolic rate (BMR) and Harris–Benedict Formula to suggest appropriate caloric intake. I would recommend whole grains, fresh or frozen fruits and vegetables, and lean choices of meat. I would also refer to an RD for further advice.

What lifestyle changes would you suggest?
I would suggest increasing activity in any way possible. I would also suggest limiting screen time. Finally, I would recommend a diet rich in fruits and vegetables.

You also draw fasting blood work on her and find the following:
Basic Metabolic Panel (BMP):
Sodium: 135
Potassium: 3.7
Chloride: 101
Carbon dioxide (CO_2): 25
Blood urea nitrogen (BUN): 22
Creatinine: 1.0
Glucose: 135

Complete Blood Count (CBC):
 White blood cells (WBCs): 6.5
 Hemoglobin (Hb): 14.7
 Hematocrit (Hct): 44.5
 Platelets: 202
Thyroid-stimulating hormone (TSH): 2.0
Fasting Lipid Panel:
 Total cholesterol: 215
 Triglycerides: 225
 High-density lipoprotein (HDL): 35
 Low-density lipoprotein (LDL): 130

Would you make any additional changes in her medications?
Not at this time. I would, however, repeat a fasting glucose level in the next 2 to 3 weeks. I would also recommend weight loss and foods low in saturated fats and cholesterol. I would repeat a fasting lipid panel in 6 to 8 weeks.

When would you repeat laboratory work?
Fasting glucose level in 2 to 3 weeks.
Lipid panel in 6 to 8 weeks.

When would you schedule her next follow-up appointment?
I would schedule a next follow-up appointment in 4 to 6 weeks.

Would you involve any other advanced practice nurses (APNs) in her care?
Not at this time. If her mood or depression worsens, I would refer her to a psychiatric mental health nurse practitioner (PMHNP).

What additional education, if any, would you provide?
I would recommend contacting the office with any further questions and/or concerns. I would also suggest routine follow-up. Further education would depend upon any patient questions.

CASE STUDY 2

Is he overweight or obese? What category does his BMI fall into? Would you use BMI in an 11-year-old?
He would be considered obese, as his weight falls in the greater than 95th percentile. I would not use BMI, as the patient is still a pediatric patient.

How would you address his weight?
With his age, I would proceed cautiously with a recommendation for weight loss. I would address his weight and tell him that he is still in the growing stage. I would explain that with this, he may grow taller, but do not want him to be at an increased risk for obesity in the future. I would encourage continued activity and advise him to decrease his screen time and to limit sedentary activities. I would also recommend that he choose healthier foods for snack time and meals. I would also recommend parental involvement in preparing and cooking meals. I would ask the parent or guardian to engage the child in helping make the shopping list and to choose healthy meals and snacks.

What has led to his obesity?
His sedentary time with video games, parental influences, and snack and meal choices.

Is he a candidate for weight loss?
He is not necessarily a candidate for weight loss, but I would recommend healthier choices and increased physical activity.

How would you present him with a plan for weight loss? What would this include?
I would not want him to become obsessed with his weight or weight loss, so I would be very careful in presentation. I would include appropriate referrals, including that of a registered dietitian (RD). I would also recommend that he make a sample shopping list to include fruits, vegetables, and healthy snacks. I would also recommend continued activities. I would discuss keeping a journal and writing down what he eats, drinks, and does for activity each day. I would also encourage parental involvement, as supervision plays an essential role in weight.

Would you make any additional referrals?
Yes, to an RD.

Would you order any testing? If yes, what testing and why?
Yes, a baseline basic metabolic panel (BMP), thyroid-stimulating hormone (TSH), and lipid panel. This would assess for fasting blood glucose, thyroid levels, and cholesterol.

What dietary advice would you provide?
I would use the basal metabolic rate (BMR) and Harris–Benedict Formula to suggest appropriate caloric intake. I would recommend a well-balanced diet rich in whole grains, fresh or frozen fruits and vegetables, low-fat dairy products, and lean choices of meat. I would also refer to an RD for further advice.

What lifestyle changes would you suggest?
I would recommend continued activity. I would recommend decreased screen and/or video time to less than 1 hour per day.

Would you recommend any family lifestyle counseling?
Yes, if the patient and/or parent would be willing to consider this.

You also draw fasting blood work on him and find the following:
Thyroid-stimulating hormone (TSH): 3.5
Fasting lipid panel:
 Total cholesterol: 215
 Triglycerides: 550
 High-density lipoprotein (HDL): 30
 Low-density lipoprotein (LDL): 150

Would you consider any medications? If yes, what?
No, not at this time.

When would you repeat laboratory work?
I would repeat a fasting lipid panel in 6 to 8 weeks.

When would you schedule his next follow-up appointment?
I would schedule a follow-up appointment in 4 to 6 weeks.

Would you involve any other advanced practice nurses (APNs) in his care?
Consideration could be made to involve a pediatric nurse practitioner (PNP) if needed.

What additional education, if any, would you provide?
I would continue to emphasize the importance of healthy choices (both good dietary and activity choices) and not focus on weight loss. I would address any additional questions.

CASE STUDY 3

Is she overweight or obese? What category does her BMI fall into?
Obese. BMI class III obesity.

How would you address her weight?
Mrs. Smith, let's talk about your weight. Your BMI, which is a combination of your height and weight, puts you at risk for increased health problems. Your weight is also dangerous because of your family history of hypertension (HTN), hypercholesterolemia, and type 2 diabetes mellitus (T2DM). Have you thought about weight loss? What can we work on today to get you started on a plan to lose weight? How can I best help you lose weight?

What has led to her obesity?
Her age, joint pain, sedentary lifestyle, depression, possible bulimia, and family history of obesity.

Is she a candidate for weight loss?
Yes! She is a great candidate for weight loss, considering her current weight, risk factors, and family history of cardiovascular risk factors.

Is her weight loss of 100 pounds in 6 months feasible? Why or why not? What would you recommend?
No, it is not feasible. This would be a quick weight loss and most likely one that could not be sustained in the long term. I would recommend a weight loss of 10% of her body weight (37 to 38 pounds) in 6 months.

How would you present her with a plan for weight loss? What would this include?
I would approach the subject carefully so as to not offend her. I would suggest keeping a daily dietary and activity journal to keep track of what she is eating and how much activity she is doing. I would recommend starting with cardiovascular exercise 15 minutes daily. This could be done in a form of activity she enjoys (walking, biking, or even swimming). I would also recommend a weight-loss goal of 1 to 2 pounds per week with a 6-month weight loss of 10% of her body weight. I would also talk about referral to a registered dietitian (RD) and an exercise specialist. I would schedule close follow-up to review her journal and set any

additional goals. Before finishing the appointment, I would address any further goals that she may have.

How would you address her "getting sick" or vomiting?
Mrs. Smith, you say that you sometimes "get sick and vomit" after eating too much. How often are you doing this? For how long have you done this? I would encourage her to avoid getting sick and advise her to listen to her body, so that she does not eat too much to feel so full. Depending on her responses, I would refer her to a specialist, such as a counselor or psychiatric mental health nurse practitioner (PMHNP).

Would you make any additional referrals?
Yes, I would refer to an RD, exercise specialist, and counselor or PMHNP.

Would you order any testing? If yes, what testing and why?
Yes, I would order a repeat fasting glucose level and lipid panel. A fasting glucose should be repeated, as the initial one is elevated. I would want to rule out any metabolic syndrome and/or T2DM. I would repeat a fasting lipid panel after she has worked on dietary and exercise changes. This would be done in approximately 8 weeks. I would also consider a sleep study, as she is significantly obese. With her age and risk factors, I would consider a resting baseline EKG and treadmill stress test before prescribing any exercise.

What dietary advice would you provide?
I would use the basal metabolic rate (BMR) and Harris–Benedict Formula to suggest appropriate caloric intake. I would recommend a well-balanced diet rich in whole grains, fresh or frozen fruits and vegetables, low-fat dairy products, and lean choices of meat. I would also refer to an RD for further advice. Again, I would stress the importance of not vomiting after meals and listening to her body.

What lifestyle changes would you suggest?
I would suggest increasing activity in any way possible. I may even suggest a support group if she would be open to this.

What physical activity would you encourage? Please include mode/type, frequency, duration, and time.
Based on her reported interests, I would recommend biking (indoor or outdoor), 5 to 7 days per week, starting out with 15 minutes at a time, progressing to 30 to 60 minutes 5 to 7 days per week lifelong. As she progresses with biking or if she complains of joint pain, swimming or water aerobics could be an alternative.

Would you recommend stretching and strengthening activities? Please include mode/type, frequency, duration, and time.
Yes, I would recommend both stretching and strengthening activities.

Stretches:

- Triceps stretch
- Biceps stretch
- Chest stretch
- Shoulder stretch

- Side stretch
- Hamstring stretch
- Quadriceps stretch
- Groin stretch
- Calf stretch

Stretches should be done daily. Each stretch should be held at least 10 to 30 seconds and repeated on both sides of the body as needed.

Strengthening:

- Chest press
- Triceps kickback
- Bent-over row
- Biceps curl
- Wall push-ups
- Seated leg extension
- Standing hamstring curl
- Hip adduction
- Hip abduction
- Hip extension
- Heel raises (calf raises)
- Squats

Strengthening activities should be done at least 3 days per week. The patient should be encouraged to start with 10 repetitions, progressing up to 15. Each strengthening activity should be repeated for a total of three sets.

Would you recommend any family lifestyle counseling?
Yes, I think this would benefit the patient if she and her family are willing to do it. It should be offered as an option.

Would you continue her current medication—Prozac? Would there be a better choice?
Prozac is considered a good option, as it is an off-use medication for the treatment of obesity. Its primary purpose as a highly selective serotonin reuptake inhibitor (SSRI) is to treat depression. However, it appears that her depression is also not under the best possible control. Depending on the provider's level of comfort with changing medications, this could be done or referred to a PMHNP. Any possibility would include bupropion (Wellbutrin).

Would you consider any additional medications? If yes, what?
I would not start medication for blood pressure (BP) yet; however, I would continue to monitor it. I would have her keep track of her BP trends at home. I would also see how her BP responds to exercise. I would hold off on any other medication changes at this time.

Would you order any other laboratory work? If yes, what?
Yes, I would order a repeat fasting glucose level and lipid panel.

I may also consider ordering a vitamin D level, as she lives in the Midwest and would be at a higher risk for vitamin D deficiency.

When would you repeat laboratory work?
I would order a fasting glucose level to be done in the next 1 to 2 weeks. I would repeat a fasting lipid panel after she has worked on dietary and exercise changes. This would be done in approximately 8 weeks.

When would you schedule her next follow-up appointment?
I would schedule a follow-up appointment in 1 to 2 weeks.

Would you involve any other advanced practice nurses (APNs) in her care?
If she would agree, I would schedule her for a follow-up appointment with a PMHNP.

What additional education, if any, would you provide?
I would recommend contacting the office with any further questions and/or concerns. I would also suggest routine follow-up. Further education would depend upon any patient questions.

CASE STUDY 4

How would you address and treat his blood pressure?
He is already on hydrochlorothiazide (HCTZ) and lisinopril to treat his blood pressure (BP). He is on the maximum dose of HCTZ. There is still room to increase his lisinopril to better treat his BP. According to the 2014 Hypertension (HTN) Guidelines, his BP should be treated to achieve a goal of systolic blood pressure (SBP) less than 140 and diastolic blood pressure (DBP) less than 90. I would encourage him to increase his activity and choose good dietary options, including a low-sodium diet. I would also increase his lisinopril to 40 mg PO daily. I would order a basic metabolic panel (BMP) to be done in 2 to 3 weeks and repeat a BP check in 4 to 6 weeks. I would advise the patient to report any symptoms of low BP (dizziness, lightheadedness, or syncope) immediately to the office.

What about his type 2 diabetes mellitus (T2DM)?
Unfortunately, his glycosylated hemoglobin (HgA1c) is not at goal either and is elevated at 9.0. He is already on metformin 1,000 mg PO BID. Technically, this medication can be titrated up to 2,500 mg PO daily; however, I do not think this would be a feasible or realistic option with an HgA1c of 9.0. Metformin is a good choice for first-line treatment of his T2DM with his obesity. I would consider adding in another agent at this time. Metformin, exenatide, amylin, pramlintide, and acarbose have been studied for the off-label use of weight loss. I would hold off on an injectable medication at this time, as he is young and this may seem too similar to insulin. I would consider an additional oral agent at this time, a sulfonylurea, glipizidem 5 mg PO daily. I would increase this, as needed, in 1 week to be determined by his self-recorded blood sugars.

How would you address his weight?
Mr. Dundee, let's talk about your weight. Your body mass index (BMI), which is a combination of your height and weight, puts you at risk for increased health problems. You're young and we are already treating you for HTN and T2DM. These conditions alone are worrisome for increasing your risk for a cardiovascular

event. Have you thought about weight loss? What can we work on today to get you started on a plan to lose weight? How can I best help you lose weight?

What would be a good weight-loss goal for him?
A good weight-loss goal in the short term would be 1 to 2 pounds per week with a 10% (27–28 pounds) weight-loss goal in 6 months.

How would you present him with a plan for weight loss? What would this include?
I would approach the subject carefully so as to not offend him. I would suggest keeping a daily dietary and activity journal to keep track of what he is eating and how much activity he is doing. I would recommend starting with cardiovascular exercise 15 minutes daily. This could be done in a form of activity he enjoys (walking, biking, or even swimming). I would also talk about referral to a registered dietitian (RD) and an exercise specialist. I would schedule close follow-up to review the journal and set any additional goals. Before finishing the appointment, I would address any further goals that he may have.

Would you make any additional referrals?
Yes, I would consider referrals to an RD and exercise specialist. Because of his age and extent of his T2DM, I could consider referral to endocrinology.

His physical examination shows the following:

General: Looks stated age, appropriate conversation, in no acute distress
Head, Eyes, Ears, Nose, Throat (HEENT): PERRLA, extraocular muscles intact. Conjunctiva normal, anicteric
Neck: Supple, no jugular vein distension (JVD)
Skin: Warm. Pink. Dry
Mucosa: No cyanosis, moist
Cardiovascular: Normal S1 and S2. No murmur
Lungs: Good bilateral air entry
Abdomen: Obese, soft, and nontender. Normal bowel sounds. No rebound pain or rigidity
Extremities: No edema, no cyanosis, no clubbing
Neurological: Alert and oriented ×3. No motor or sensory deficit

After talking with the patient further, he said that over the past 2 months when he has been exercising he has noticed more instances of shortness of breath. He also reports that he has occasional chest tightness. It is present with activity and resolved with sitting down and resting. At times, he also feels that his jaw is sore, but he does not know why. Reluctantly, he also mentions that his wife is worried about his snoring. He reports that she states it is so bad that sometimes she gets up and goes into another room to sleep. The patient admits to feeling more tired, but thinks it is due to the extra hours he is picking up at work. He also reports that he has been under more stress because of his long working hours. He reports that smoking is his stress relief. He is now smoking a half pack per day.

In reviewing his family history, one notices that his father is deceased secondary to sudden cardiac death at the age of 45.

Would you order any additional testing? If yes, what testing and why?
Yes, I would order a resting baseline EKG and treadmill stress test. This would be pertinent because of his current symptoms of chest pain, strong family history of

coronary artery disease (CAD), personal risk factors, and current stress level. I may also refer to cardiology for further workup. I would also consider referral for a sleep study because of his neck size, symptoms, and body habitus.

What dietary advice would you provide?
I would use the basal metabolic rate (BMR) and Harris–Benedict Formula to suggest appropriate caloric intake. I would recommend a well-balanced diet rich in whole grains, fresh or frozen fruits and vegetables, low-fat dairy products, and lean choices of meat. I would also refer to an RD for further advice.

What lifestyle changes would you suggest?
I would suggest increasing activity in any way possible. A diabetes support group may also be offered to the patient.

What physical activity would you encourage? Please include mode/type, frequency, duration, and time.
Again, because of his current symptoms, I would get an EKG and treadmill stress test done. I may even consider referral to a cardiologist before giving exercise recommendations. Once he is okay to proceed with exercise, I would first inquire about his activity interests. If he does not have a particular favorite, I would suggest walking (indoor or outdoor), 5 to 7 days per week, starting out with 15 minutes at a time, progressing to 30 to 60 minutes 5 to 7 days per week lifelong. If he gets bored with walking, biking or swimming could be other alternatives.

Would you recommend stretching and strengthening activities? Please include mode/type, frequency, duration, and time.
Yes, I would recommend both stretching and strengthening activities.

Stretches:

- Triceps stretch
- Biceps stretch
- Chest stretch
- Shoulder stretch
- Side stretch
- Hamstring stretch
- Quadriceps stretch
- Groin stretch
- Calf stretch

Stretches should be done daily. Each stretch should be held at least 10 to 30 seconds and repeated on both sides of the body, as needed.

Strengthening:

- Chest press
- Triceps kickback
- Bent-over row
- Biceps curl
- Wall push-ups
- Seated leg extension
- Standing hamstring curl
- Hip adduction

- Hip abduction
- Hip extension
- Heel raises (calf raises)
- Squats

Strengthening activities should be done at least 3 days per week. The patient should be encouraged to start with 10 repetitions, progressing up to 15. Each strengthening activity should be repeated for a total of three sets.

Would you consider any additional medications? If yes, what?
Yes, according to the cholesterol guidelines, there are five recommendations under primary prevention for those without diabetes mellitus (DM) and low-density lipoprotein cholesterol (LDL-C) of 70 to 189. Statin therapy initiation should be based on the atherosclerotic cardiovascular disease (ASCVD) risk score for those without ASCVD to further determine therapy. Moderate- to high-intensity statin therapy should be used for adults aged 40 to 75 with an ASCVD risk score greater than or equal to 7.5%.

ASCVD Risk Estimator: (Since race is not identified, I used White).

- 10-year ASCVD risk: 21.9%
- Lifetime ASCVD risk: 69%

Because of his significant 10-year ASCVD risk, I would initiate high-intensity statin therapy. Options could include the following medications:

- High-intensity statins
  - Atorvastatin 40 to 80 mg
  - Rosuvastatin 20*(40)* mg

I would also consider adding aspirin 81 mg PO daily because of his current complaints of chest pain and significant risk factors. A prescription for sublingual nitroglycerin 0.4 mg could also be considered.

Would you order any other laboratory work? If yes, what?
I would order a thyroid-stimulating hormone (TSH) and C-reactive protein (CRP).

When would you repeat laboratory work?
After initiating statin therapy, I would repeat a fasting lipid and liver panel in 8 weeks. I would also order a repeat HgA1c level in 3 months.

When would you schedule his next follow-up appointment?
I would consider a once-weekly follow-up for his weight for at least 1 month.

Would you involve any other advanced practice nurses (APNs) in his care?
Referral could be considered to endocrinology and cardiology.

What additional education, if any, would you provide?
I would recommend contacting the office with any further questions and/or concerns. I would also suggest routine follow-up. Further education would depend upon any patient questions.

CASE STUDY 5

Is he overweight or obese? What category does his BMI fall into?
Obese, class III obesity.

How would you address his weight?
Mr. Jones, let's talk about your weight. Your BMI, which is a combination of your height and weight, puts you at risk for increased health problems. You also have a history of hypertension (HTN) and sleep apnea; these conditions alone are worrisome for increasing your risk for a cardiovascular event. What can we work on today to get you started on a plan to lose weight? How can I best help you lose weight?

Is he a candidate for weight loss?
Yes, he is a great candidate for weight loss!

Would you consider medication for weight loss?
Yes, especially since it has worked for him in the past.

Would you restart Phentermine or try a new medication?
Since Phentermine worked for him previously, I would restart this medication, but would recommend a trial of dietary and exercise changes first.

How would you present him with a plan for weight loss? What would this include?
I would approach the subject carefully so as to not offend him. I would suggest keeping a daily dietary and activity journal to keep track of what he is eating and how much activity he is doing. I would recommend starting with cardiovascular exercise 15 minutes daily. This could be done in a form of activity he enjoys (walking, biking, or even swimming). I would also talk about referral to a registered dietitian (RD) and an exercise specialist. I would schedule close follow-up to review the journal and set any additional goals. Before finishing the appointment, I would address any further goals that he may have. I would tell him that I prefer to try this method for weight loss first, but then if he continues to struggle with his weight, I would consider medication therapy.

What about his blood pressure (BP)? How would you treat this?
His BP is elevated today, but this is my first time of meeting him. I would hold off on medication and recommend medical treatment with dietary changes and exercise. I would ask him to monitor his BP at home.

With his recent stress, you decide to suggest stress management and medical treatment. Since it is your first time of meeting him, you want to give him a chance to try and lose weight without medication and devise a treatment plan together. This includes a healthy diet and routine exercise. A referral to a registered dietitian (RD) was offered, but he declined. You give him a weight-loss goal of 10 pounds in 1 month. You decide to see if weight loss helps control his BP and hold off on any medication at this point. A follow-up appointment is set up for 1 month.

He comes back 1 month later and tells you that he did well with the changes for about a week, but then "fell apart." He reports that with his new job, he is trying to work extra and just did not have the time to continue "all of these changes."

His vitals today are as follows:

Blood pressure: 150/90
Pulse: 66 bpm
Respirations: 12
Height: 6 feet, 2 inches
Weight: 364 pounds
Body mass index (BMI): 46.7 kg/m^2
Pulse oximetry: 96% on room air
Neck circumference (NC): 18 inches

His physical examination is within normal limits (WNL).
You also have fasting laboratories drawn before his appointment today. They are as follows:

Basic Metabolic Panel (BMP):
    Sodium: 139
    Potassium: 3.7
    Chloride: 101
    CO_2: 25
    Blood urea nitrogen (BUN): 18
    Creatinine: 0.7
    Glucose: 110
Complete Blood Count (CBC):
    White blood cells (WBCs): 6.5
    Hemoglobin (Hb): 14.7
    Hematocrit (Hct): 44.5
    Platelets: 180
Thyroid-stimulating hormone (TSH): 2.7
Fasting Lipid Panel:
    Total cholesterol: 200
    Triglycerides: 250
    High-density lipoprotein (HDL): 36
    Low-density lipoprotein (LDL): 130

How would you address his weight (which is up by 20 pounds)?
Mr. Jones, I see that your weight is up by 20 pounds. Why and how do you think you've gained this weight? I'm worried about your weight gain as well as your BP and cholesterol levels. You're young. We need to get ahead of this now.

Would you consider medication at this time for weight loss?
Yes, I would consider medication.

Would you restart Phentermine or try a new medication?
I would start Phentermine 37.5 mg PO daily.

How would you present him with a plan for weight loss? What would this include?
I would approach this similarly as I had at his first appointment—carefully so as to not offend him. I would inquire about his keeping a daily dietary and activity journal. I would also recommend restarting with cardiovascular exercise 15

minutes daily. I would readdress referral to an RD and an exercise specialist. I would schedule close follow-up to review the journal and set any additional goals. Before finishing the appointment, I would address any further goals that he may have.

What about his BP? How would you treat this?
Because his BP today is still high and his weight is up by 20 pounds, I would treat this. I would start hydrochlorothiazide (HCTZ) 12.5 mg PO daily along with recommended dietary and exercise efforts.

What would you do about his cholesterol?
I would first calculate his atherosclerotic cardiovascular disease (ASCVD) risk (since there was no mention of his race, I used White, nondiabetic, and non-smoker). Since he is only 35 years old, I could not calculate his 10-year ASCVD risk; however, I could assess his lifetime ASCVD risk. This is estimated at 50%. I would hold off on medication at this time for treatment of his cholesterol. I will continue to treat this medically and continue to monitor him.

Would you make any additional referrals?
Yes, to an RD and exercise specialist. He may also benefit from seeing a counselor or psychiatric mental health nurse practitioner (PMHNP) because of his divorce and stress.

Would you order any testing? If yes, what testing and why?
Yes, I would order a sleep study, as he has a history of sleep apnea. I would also order a repeat fasting BMP in 1 to 2 weeks to assess the glucose level as well as electrolyte and kidney status secondary to the initiation of HCTZ.

What dietary advice would you provide?
I would use the basal metabolic rate (BMR) and Harris–Benedict Formula to suggest appropriate caloric intake. I would recommend a well-balanced diet rich in whole grains, fresh or frozen fruits and vegetables, low-fat dairy products, and lean choices of meat. I would also refer to an RD for further advice.

What lifestyle changes would you suggest?
I would suggest increasing activity in any way possible. A weight-loss support group may also be offered to the patient.

What physical activity would you encourage? Please include mode/type, frequency, duration, and time.
I would first inquire about his activity interests. If he does not have a particular favorite, I would suggest walking (indoor or outdoor), 5 to 7 days per week, starting out with 15 minutes at a time, progressing to 30 to 60 minutes 5 to 7 days per week lifelong. If he gets bored with walking, biking or swimming could be other alternatives.

Would you recommend stretching and strengthening activities? Please include mode/type, frequency, duration, and time.
Yes, I would recommend both stretching and strengthening activities.

Stretches:

- Triceps stretch
- Biceps stretch
- Chest stretch
- Shoulder stretch
- Side stretch
- Hamstring stretch
- Quadriceps stretch
- Groin stretch
- Calf stretch

Stretches should be done daily. Each stretch should be held at least 10 to 30 seconds and repeated on both sides of the body as needed.

Strengthening:

- Chest press
- Triceps kickback
- Bent-over row
- Biceps curl
- Wall push-ups
- Seated leg extension
- Standing hamstring curl
- Hip adduction
- Hip abduction
- Hip extension
- Heel raises (calf raises)
- Squats

Strengthening activities should be done at least 3 days per week. The patient should be encouraged to start with 10 repetitions, progressing up to 15. Each strengthening activity should be repeated for a total of three sets.

Would you consider any additional medications? If yes, what?
Not at this time.

Would you order any other laboratory work? If yes, what?
Yes, I would repeat a BMP.

When would you repeat laboratory work?
In 1 to 2 weeks.

When would you schedule his next follow-up appointment?
Because I am starting him on two new medications, I would like to see him back in 2 weeks.

Would you involve any other advanced practice nurses (APNs) in his care?
Yes, referral could be made to a PMHNP.
You decide to try him on Phentermine 37.5 mg PO daily, as he told you this had worked well for him. You set him up for a return appointment in 1 month. You also start him on low-dose hydrochlorothiazide (HCTZ) 12.5 mg PO daily for his BP. You repeat a fasting glucose test at his next appointment.

He presents 1 month later for his follow-up appointment and is very happy. He is down 20 pounds and reports that he is trying to make better choices. His vitals today are as follows:

Blood pressure: 130/84
Pulse: 68 bpm
Respirations: 12
Height: 6 feet, 2 inches
Weight: 344 pounds
Body mass index (BMI): 44.2 kg/m^2
Pulse oximetry: 96% on room air
Neck circumference: 17.5 inches

His physical examination is WNL.
His fasting glucose is 100.

What would you suggest next for this patient? Would you continue medication? For how long?
I would continue his current medication for a total of 3 months. I would continue to see this patient every 2 weeks.

You continue his Phentermine for a total of 3 months. He is followed up monthly in the clinic. After the 3-month period, he has a weight loss of 45 pounds. You discontinue his Phentermine at that time and advise good dietary and exercise choices. You scheduled his next appointment, but he called to cancel. You do not see him again for 6 months. When he presents again, his weight is at an all-time high, 380 pounds, and a BMI of 48.8 kg/m^2. He reports that he ran out of HCTZ a month ago and his BP is elevated today at 152/96.

When would you want to set up his next appointment?
Two weeks.

How would you treat this patient?
Again, I would bring up his weight and risk factors as well as elevated BP. I would have a discussion with him about his appointment and medication compliance. I would tell him that it is very important to keep his scheduled appointments as well as continue current medications. I would renew his prescription for HCTZ 12.5 mg PO daily and repeat fasting laboratory work.

Would you discuss or consider referral to a bariatric surgeon? Why or why not?
Yes, I would refer the patient to a bariatric surgeon. I think he would be a good candidate for weight loss, but would like to see more compliance from him to promote overall success with weight loss. I would continue to follow up this patient routinely while waiting for referral and the surgery process.

What referrals would you suggest?
Bariatric surgery, RD, exercise specialist, and PMHNP.

What other education would you provide at this time?
I would recommend contacting the office with any further questions and/or concerns. I would also advise routine follow-up. Further education would depend upon any patient questions.

Weight Management Tools and Resources

This section provides resources on obesity and weight management tools and is divided into categories to make it easier to view.

Bariatric Surgery

- American Society for Metabolic and Bariatric Surgery
  https://asmbs.org

- Mayo Clinic—Gastric Bypass Surgery
  www.mayoclinic.org/tests-procedures/bariatric-surgery/in-depth/gastric-bypass-diet/art-20048472?p=1

- Medline Plus—Weight-Loss Surgery
  www.nlm.nih.gov/medlineplus/weightlosssurgery.html

- Obesity Action Coalition—Bariatric Surgery
  www.obesityaction.org/obesity-treatments/bariatric-surgery

Body Mass Index

- Centers for Disease Control and Prevention
  www.cdc.gov/healthyweight/assessing/bmi/index.html

Childhood Obesity

- Alliance for a Healthier Generation
  www.healthiergeneration.org

- Barbara Bush Children's Hospital at Maine Medical Center
  www.letsgo.org/partners/sponsors

- Centers for Disease Control and Prevention
  www.cdc.gov/healthyweight/children/index.html

- healthychildren.org
  www.healthychildren.org/English/health-issues/conditions/obesity/Pages/default.aspx

- National Initiative for Children's Healthcare Quality—Collaborate for Healthy Weight
  http://obesity.nichq.org

- The Nemours Foundation—Child Care Provider's Guide: Helping Kids Eat Right and Stay Active in a Child Care Setting
http://healthykidshealthyfuture.org/content/dam/hkhf/filebox/khchildcareguide.pdf

Cooking Skills

- BBC—Food Techniques
www.bbc.co.uk/food/techniques

- Cooking Light—Simple Cooking Techniques
http://www.cookinglight.com/healthy-living/healthy-habits/simple-cooking-techniques

- Jamie's Home Cooking Skills
www.jamieshomecookingskills.com/international

- New York Times Video—Cooking Techniques
www.nytimes.com/video/cooking-techniques

- Stella Culinary
www.stellaculinary.com/knife-skill-video-techniques-hd

- Wiki How—Basic Cooking Skills
www.wikihow.com/Category:Basic-Cooking-Skills

Definitions of Overweight and Obesity

- American Heart Association
www.heart.org/HEARTORG/GettingHealthy/WeightManagement/Obesity/Obesity-Information_UCM_307908_Article.jsp

- Centers for Disease Control and Prevention
www.cdc.gov/obesity/adult/defining.html

- National Heart, Lung, and Blood Institute
www.nhlbi.nih.gov/health/health-topics/topics/obe

Dietary Recommendations and Nutrition Tools

- Academy of Nutrition and Dietetics
www.eatright.org

- American Heart Association—Menu Labeling Fact Sheet
www.heart.org/idc/groups/heart-public/@wcm/@adv/documents/downloadable/ucm_304378.pdf

- Calorie Control Council
www.caloriecontrol.org

- Choose My Plate
www.choosemyplate.gov

- Health Care Without Harm—Healthy Food in Health Care
https://noharm-uscanada.org/issues/us-canada/healthy-food-health-care

- HelpGuide.org
www.helpguide.org/articles/healthy-eating/healthy-eating.htm

- National Heart, Lung, and Blood Institute—Eating Healthy at Home or Dining Out
  www.nhlbi.nih.gov/health/educational/lose_wt/eat/tips.htm

- Nourish Interactive
  www.nourishinteractive.com/nutrition-tools-healthy-family

- Nutrition
  www.nutrition.gov

- U.S. Department of Agriculture
  www.choosemyplate.gov

- What to EAT! Basic Nutrition, Weight Loss, Healthy Diet, Best Foods Tips—Virtual Health Coach
  www.youtube.com/watch?v=ccn6IHivD5M

- Yale Rudd Center for Food Policy and Obesity—Fast Food FACTS
  www.fastfoodmarketing.org

- Yale Rudd Center for Food Policy and Obesity—Sugary Drink FACTS
  www.sugarydrinkfacts.org

Diseases Associated With Obesity

- Centers for Disease Control and Prevention
  www.cdc.gov/healthyweight/effects/index.html

Food Addiction

- Food Addiction Institute
  http://foodaddictioninstitute.org

- Food Addiction Research Foundation
  http://foodaddictionresearch.org

- Food Addicts in Recovery Anonymous
  www.foodaddicts.org

General Websites

- American Academy of Family Physicians (AAFP)
  www.aafp.org/home.html

- American Board of Medical Specialties (ABMS)
  www.abms.org

- American College of Cardiology (ACC)
  www.acc.org

- American College of Obstetricians and Gynecologists (ACOG)
  www.acog.org

- American College of Physicians (ACP)
  www.acponline.org

- American College of Preventive Medicine (ACPM)
  www.acpm.org

- American Diabetes Association
  www.diabetes.org

- American Gastroenterological Association (AGA)
  www.gastro.org

- American Heart Association
  www.heart.org

- The Endocrine Society (ENDO)
  www.endocrine.org

- Harvard School of Public Health—Obesity Prevention Source
  www.hsph.harvard.edu/obesity-prevention-source

- Mayo Clinic
  www.mayoclinic.org

- WebMD
  www.WebMD.com

Healthy Recipes

- All Recipes: Healthy Recipes
  http://allrecipes.com/recipes/healthy-recipes

- American Diabetes Association—My Food Advisor: Recipes for Healthy Living
  www.diabetes.org/mfa-recipes/recipes

- Cooking Light—Quick and Healthy Recipes
  www.cookinglight.com/food/quick-healthy-recipes

- Eating Well
  www.eatingwell.com/recipes_menus

- Food Network—Healthy Eating
  www.foodnetwork.com/healthy.html

- My Recipes: Healthy Diet
  www.myrecipes.com/healthy-diet

- NewStart Lifestyle Club
  newstartclub.com/recipes

- VeganEasy.org
  www.veganeasy.org/recipes

- Whole Food Market
  www.wholefoodsmarket.com/recipes

How to Organize a Healthy Menu Plan

- Nourish Interactive
  www.nourishinteractive.com/nutrition-tools-healthy-family

- Organize Yourself Skinny
  www.organizeyourselfskinny.com/category/weekly-menu-plans

- Plan to Eat
  www.plantoeat.com

- Well Right—Healthy Meal Planning
  http://wellright.com/university-courses/healthy-meal-planning

How to Organize Your Kitchen to Eat Healthy

- Eating Well—Kitchen Intervention Video
  www.eatingwell.com/videos/kitchen-intervention-how-to-eat-healthy.htm?showVideo=true

- WebMD Diet—Guide to a Healthy Kitchen
  www.webmd.com/diet/healthy-kitchen-11

Nursing

- American Association of Nurse Practitioners
  www.aanp.org

- American Nurses Association
  www.nursingworld.org

- National Association of Pediatric Nurse Practitioners (NAPNAP)
  www.napnap.org

- Preventive Cardiovascular Nurses Association
  www.pcna.net

Obesity Organizations

- American Society for Metabolic and Bariatric Surgery (ASMBS)
  https://asmbs.org

- American Society of Bariatric Physicians (ASBP)
  www.asbp.org

- Canadian Obesity Network (CON)
  www.obesitynetwork.ca

- Cardiometabolic Health Congress (CMHC)
  www.cardiometabolichealth.org

- Cardiometabolic Risk Summit (CRS)
  www.primarycarecardiometabolic.com

- Cleveland Clinic Obesity Summit
  www.clevelandclinicmeded.com/live/courses/obesity/default.asp?sessionid=YVN2VPY5TT

- Columbia University Institute of Human Nutrition
  www.cumc.columbia.edu/ihn

- Global Obesity Prevention Center (GOPC) at Johns Hopkins
  www.globalobesity.org

- Harvard Medical School Blackburn Course in Obesity Medicine
  http://obesity.hmscme.com

- Massachusetts General Hospital—Obesity, Metabolism, and Nutrition Institute (OMNI)
  www.massgeneral.org/omni

- Mayo Clinic: Nutrition and Wellness in Health and Disease
  https://ce.mayo.edu/nutrition/node/1276

- Obesity Action Coalition (OAC)
  www.obesityaction.org

- The Obesity Society (TOS)
  www.obesity.org

- STOP Obesity Alliance
  www.stopobesityalliance.org/wp-content/themes/stopobesityalliance/pdfs/
  NEW_STOP_Obesity_Alliance_Recommendations.pdf

- Trust for America's Health
  http://healthyamericans.org

- World Congress on Insulin Resistance, Diabetes, and Cardiovascular Disease
  (WCIRDC)
  http://wcir.org

Pediatrics

- American Academy of Pediatrics (AAP)
  www.aap.org/en-us/Pages/Default.aspx

- National Association of Pediatric Nurse Practitioners (NAPNAP)
  www.napnap.org

Physical Activity

- Americans in Motion-Healthy Interventions (AIM-HI) American Academy of
  Family Physician
  www.aafp.org/online/en/home/clinical/publichealth/aim.html

- Exercise, Nutrition, and Weight Management Toolkit—Healthy Living
  https://Healthnetfederalservices.com/content/hnfs/home/tn/prov/res/prov_well
  ness/hetoollanding/hetoolexercise.html

- MOVE! Physical Activity Handouts
  www.move.va.gov/handouts.asp?physical

- Physical Activity Guidelines for Americans. U.S. Department of Health and
  Human Services
  http://health.gov/paguidelines/

School Curriculum Resources

- Centers for Disease Control and Prevention—Physical Education Curriculum
  Analysis Tool (PECAT)
  www.cdc.gov/healthyyouth/PECAT/index.htm

- Harvard School of Public Health—Eat Well and Keep Moving
  www.hsph.harvard.edu/prc/projects/school-research/eat-well-keep-moving

- Harvard School of Public Health—Planet Health
  www.hsph.harvard.edu/prc/projects/school-research/planet

- WellSAT2.0—Wellness School Assessment Tool
  http://wellsat.org/default.aspx

School Resources

- Alliance for a Healthier Generation—Healthy Schools Program
  https://schools.healthiergeneration.org

- California Food Policy Advocates—Water in Schools
  http://cfpa.net/water-in-schools

- Cornell Food and Brand Lab—Smarter Lunchrooms
  http://smarterlunchrooms.org

- Let's Move—Schools
  www.letsmove.gov/schools

- Massachusetts and USDA Competitive Foods and Beverage Nutrition Standards
  "At-a-Glance"
  http://www.mass.gov/eohhs/docs/dph/mass-in-motion/school-nutrition-glance
  .pdf

- National Center for Safe Routes for School
  www.saferoutesinfo.org

Sleep Information

- American Association of Sleep Medicine
  www.aasmnet.org

- American Board of Sleep Medicine
  www.absm.org

- American Sleep Association
  www.sleepassociation.org

- Centers for Disease Control and Prevention—Sleep and Sleep Disorders
  www.cdc.gov/sleep

- Healthy Sleep, Division of Sleep Medicine, Harvard Medical School
  http://healthysleep.med.harvard.edu

- National Sleep Foundation
  http://sleepfoundation.org

- Sleep for Kids, National Sleep Foundation
  http://sleepfoundation.org/sleep-topics/children-and-sleep

Weight Control

- Shape Up America!
  www.shapeup.org

- Weight-Control Information Network
  http://win.niddk.nih.gov/publications/understanding.htm

- Weight Watchers
  https://welcome.weightwatchers.com

Center for Lifestyle Medicine Sample Business Plan

Center for Lifestyle Medicine (CLM)
Clinic Address
Clinic Phone Number
Clinic Website

The CLM provides individualized weight-loss counseling, dietary advice, and exercise strategies without the use of any medications or supplements. This clinic provides a natural approach to weight loss, the ease and availability of cardiac testing and exercise equipment, structured nutrition advice provided by a registered dietitian (RD), a new facility, and one-on-one guidance by a doctorate-prepared nurse practitioner (NP). The target of this clinic is to educate and treat overweight and obese patients. This clinic uses the knowledge of multidisciplinary experts to help achieve goals through diet, exercise, and healthy eating habits.

Mission

Our mission is to provide our patients with the highest level of excellence in weight loss and lifestyle medicine. We strive to create an atmosphere that supports education, compassionate care, and commitment to the communities in which we serve.

Goal

The goal of the CLM is to be the leading facility serving all your weight-loss needs.

Vision

- To provide for a mechanism of utilization review, continuous quality improvement, outcomes research, and practice guidelines to ensure the delivery of the highest quality patient care
- To create practice opportunities for other fields and specialties in the area, and provide for greater subspecialization within existing specialties
- To provide for a means of increasing patient education and public awareness of issues pertaining to health care
- To promote cooperation, communication, and coordinated care across all specialties

- To earn the right to "remain" into the future—become indispensable to patients and their third-party payers (e.g., by attention to cost, quality, access)
- To better serve patients by remaining professionally managed

Objectives

The CLM is set to accomplish the following:

- To provide superior patient care
- To promote patient education
- To reach out toward communities to provide weight loss and lifestyle medicine
- To educate health care providers, nurses, and medical staff
- To promote healthy lifestyle choices
- To respect patients and their families and work together with them in providing care

Business Philosophy

The business philosophy of the CLM is to build patient and provider trust and loyalty by providing quality care and service.

Target Market

The CLM's initial target market is those overweight and obese people with cardiac disease and multiple comorbid medical diseases who are struggling to lose weight. Long-term targets are overweight and obese people who are interested in weight loss.

Core Strengths

The CLM's core strengths are the providers and quality patient services. The providers have education in internal medicine, family practice, cardiology, basic weight-loss practices, wellness, exercise science, and nutrition. Great patient care starts with our providers, nursing staff, front desk, and supporting office staff. The CLM specializes in treating overweight and obese patients with multiple comorbidities. Serving a wide variety of insurance plans, including Medicare and Medicaid, as well as a payment plan option, the CLM offers flexible options to attend to all patient populations.

Located in _____, close to _____ Hospital, the CLM provides service to those patients in the area and in surrounding communities. The clinic and staff understand care, compassion, and confidentiality and provide a warm, friendly environment.

Competitive Advantage

The CLM's competitive advantage is the multidisciplinary approach with a lifestyle medicine focus. The competitive advantage also includes one-on-one patient and provider time, counseling, and individualized nutrition and exercise advice in a comfortable environment.

Business Background

Obesity is a growing epidemic—one that is undertreated and misunderstood by many medical professionals. According to the WHO, "obesity is reaching epidemic proportions with more than 1 billion adults who are overweight, 300 million who have class I or II obesity and 30 million who have class III obesity, defined as a body mass index (BMI) greater than 40 kg/m^2 (also referred to as morbid obesity)" (Christou & Efthimiou, 2009, p. 250). *BMI* is defined as the total body mass (in kilograms) divided by the height squared (in meters) (Kemper, Stasse-Wolthuis, & Bosman, 2004). In more recent years, alarms have sounded regarding the pervasiveness of obesity in the United States, mostly because of the researched links found between obesity and increased health risks. This concern was the impetus for the development of guidelines for clinical practice. Christou and Efthimiou (2009) also state that some view obesity as the highest disease killer in the United States. Establishing an obesity clinic will spotlight prevention and treatment of obesity, with goals toward improving the overall quality of life.

Literature Review

Prevention   Appropriate identification and recognition is essential with pending treatment and management of obesity. Greater than 30% of people are not recognized as obese, whereas a minimal number are offered treatment. Preventative health care and treatment continue to encounter many barriers; however, these barriers are predicted to lessen, as further treatment options and knowledge continue to grow (Fujioka & Bakhru, 2010).

Determining basal metabolic index (BMI), as well as discussing weight and weight loss in routine office visits, can lead to prevention and determine treatment of obesity (Thompson, Cook, Clark, Barida, & Levine, 2007). Kemper et al. (2004) discuss the report produced by the Health Council of the Netherlands. In this report, prevention and a weight-loss goal of approximately 10% were shown to aid in sustained long-term weight loss. Ward-Smith (2010) and Robinson and Butler (2011) also discuss the need for recognizing and calculating BMI, with the latter article focusing specifically on the treatment of women. These articles determine the need for recognizing patients at risk for obesity and also identify the need for the establishment and maintenance of a weight-loss clinic.

Behaviors, Addiction, and Eating Disorders   Establishing a weight-loss clinic and focusing on the treatment of obesity includes a vast understanding of behaviors, addiction, and eating disorders. Discussing the need and assessing for any type of addiction to food, underlying psychological behavior, and/or eating disorder prior to treatment is also essential (Palmeira et al., 2009; Sonntag, Renneberg, Bockelbrink, Braun, & Heintze, 2010; Wilson, 2010). Adam and Epel (2007) and Zellner et al. (2006) also address the relationship between stress and eating—another form of food addiction. Further research and referrals, as appropriate, to a psychologist/psychiatrist may be warranted. This research and understanding is essential in establishing this clinic.

Medical Therapy   Medical therapy, including assessing dietary and exercise patterns, will also play a necessary role in this clinic. Evaluating pharmacotherapy and determining its appropriateness will be addressed in establishing this clinic. No single diet proves to be the best; however, the reduction in caloric need produces weight loss (Bray, 2010; Dubnov-Raz & Berry, 2010; Redman & Ravussin, 2010). The aforementioned studies focus on reduced caloric consumption, whereas the study by Hainer, Toplak, and Mitrakou (2008) focuses on individualized treatment and a combination of dietary choices and pharmacological therapy.

Surgical Therapy   "Although surgical procedures more reliably produce large initial weight losses, it is not clear whether surgical patients are more successful at maintaining their weight losses than individuals who have lost comparable amounts of weight through nonsurgical means" (Bond, Phelan, Leahey, Hill, & Wing, 2009, p. 173). Providers need to present patients with the most accurate, up-to-date information to aid in decision making and the treatment plan. Cannon and Kumar (2009) determine a combination of medical therapy—dietary changes and pharmacotherapy—along with referral for bariatric surgery, as needed, to be the best individualized treatment.

However, the four studies by Bond et al. (2009), Bult, van Dalen, and Muller (2008), Dixon et al. (2008), and O'Brien et al. (2006) reviewed sustained weight loss in surgical versus nonsurgical patients and found surgical means to be more beneficial in sustaining weight loss for a longer period. O'Brien et al. demonstrated initial weight loss (13.8%) in both the surgical and nonsurgical groups at 6 months, as evidenced by changes in BMI and overall weight loss. Bond et al. were similar to O'Brien et al. in that they evaluated weight loss of both surgical and nonsurgical patients. Surgical and nonsurgical groups reported weight regains within the first year, but results did not differ significantly between the two groups (Bond et al., 2009). The study by Dixon et al. was slightly different and primarily focused on diabetes treatment and reduction between surgical and nonsurgical participants. Seventy-three percent of the surgical group and 13% of the conventional therapy group achieved remission of type 2 diabetes (T2DM) for a total of 43% (Dixon et al., 2008). These articles support surgical therapy means as an option for weight-loss therapy. In those with multiple comorbidities, surgical means is a good option for weight loss, as supported earlier.

Clinic Establishment   Financial savvy and business experience are stated as two indispensable skills needed to establish a clinic or practice (Frezza & Wachtel, 2008). Along with business expertise, a team approach, counseling, and flexibility are key aspects in establishing a successful weight-loss or obesity clinic (Frezza & Wachtel, 2008; Fujioka & Bakhru, 2010). A positive attitude is also essential when treating obese patients. Many patients feel providers are discriminatory about weight and pass prior judgment when treating obesity (Chang, Asch, & Werner, 2010; Ferrante, Piasecki, Ohman-Strickland, & Crabtree, 2009; Wadden et al., 2000). Increasing the number of patient referrals is crucial for further productivity (Frezza & Wachtel, 2008).

Along with the skills stated earlier, one must look at insurance reimbursement. Both Frezza and Wachtel (2008) and Fujioka and Bakhru (2010) stress the importance of understanding what insurance companies will reimburse in terms of office visits and treatment options. "Oftentimes, the most challenging aspect of practicing obesity medicine is obtaining insurance coverage for treatment options. However, there are situations where insurance coverage can be successfully attained in many obese patients. To find these situations, one should treat obesity like any other medical condition and define the comorbid conditions" (Fujioka & Bakhru, 2010, p. 470). Comorbid conditions, including diabetes, are readily used in combination with an obesity ICD-9 code.

Principal Owners

The CLM is locally owned and operated as a subdivision of _____.
This clinic is a separate entity and is owned _____.

Providers and Staff

Lisa L. M. Maher, DNP, ARNP, FNP-BC

Lisa Maher is the primary medical provider for the CLM. Dr. Maher is a graduate of the University of Iowa, Iowa City, Iowa, DNP program and received her training in family practice nursing. She has a master's in nursing from Graceland University, Independence, Missouri, and has undergraduate degrees in both nursing and wellness. She provides general medical knowledge and has taken special interest in weight loss, lifestyle medicine, sleep apnea, and prevention and treatment of cardiovascular disease (CVD).

Legal Form of Ownership

The CLM is a partnership with its parent company, _____.

Products and Services

Product
The current product of the CLM is servicing the clinic area with quality patient care with a specific focus on weight loss in addition to multiple comorbid diseases.

Future plans include the addition of more exercise equipment and a larger workout room. Classes specializing in weight loss, diet, and exercise will also be added. Screening for obesity, CVD, sleep apnea, diabetes, and peripheral vascular disease (PVD), as well as company health screenings, is also included in future plans.

REFERENCES

Adam, T. C., & Epel, E. S. (2007). Stress, eating and the reward system. *Physiology & Behavior, 91,* 449–458. doi:10.1016/j.physbeh.2007.04.011

Bond, D. S., Phelan, S., Leahey, T. M., Hill, J. O., & Wing, R. R. (2009). Weight-loss maintenance in successful weight losers: Surgical vs non-surgical methods. *International Journal of Obesity, 33,* 173–180. doi:10.1038/ijo.2008.256

Bray, G. A. (2010). Medical therapy for obesity. *Mount Sinai Journal of Medicine, 77,* 407–417. doi:10.1002/msj.20207

Bult, M. J. F., van Dalen, T., & Muller, A. F. (2008). Surgical treatment of obesity. *European Journal of Endocrinology, 158,* 135–145.

Cannon, C. P., & Kumar, A. (2009). Treatment of overweight and obesity: Lifestyle, pharmacologic, and surgical options. *Clinical Cornerstone, 9*(4), 55–71.

Chang, V. W., Asch, D. A., & Werner, R. M. (2010). Quality of care among obese patients. *Journal of the American Medical Association, 303*(13), 1274–1281. doi:10.1001/jama.2010.339

Christou, N., & Efthimiou, E. (2009). Five-year outcomes of laparoscopic adjustable gastric banding and laparoscopic Roux-en-Y gastric bypass in a comprehensive bariatric surgery program in Canada. *Canadian Journal of Surgery, 52*(6), E259–E258.

Dixon, J. B., O'Brien, P. E., Playfair, J., Chapman, L., Schachter, L. M., Skinner, S., . . . Anderson, M. (2008). Adjustable gastric banding and conventional therapy for type 2 diabetes: A randomized controlled trial. *Journal of the American Medical Association, 299*(3), 316–323. doi:10.1001/jama.299.3.316

Dubnov-Raz, G., & Berry, E. M. (2010). Dietary approaches to obesity. *Mount Sinai Journal of Medicine, 77,* 488–498. doi:10.1002/msj.20210

Ferrante, J. M., Piasecki, A. K., Ohman-Strickland, P. A., & Crabtree, B. F. (2009). Family physicians' practices and attitudes regarding care of extremely obese patients. *Obesity, 17*, 1710–1716. doi:10.1038/oby.2009.62

Frezza, E. E., & Wachtel, M. S. (2008). A successful model of setting up a bariatric practice. *Obesity Surgery, 18*, 877–881. doi:10.1007/s1169-007-9377-7

Fujioka, D., & Bakhru, N. (2010). Office-based management of obesity. *Mount Sinai Journal of Medicine, 77*, 466–471. doi:10.1002/msj.20201

Hainer, V., Toplak, H., & Mitrakou, A. (2008). Treatment modalities of obesity. *Diabetes Care, 31*(2), S269–S277. doi:10.2337/dc08-s265

Kemper, H. C. G., Stasse-Wolthuis, M., & Bosman, W. (2004). The prevention and treatment of overweight and obesity: Summary of the advisory report by the Health Council of the Netherlands. *Journal of Medicine, 62*(1), 10–17.

O'Brien, P. E., Dixon, J. B., Laurie, C., Skinner, S., Proietto, J., McNeil, J., . . . Anderson, M. (2006). Treatment of mild to moderate obesity with laparoscopic adjustable gastric banding or an intensive medical program: A randomized trial. *Annals of Internal Medicine, 144*(9), 625–633. Retrieved from http://annals.org/article.aspx?articleid=722580

Palmeira, A. L., Markland, D. A., Silva, M. N., Branco, T. L., Martins, S. C., Minderico, C. S., . . . Teixeira, P. J. (2009). Reciprocal effects among changes in weight, body image, and other psychological factors during behavioral obesity treatment: A mediation analysis. *International Journal of Behavioral Nutrition and Physical Activity, 6*(9), 1–12.

Robinson, K. T., & Butler, J. (2011). Understanding the causal factors of obesity using the international classification of functioning, disability and health. *Disability and Rehabilitation, 33*, 643–651.

Sonntag, U., Henkel, J., Renneberg, B., Bockelbrink, A., Braun, V., & Heintze, C. (2010). Counseling overweight patients: Analysis of preventive encounters in primary care. *International Journal for Quality in Health Care Advance Access, 22*, 486–492. doi:10.1093/intqhc/mzq060

Thompson, W. G., Cook, D. A., Clark, M. M., Bardia, A., & Levine, J. A. (2007). Treatment of obesity. *Mayo Clinic Proceedings, 82*(1), 93–102. doi:10.4065/82.1.93

Wadden, T. A., Anderson, D. W., Foster, G. D., Bennett, A., Steinberg, C., & Sarwer, D. B. (2000). Obese women's perceptions of their physicians' weight management attitudes and practices. *Archives of Family Medicine, 9*, 854–860. Retrieved from http://archfammed.com

Ward-Smith, P. (2010). Obesity—America's health crisis. *Urologic Nursing, 30*(4), 242–245. Retrieved from http://ehis.ebscohost.com.proxy.lib.uiowa.edu/ehost/pdfviewer/pdfviewer?vid=2&hid=115&sid=ca223642-3da7-4adf-93ef-3b0365968eff%40sessionmgr113

Wilson, G. T. (2010). Eating disorders, obesity and addiction. *European Eating Disorders Review, 18*, 341–351. doi:10.1002/erv.1048

Zellner, D. A., Loaiza, S., Gonzalez, Z., Pita, J., Morales, J., Pecora, D., & Wolf, A. (2006). Food selection changes under stress. *Physiology & Behavior, 87*, 789–793. doi:10.1016/j.physbeh.2006.01.014

Appendices

Appendix A: Strengths, Weaknesses, Opportunities, and Threats

Strengths	Opportunities
• Staffed with a nurse practitioner (NP) and cardiologist. • New facility and equipment, including EKG, treadmill/nuclear stress test, echocardiogram (ECG), Holter monitor, and Ankle-Brachial Index (ABI), all in the same building. • Dedicated support staff and administration. • Internal patient referrals. • Team establishment and collaborative care—NP, cardiologist, nurse, dietitian, exercise specialist, counselor, and office support staff.	• In 2009, 25% to 29% of Iowa's population had a body mass index (BMI) greater than 30. • Up to 25% of patients with a BMI greater than or equal to 30 are not appropriately identified by primary care physicians as being obese. • Opportunity to improve overall cardiac care and reduce chronic disease.
Weaknesses	**Threats**
• Lack of formal obesity training.	• Another weight-loss clinic located in the Cedar Valley. • Close proximity of a bariatric surgeon located within the clinic area. • Pending cuts to cardiology and cardiac testing. • Limited funding for prevention, obesity treatment, and disease management. • Lack of formal advertisement. • Limited number of outside patient referrals.

Appendix B: Implementation Plan/Theory Outcomes Model

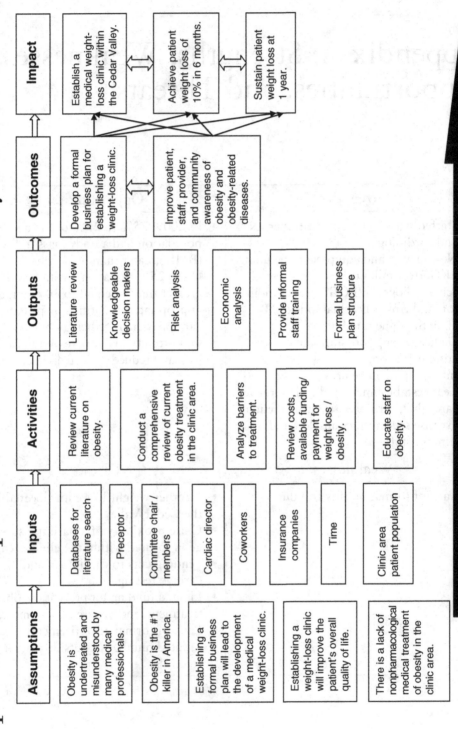

Assumptions	Inputs	Activities	Outputs	Outcomes	Impact
Obesity is undertreated and misunderstood by many medical professionals.	Databases for literature search	Review current literature on obesity.	Literature review	Develop a formal business plan for establishing a weight-loss clinic.	Establish a medical weight-loss clinic within the Cedar Valley.
	Preceptor		Knowledgeable decision makers		
Obesity is the #1 killer in America.	Committee chair / members	Conduct a comprehensive review of current obesity treatment in the clinic area.	Risk analysis		Achieve patient weight loss of 10% in 6 months.
Establishing a formal business plan will lead to the development of a medical weight-loss clinic.	Cardiac director				
	Coworkers	Analyze barriers to treatment.	Economic analysis	Improve patient, staff, provider, and community awareness of obesity and obesity-related diseases.	
Establishing a weight-loss clinic will improve the patient's overall quality of life.	Insurance companies	Review costs, available funding/payment for weight loss / obesity.	Provide informal staff training		Sustain patient weight loss at 1 year.
	Time				
There is a lack of nonpharmacological medical treatment of obesity in the clinic area.	Clinic area patient population	Educate staff on obesity.	Formal business plan structure		

354

Appendix C: Timeline

Assumptions	Inputs	Activities	Outputs	Outcomes	Impact
Obesity is undertreated and misunderstood by many medical professionals.	Databases for literature search	Review current literature on obesity. *Prevention; behaviors, addiction, and eating disorders; medical therapy; surgical therapy; clinic establishment*	Literature review *Final paper*	Develop a formal business plan for establishing a weight-loss clinic.	Establish a medical weight-loss clinic within the Cedar Valley.
Obesity is the #1 killer in America.	Preceptor		Knowledgeable decision makers *-Myself* *-Inputs*	Improve patient, staff, provider, and community awareness of obesity and obesity-related diseases.	Achieve patient weight loss of 10% in 6 months.
Establishing a formal business plan will lead to the development of a medical weight-loss clinic.	Committee chair / members	Conduct a comprehensive review of current obesity treatment in the clinic area. *-Bariatric center lap band, gastric bypass surgery* *-Pharmacological Tx Phentermine, HCG* *-VLCD (600-800 kcal)*	Risk analysis *-SWOT* *-Risk management matrix*		Sustain patient weight loss at 1 year.
	Cardiac director				
Establishing a weight-loss clinic will improve patient's overall quality of life. *Reduce risks for: CAD, Type 2 DM, HTN, Hyperlipidemia, OSA*	Coworkers		Economic analysis *-Start-up costs* *-Cash flow projections* *-Break-even analysis*		
	Insurance companies *Medicare, medicaid, BCBS, United Health*	Analyze barriers to treatment. *Time; money; insurance reimbursement; support; existing medical problems; transportation; motivation*	Provide informal staff training *-Providing reading material* *-Informal training* *-Practice session*		
There is a lack of nonpharmacological medical treatment of obesity in the Cedar Valley area. *- Bariatric center* *- Pharmacological Tx* *- Very low-calorie diet*	Time	Review costs, available funding/ payment for weight-loss/obesity. *Insurance coverage; self-pay; grants; billable ICD-9 codes*	Formal business plan structure 1. Executive summary 2. Business description 3. Market strategies 4. Competitive analysis 5. Design and development plan 6. Operations and management plan 7. Financial factors		
	Clinic area patient population	Educate staff on obesity.			

Key:
Words in Roman = statements from Logic Outcomes Model
Words in italics = a more specific description

Appendix D: Risk Management Matrix

RISK MANAGEMENT WORKSHEET

Type of Risk	Jeopardy	Description of Risk	Expectation of the Risk (1–5)	Impact of the Risk (1–5)	Severity of the Risk (Expectation × Impact)	Contingency Plan of Action
Market—risk of competition	Schedule	Another weight-loss clinic exists within the clinic area.	2	4	8	Promote staffing, including an NP and a cardiologist. Internal patient referrals. Team establishment and collaborative care—NP, cardiologist, nurse, dietitian, exercise specialist, counselor, and office support staff. New facility and equipment, including EKG, treadmill/nuclear stress test, ECG, Holter monitor, and ABIs, all in the same building.
Liquidity—questionable funding/billing	Budget	There are existing cuts to primary care and specialty practices and testing. Also, lack of funding for preventative programs.	4	5	20	In 2009, 25% to 29% of Iowa's population had a BMI greater than 30. Up to 25% of patients with a BMI of greater than or equal to 30 are not appropriately identified by primary care physicians as being obese.
Operational—inadequate training	Reputation, patient risk	The staff has had no formal obesity/weight-loss training.	2	3	6	Conduct formal research on weight loss and obesity. Provide staff education.
Legal—appropriate certification or accreditation	Practice and clinic credibility	The clinic has no existing licensure or certification for weight loss or obesity.	3	3	9	Develop a formal business plan. Conduct research to see what certifications or accreditations exist.
Reputational—specialty practice	Negative publicity	New development of weight loss/obesity clinic.	2	2	4	Team establishment and collaborative care—NP, cardiologist, nurse, dietitian, exercise specialist, counselor, and office support staff. Determine and develop an advertising plan.

Key: 1—lowest impact or likelihood of occurrence to 5—highest impact or likelihood of occurrence.
(Baker, Baker, & Campbell, 2003, p. 83).

Appendix E: Center for Lifestyle Medicine Patient Letter

Center for Lifestyle Medicine (CLM)
Clinic Address
Clinic Phone Number

Dear _____,

Thank you for your interest in the CLM! We look forward to and are excited to share in your weight-loss and lifestyle changes!

On your first visit to the clinic, please bring your insurance cards, list of medications, and a positive attitude! Expect the first visit to be approximately 1 hour, as we ask detailed questions about your health and weight history. Measurements and weight, as well as a comprehensive body analysis, will also take place. We provide a warm atmosphere and ensure your privacy. The first visit will also entail plenty of time for discussion, questions, and answers. You will receive a patient journal to track your progress, exercise, and food choices throughout your time with us.

After your first visit, there are several options on how to proceed with your weight loss. Each session is tailored to fit your personal needs and goals. Our goal is to provide you with the knowledge and life skills for healthy, happy days.

We look forward to working with you. We will contact you in July to follow up and see if you are still interested in working with us. In the meantime, please feel free to contact us with any questions or concerns!

Sincerely,

Clinic Team Member Names and Credentials

Appendix F: Center for Lifestyle Medicine Provider Letter

CLM
Clinic Address
Clinic Phone Number

Dear _____,

We would like to take the opportunity to inform you about our new clinic—the CLM—located _____
_____. We are excited to announce that we will begin seeing patients as of _____.

This clinic will focus on treatment for those struggling with overweight and obesity through medical management. Individualized care through one-on-one visits with our provider _____ and specialists _____ and _____ will focus on personalized treatment methods. Detailed questions about your patient's health and weight history, measurements, and weight, as well as a comprehensive body analysis, will also take place. The first visit will also entail plenty of time for discussion, questions, and answers. Each patient will receive a patient journal to track progress, exercise, and food choices.

After your first visit, there are several options on how to proceed with weight loss. Each session is tailored to fit personal needs and goals. Our goal is to provide your patient with the knowledge and life skills for healthy, happy days.

Thank you for your interest in the CLM! We look forward and are excited to share in your patient's weight-loss and lifestyle changes! Please feel free to contact us with any questions or concerns!

Sincerely,

Clinic Team Member Names and Credentials

Appendix G: Center for Lifestyle Medicine Description of Services

The CLM offers dietary and exercise programs for weight and stress management.

By making small changes to current habits, we will help you establish a healthier lifestyle that is sustainable for a lifetime! Insurance may cover your participation in the weight management program. Fitness assessments, supervised exercise sessions, and group fitness classes are also available.

It is our mission to provide educational tools and resources to promote health habits and lifestyle modification through nutrition, exercise, stress management, and smoking cessation with the focus on preventative medicine.

Goals

- Provide quality care to all patients
- Promote healthy lifestyles
- Educate the community on healthy lifestyle choices to prevent and treat disease
- Respect patients and work with them to establish healthier sustainable habits
- Improve the quality of life for people of all ages

Why choose the CLM?

- We have an advanced practice nurse (APN), exercise specialist, and registered dietitian (RD) ready to work together with you.
- For those at risk or with known heart disease, an APN will follow you through your program and manage your medications.
- Our programs are designed to be tailored to each patient to ensure maximum success. Since no two people are alike, your program and the professional advice you receive will be uniquely focused on you.
- We offer individualized one-on-one nutrition, exercise, stress management, and smoking cessation counseling as well as group exercise opportunities and group education classes.

Services Offered

- Fitness assessments for those beginning exercise who want to ensure it is safe
- Weight management counseling

- Nutrition counseling
- Supervised weight sessions
- Group exercise classes for all fitness levels
- Group education classes
- Support groups for weight loss

Who will benefit from the CLM?

- Those who have tried to lose weight or quit smoking, but have been unsuccessful on their own
- People with a need to manage stress
- Those who need to lose weight before a medical procedure
- Anyone who is overweight
- Those at risk for or with known heart disease
- People with comorbidities such as high blood pressure (BP), diabetes, or high cholesterol
- Anyone who wants to establish healthier habits
- Anyone who plans to start exercise and wants to ensure it is safe or just needs basic advice of how to get started on their own

Weight Management Program

- Services provided by an APN, exercise specialist, and RD
- Our APN will follow your health, listen to your heart and lungs, and manage medication therapy
- You will complete a baseline assessment that will allow the exercise specialist to prescribe appropriate exercise
- The RD will assess your current eating habits and is knowledgeable in diet recommendations for medical conditions (diabetes, high BP, high cholesterol, and/or cardiac disease)
- Small short-term goals are set during each visit with the end result of healthier habits and an overall general healthier lifestyle
- The number of visits and length between visits are individualized and based on each person's needs and requests

Group Nutrition and Exercise Educational Presentation

Educational classes are open to anyone who is interested. To sign up, call the office at _____. Cost is $5 and is paid the day of the class. Cost of classes may change depending on the materials provided.

For a schedule of upcoming topics, please visit _____ or call our office.

To learn more about all the services offered at the CLM or to schedule an appointment, please call the office at _____.

We look forward to working with you,

Clinic Team Member Names and Credentials

Appendix H: Staff Education

- This informal staff training will include nursing staff, front desk staff, NPs, and the cardiac director.
- This will involve a plan to review current literature on obesity and an informal training and practice session.
- Each session will provide information on obesity and its comorbidities with emphasis on calculating body mass index (BMI), Harris–Benedict Formula, and basal metabolic rate (BMR). It will also focus on correct weighing and taking body measurements (neck circumference [NC], waist circumference [WC], and hip circumference [HC]).
- To ensure that the staff have received adequate training and comprehend the information taught, they will be asked to calculate BMI, the Harris–Benedict Formula, and BMR. They will also be asked to demonstrate correct measurements.
- Monthly article reviews will also be done and will be shared among providers. This will be an ongoing process to promote increased knowledge and will help increase internal referrals.
- This output and training will take place after the project is completed, as the development of a formal business plan has to be approved before the establishment of a medical weight-loss clinic and staff training will be implemented.

Appendix I: Nutrition and Exercise Journal

CLM

Nutrition & Exercise

Journal

Name: _____

Start Date: _____

Today's Date: _____
Nutrition Goal: _____

Time	What you ate	Why you ate/How you feel	Food group
7:00 a.m. 2:00 p.m.	1 cup Cheerios w/ banana and 1 cup skim milk 5 oz regular club crackers	Satisfied, not too full, bored, stuffed, guilty	Grain, fruit, and dairy; grain, fats/ sweets

Physical Activity Goal: _____

Time	What you did	Duration	How you felt (during/after)
7:00 p.m.	Cleaned house: dusted, vacuumed, swept, laundry, scrubbed bathroom	2.5 hrs	Good/energized while cleaning, tired afterward

Today's Date: _____
Nutrition Goal: _____

_____

Time	What you ate	Why you ate/How you feel	Food group

Physical Activity Goal: _____

_____

Time	What you did	Duration	How you felt (during/after)

Appendix J: Baseline Assessment

Patient Name: _____ Date: _____

Age: _____ Sex: _____ DOB: _____ Height: _____ Weight: _____

Body mass index: _____ Neck circumference: _____

Waist circumference: _____ Hip circumference: _____

Waist-to-hip ratio (WHR): _____ WHR classification: _____

Previtals

BP: _____ Heart Rate (HR): _____ Resp: _____ SpO$_2$: _____

Cardiorespiratory Endurance

Protocol used: _____ Score (m/# marched) _____

Reason for termination: _____ Classification: _____

BORG score: Prefatigue _____ Shortness of breath _____

Postfatigue _____ Shortness of breath _____

Muscular Endurance

Wall pushups: _____ # Completed/Classification: _____

Seated crunch: _____ # Completed/Classification: _____

Muscular Strength

Bicep curl: _____ Classification: _____

Chair to stand: _____ Classification: _____

Flexibility

Sit and reach distance (inches): Right _____ Classification: _____

Left _____ Classification: _____

Agility

8' up and go time: _____ Classification: _____

Postvitals

BP: _____ HR: _____ Resp: _____ SpO$_2$: _____

Appendix K: The Borg Rating of Perceived Exertion (RPE) Scale

0: Nothing at all
0.5: Very, very slight (just noticeable)
1: Very slight
2: Slight (light)
3: Moderate
4: Somewhat severe
5: Severe (heavy)
6:
7: Very severe
8:
9:
10: Very, very severe (maximal)

Appendix L: Insurance-Based Package

Cardiac Patient: (Insurance Based)

The length between visits will depend on individual needs and success in a program. We will start by seeing patients every 2 weeks until there is weight loss at two consecutive visits. When patient and provider are comfortable, visits will first be pushed back to every 3 to 4 weeks, then 6 to 8 weeks, and finally 3 months.

Repeat Baseline Assessment Every 3 Months

First visit—Introduction to program, personal and medical background, short-term goals: start food and exercise journal, 1 to 2 pounds weight loss/week, slightly increase physical activity (PA); long-term goal: (realistic weight, medical improvements, etc.)

Second visit (2 weeks later)—Baseline assessment, exercise suggestions, set short-term goals. Orientation to fitness center and equipment. Introduction to stretches and resistance bands

Third visit—Refine goals. Meet with registered dietitian (RD)

Fourth visit (2 weeks later)—Stress management technique, nutrition material/lesson (tips/suggestions, education, etc.)

Fifth visit—Demonstrate exercise form: more bands and body weight exercises (wall squats, triceps dips, etc.), nutrition (basic info/small modification)

(Fourth and fifth visits can be interchanged depending on patient needs.)

Sixth visit—Stress management techniques, exercise session

Seventh visit—Nutrition and exercise counseling

Eighth visit—Nutrition and exercise counseling, stress management techniques

After the eighth visit, the appointment will be structured to best fit the patient's needs; therefore, nutrition, exercise, or stress management may become more of a focus.

Appendix M: Noninsurance-Based Package Options

Patients (Not Insurance Based):

Weight-Loss Packages (Nutrition and Exercise):

The weight-loss packages focus on nutrition and PA behavior modification through professional advisement, patient education using handouts, counseling, and hands-on training.

Basic Beginning Package (1 month)
$200 for 3 visits
Description: This starter package provides basic information and recommendations to jump-start healthier habits. The package includes a fitness assessment to ensure that exercise is safe and appropriate, orientation to fitness equipment and exercises to ensure proper form and injury prevention, and basic nutrition counseling for educated food selection.

Jump Start Package (3 months)
$375 for 6 visits (includes group information classes and reassessment)
Description: This jump start package provides everything from the basic package, but takes it a step further by offering a personalized exercise session, access to group education classes, and a reassessment to take your PA prescription one step further.

Weight-Loss Counseling and Education (6 months)
$575 for 9 visits (includes stress management, group information classes, and reassessments)
Description: The counseling and education package takes the weight-loss effort to the next level. In addition to the jump start package, this package offers stress management techniques to help control emotional eating, even more one-on-one nutrition, and exercise counseling and group information sessions.

Start to Finish: Lifestyle Modification (1 year)
$775 for 13 visits (includes stress management, group information and group fitness classes, every 3-month reassessment and postassessment, and weight check once/month)
Description: This package takes you from start to finish in your weight management efforts. The package offers access to group fitness classes, a full year of nutrition and exercise guidance, and will leave you physically and mentally healthier,

and feeling better about yourself and life. Before the year is up, you will have a healthier lifestyle, which will enable you to maintain your weight-loss success.

First visit (1.5 hours)—Fitness assessment (stress test), nutrition and exercise journal, learn about the weight-loss program if applicable, general advice on home exercise routine/program, and set long- and short-term goals.

Balke Treadmill Test, sit and reach, 1-minute crunches, push-ups (possibly biceps and bench press).

Second visit (2 weeks later) (1 hour)—Orientation to fitness equipment and resistance bands for home exercise routine (demonstration for proper form), nutrition suggestions, goals, and review journal for advice on modifications.

Third visit (2 weeks later) (30 minutes)—Q&A nutrition and exercise counseling.

Fourth visit (2 weeks later) (30–45 minutes)—Exercise session.

Fifth visit (3 weeks later) (30 minutes)—Nutrition and exercise counseling (Q&A).

Sixth visit (3 weeks later) (45 minutes)—Reassess and update exercise routine.

Seventh visit (4 weeks later) (30 minutes)—Stress management techniques, nutrition counseling.

Eighth visit (4 weeks later) (30 minutes)—Stress management techniques, nutrition counseling.

Ninth visit (4 weeks later) (45 minutes)—Reassessment and stress management techniques.

10th visit (6 weeks later) (30 minutes)—Stress management, nutrition, and exercise counseling.

11th visit (6 weeks later) (45 minutes)—Reassess and update exercise prescription.

12th visit (7 weeks later) (30 minutes)—Stress management, nutrition, and exercise counseling.

13th visit (8 weeks later) (30 minutes)—Postassessment, review of progress (health status).

Appendix N: Group Fitness Class Prices

1–2×/week for 1 month	$10/session
1–2×/week for 4 months	$8/session

Index

abdominal obesity, 20–21
acarbose (Precose), 261
Accreditation Commission for Midwifery
  Education (ACME), 30
ACLM. *See* American College of Lifestyle
  Medicine
ACME. *See* Accreditation Commission for
  Midwifery Education
ACNP. *See* acute care nurse practitioner
ACSM. *See* American College of Sports
  Medicine
action plan, 292–293
activities of daily living (ADLs), 22
activity thermogenesis (AT), 21
acute care nurse practitioner (ACNP),
  29
additional eating disorders, 104
adipocytes, 21, 95
ADLs. *See* activities of daily living
adult nurse practitioner (ANP), 29
advanced practice nurses (APNs), 22, 39,
  49, 53, 111, 113, 179–182
advanced practice registered nurses
  (APRNs), 27–29
air displacement, 109
Albright's hereditary osteodystrophy, 93
Alli, 262
alpha-1 acid glycoprotein, 95
alpha-melanocyte-stimulating hormone
  (α-MSH), 92
α-MSH. *See* alpha-melanocyte-stimulating
  hormone
Alstrom syndrome, 93
AMA. *See* American Medical
  Association
AMCB. *See* American Midwifery
  Certification Board
American College of Lifestyle Medicine
  (ACLM), 287
American College of Sports Medicine
  (ACSM), 107, 108

*The American Journal of Clinical
  Nutrition*, 21
American Medical Association (AMA), 3
American Midwifery Certification Board
  (AMCB), 30
American Nurses Association (ANA),
  28, 49
American Nurses Credentialing Center
  (ANCC), 29
amylin, 261
ANA. *See* American Nurses Association
ANCC. *See* American Nurses
  Credentialing Center
anorexia nervosa, 101–102, 249–251
ANP. *See* adult nurse practitioner
anthropometry, 109
antidepressants, 260
antidiabetic drugs, 260–261
antiseizure medications, 261–262
APNs. *See* advanced practice nurses
APRNs. *See* advanced practice registered
  nurses
arrhythmia, 96
asthma, 179
  basics of, 222
  diagnostic tests, 223
  pathophysiology, 222–223
  patient education, 224
  pediatric patients, 222–224
  signs and symptoms, 223
  treatment, 223–224
AT. *See* activity thermogenesis
atheroma, 96
autonomy, 24

Bardet–Biedl syndrome (BBS), 93
bariatric surgery
  candidates for, 265–266
  medical clearance, 266–267
  pediatric obesity, 284–285

osteoarthritis (OA), 204
polycystic ovary syndrome (PCOS), 207
dietary assessment and patient recommendations
daily food record or journal, 159–161
diet composition, 162–163
eating patterns and habits, 158–159
improve behavior change, 164–165
new patient, 158
nutrition screening, 158
portion control, 163
recommendations, 163–164
weight loss, needs for, 161–162
dietary supplements, 262–263
diethylpropion (Tenuate), 255–256
disease management, 179–182
DM. *See* diabetes mellitus
dual-energy X-ray absorptiometry (DEXA), 109
dyslipidemia, 4, 23
basics, 189, 216–217
diagnostic tests, 190, 217
pathophysiology, 189–190, 217
patient education, 193, 218
pediatric patients, 216–218
signs and symptoms, 190, 217
treatment, 190–193, 218

eating disorders, 101
EBW. *See* excess body weight
EKG. *See* electrocardiogram
electrocardiogram (EKG), 23
end-stage renal disease (ESRD), 213
energy requirements, 22
ESRD. *See* end-stage renal disease
excess body weight (EBW), 20
exenatide, 261
exercise
programming, 135
response and training, 132–133
special considerations, 156
testing, 133–135
exercise programming
bent-over row, 146
biceps curl, 147
bicep stretch, 137
calf stretch, 143
chest press, 144
chest stretch, 138
groin stretch, 142
hamstring stretch, 140
heel raises, 154
hip abduction, 152

hip adduction, 151
hip extension, 153
quadriceps stretch, 141
seated leg extension, 149
shoulder stretch, 138
side stretch, 139
squats, 155–156
standing hamstring curl, 150
triceps kickback, 145
triceps stretch, 136
wall push-ups, 148

family nurse practitioner (FNP), 29
fat substitutes, 263
fatty liver disease (FLD), 95
FDA. *See* Food and Drug Administration
feeding disorders, 104
fidelity, 24
FLD. *See* fatty liver disease
fluoxetine (Prozac), 260
FNP. *See* family nurse practitioner
food addiction treatment, 247–249
Food and Drug Administration (FDA), 255–259, 260, 261, 262–263
Fragile X syndrome, 93

gastric banding, 23
gastric bypass, 23
gene variants, 10
genetics
energy balance, 91–92
environmental and genetic factors, 92–93
gene and protein function, 93–94
genetic syndromes, 93
pathophysiology, 94–96
genetic syndromes, 93
gerontological nurse practitioner (GNP), 29
GNP. *See* gerontological nurse practitioner
group fitness class prices, 370

Harris–Benedict formula, 21, 22
Health and Human Services (HHS), 7–8
HHS. *See* Health and Human Services
history of present illness (HPI), 113
HPI. *See* history of present illness
HTN. *See* hypertension
human obese (OB) gene, 91
hydrostatic weighing, 109

Printed in the United States
By Bookmasters